Atlas of Normal and Pathological Findings in Otoneuroradiology

Giorgio Conte • Fabio Triulzi
Elisa Scola
Editors

Atlas of Normal and Pathological Findings in Otoneuroradiology

Springer

Editors
Giorgio Conte
Neuroradiology Unit, Fondazione
IRCCS Ca' Granda Ospedale Maggiore
Policlinico
Department of Pathophysiology and
Transplantation, University of Milan
Milan, Italy

Fabio Triulzi
Neuroradiology Unit, Fondazione
IRCCS Ca' Granda Ospedale Maggiore
Policlinico
Department of Pathophysiology and
Transplantation, University of Milan
Milan, Italy

Elisa Scola
Neuroradiology Unit, Fondazione
IRCCS Ca' Granda Ospedale Maggiore
Policlinico
University of Milan
Milan, Italy

ISBN 978-3-032-08231-2 ISBN 978-3-032-08232-9 (eBook)
https://doi.org/10.1007/978-3-032-08232-9

This Springer imprint is published by the registered company Springer Nature Switzerland AG
The registered company address is: Gewerbestrasse 11, 6330 Cham, Switzerland

Acknowledgements

We would like to express our heartfelt gratitude and deepest appreciation to the entire staff of the Neuroradiology Department of IRCCS Fondazione Ca' Granda Ospedale Maggiore Policlinico of Milan, including all physicians, technicians, nurses and administrative personnel, for their daily and tireless dedication, professionalism and invaluable support. Their commitment makes a meaningful difference in the lives of so many.

We are also profoundly grateful to our colleagues from the Departments of Audiology, Otolaryngology, Maxillofacial surgery, Neurosurgery, Neurointensive Care and Neurology for their continued collaboration and dedication to excellence in patient care.

We look forward to continuing this shared journey.

Milan, Italy

Giorgio Conte
Fabio Triulzi
Elisa Scola

Contents

1 Imaging Technique

Principles of Computed Tomography (CT) and Magnetic Resonance (MR) Imaging of the Temporal Bone

Giorgio Conte, Annamaria Gregorio, Eliana Schifano, Luciano Lombardi, Clara Sina, Elisa Scola, and Fabio Triulzi

1.1 Introduction

Radiological imaging techniques of the temporal bone are essential for diagnosing a range of conditions affecting the ear and surrounding structures. The temporal bone is anatomically complex and houses critical components of the auditory and vestibular systems. Given this complexity, various imaging modalities are employed, each with its unique advantages and drawbacks [1]. The commonly used imaging techniques include computed tomography (CT) and magnetic resonance (MR) imaging, with each modality playing a distinct role depending on the clinical scenario.

G. Conte (✉) · F. Triulzi
Neuroradiology Unit, Fondazione IRCCS Ca' Granda Ospedale Maggiore Policlinico, Milan, Italy

Department of Pathophysiology and Transplantation, University of Milan, Milan, Italy
e-mail: giorgio.conte@policlinico.mi.it; fabio.triulzi@policlinico.mi.it

A. Gregorio · L. Lombardi · C. Sina · E. Scola
Neuroradiology Unit, Fondazione IRCCS Ca' Granda Ospedale Maggiore Policlinico, Milan, Italy
e-mail: annamaria.gregorio@policlinico.mi.it; luciano.lombardi@policlinico.mi.it; elisa.scola@policlinico.mi.it

E. Schifano
School in Radiodiagnostics, Università degli Studi di Milano, Milan, Italy

CT is the preferred imaging modality when detailed bony architecture is required. Its ability to provide high-resolution images makes it invaluable for assessing conditions such as cholesteatoma, otosclerosis, and temporal bone fractures. A CT scan is often the first imaging modality employed in cases of ear complaints, particularly when there is a suspicion of middle ear disease. Moreover, CT imaging excels in evaluating the complex air-filled spaces and the bony labyrinth, rendering it indispensable for planning surgical approaches in otologic procedures. It offers a reliable evaluation of bony integrity prior to surgery, allowing clinicians to determine the extent of disease involvement, particularly in the mastoid and middle ear regions. In contrast to CT, MR is invaluable to characterise soft tissues and assess fluid-filled structures within the temporal bone, including the labyrinth, the internal auditory canal, and the cerebellopontine angle [2].

It is essential to consider the implications of imaging techniques on patient management. The choice of imaging modality should be guided by the clinical context and the specific questions the physician seeks to answer. In many cases, a multi-modality approach is warranted; for example, a CT scan may be performed initially to assess bony abnormalities, followed by MR imaging to characterise soft tissues. The integration of findings from different imaging modali-

G. Conte et al. (eds.), *Atlas of Normal and Pathological Findings in Otoneuroradiology*,
https://doi.org/10.1007/978-3-032-08232-9_1

ties can enhance diagnostic confidence and inform management decisions effectively.

1.2 CT of the Temporal Bone

Multi-slice CT (MSCT) has been the only technology used for assessing temporal bone for many years; however, in the last time the flat-panel CT, also known as cone beam CT (CBCT), is taking over that role.

1.2.1 CBCT of the Temporal Bone

CBCT uses a rotating gantry where an X-ray tube and a flat-panel detector go around a supine patient. The main difference with MSCT is the use of a cone-shaped radiation beam which allows each exposure to cover the entire field of view (FOV), acquiring a series of complete two-dimensional images of the temporal bone in different projections during a single 360° turn. Furthermore, the radiation emission is not continuous but pulsed, limiting the dose to the patient. The data acquired by the flat-panel detector are then analysed and processed [1, 3].

We performed CBCT using the angiographic C-arm unit equipped with a flat panel detector. Fixation of the patient's head is done to prevent motion artefacts in a supine position. We used the following parameters: FOV = 22 cm, 110 kV, 140 mAS, 30 frames per second, reconstructed voxel size = $0.14 \times 0.14 \times 0.14$ mm^3, and scan time = 22 s. The isotropic voxel allows multi-planar reconstructions without losing spatial resolution. The axial images are reconstructed along the plane parallel to the lateral semicircular canal, the coronal images perpendicular to this axial set of images. This procedure is repeated for both the right and left temporal bones separately. The volume of acquisition includes mastoid apex up to the sella.

1.2.2 MSCT of the Temporal Bone

MSCT uses an X-ray tube that turns while the table is moving and multiple rows of detectors capture data to obtain cross-sectional images of the body. The patient is supine, and the gantry of the scanner is not tilted. The images are acquired in a single imaging plane, requiring multiple spiral turns by X-ray tube to cover all fields of study [4].

We use the following parameters for adult patients: FOV = 5 cm, 120 kV, 200 mAS, pitch = 0.85, matrix 512 × 512, and scan time = 5 s. Post-processing is done in a similar way as data acquired with CBCT. The voxel is isotropic and permits reconstruction in the axial and coronal planes with a slice thickness of 0.5–1 mm. The volume of acquisition includes mastoid apex up to the sella.

1.2.3 CBCT Versus MSCT

CBCT allows higher spatial resolution with an isotropic voxel (up to 0.1 mm^3) compared to MSCT (up to 0.4 mm of slice thickness). The pulsed emission of radiation permits lower radiation exposure; in addition it is less sensitive for metallic and beam hardening artefacts because the image acquisition is based on conventional radiographic images. However, CBCT has different technical disadvantages compared with MSCT: (a) it cannot provide a correlation between grey levels and absolute tissue density values (Hounsfield scale) for the lower signal/noise ratio; (b) it has lower contrast resolution resulting a suboptimal technique for soft tissue characterisation both without and with intravenous administration of contrast agent; and (c) it has longer acquisition time, approximately 20 s versus 5 s of the MSCT, resulting in more susceptibility to motion artefacts [1, 3].

It is therefore important to define when the use of FPCT is preferable to MSCT for the cross-sectional imaging of the temporal bone. FPCT is almost always preferred to MSCT in the assessment of the external and middle and inner ear because of its better image quality in depicting almost all bony structures of diagnostic interest. FPCT is highly recommended in the assessment of cochlear implants and metallic prostheses after middle ear reconstructive surgery. In contrast,

FPCT is not recommended for the assessment of pathologies that can involve the soft tissues around the temporal bone, sometimes even requiring the administration of contrast agent, and when angiographic studies are needed. Furthermore, MSCT is recommended in the case of uncooperative patients, including paediatric patients who cannot be sedated, due to the faster acquisition time [1, 3].

1.3 MR Imaging of the Temporal Bone

The temporal bone can be studied with both 1.5 and 3 Tesla (T) MR scanners. The spatial and temporal resolutions given by 3T are clearly superior to 1.5T. The magnetic susceptibility artefact due to the air/bone interface of the temporal bone and the artefact on images due to hearing aid implants can limit the use of 3T MR scanner.

Essential requirements are the use of 2D sequences with minimal slice thickness (less than 2 mm is preferable) and high in-plane resolution, high-resolution isotropic 3D sequences (less than 0.8^3 mm^3 is preferable) from which multi-planar reconstructions can be obtained. These requirements are more achievable with a 3T MR scanner equipped with image acceleration algorithms (parallel imaging and compressed sensing).

Several MR sequences are critical for imaging the temporal bone (see Table 1.1 for details about sequences parameters and Table 1.2 for MR protocols in ear disorders), each offering unique benefits:

T1-Weighted Imaging It is essential for identifying bone marrow of the temporal bone, the methaemoglobin in case of haemorrhage or cholesterol granuloma, fat-containing lesions, and post-contrast enhancing lesions. The use of pre- and post-contrast 3D DIXON T1 weighted should be preferred since it was found to produce a higher image quality and fat suppression efficiency than the hybrid techniques such as spectral presaturation with inversion recovery (SPIR) and spectral attenuated inversion recovery (SPAIR), it provides both fat-only and water-only images, and the water-only images are used for fat suppression. We acquire 2D pre-contrast turbo spin echo (TSE) T1-weighted sequence only in the assessment of sudden sensorineural hearing loss because it appears more sensitive in detecting methaemoglobin than 3D sequences and in the assessment of chronic otitis media in order to have a perfect co-registration with 2D TSE T2-weighted images and non-echo planar diffusion-weighted images (TSE DWI), being acquired with the same orientation in the coronal plane, slice thickness, and gap.

3D T1-weighted black-blood sequence also provides optimal fat suppression increasing the sensibility and diagnostic confidence of abnormal intracranial enhancements after intravenous contrast agent administration. In particular, we consider it useful for the assessment of nerves and intralabyrinthine enhancement lesions such as neurinoma [5, 6].

T2-Weighted Imaging The use of high-resolution 3D turbo spin echo (TSE) sequence images with driven equilibrium radio frequency reset pulse (DRIVE) or 3D FFE or TSE constructive interference in steady state (CISS) is particularly useful for visualising fluid-filled structures such as the labyrinth, the internal auditory canal, and the cerebellopontine angle. 2D TSE T2-weighted images are used in the assessment of soft-tissue lesions of the external and middle ear and for bony lesions. 2D-DIXON T2-weighted sequence is often preferred since it provides both fat-only and water-only images, the latter being used for fat suppression [5, 6].

Fluid-Attenuated Inversion Recovery (FLAIR) It suppresses intralabyrinthine fluid signal enhancing the visibility of changes in content as in the case of intralabyrinthine haemorrhage or inflammation. Post-contrast 3D FLAIR is acquired approximately 10 min after administration of the contrast agent and is more sensitive than a T1-weighted sequence in detecting mild intralabyrinthine contrast enhancement related to blood-labyrinthine barrier breakdown,

Table 1.1 Scanning parameters of sequences on 3T scanner (Achieva, Philips Healthcare, Eindhoven NL)

Sequences	Orientation	FOV (AP*RL)	Slice thickness (mm)	ACQ voxel size (mm)	REC voxel size (mm)	TR/TE-TI (ms)
2D TSE T1W[a]	Coronal or axial	180*160	1.5	0.7*0.9*1.5	0.35*0.35*1.5	500/10
2D TSE T2W[b]	Coronal or axial	160*160	2	0.5*0.6*2.0	0.35*0.35*2.0	3500/100
3D FFE T1W[b]	3D	120*150	0.9	0.9*0.9*0.9	0.45*0.45*0.45	5.9/1.99/3.7
3D TSE T1W BB	3D	180*183	0.8	0.8*0.8*0.8	0.36*0.36*0.36	700/35
3D FLAIR	Axial	160*160	1.0	1.0*1.0*1.0	0.48*0.48*0.48	6000/350–1850
3D TSE T2W[c]	Axial	140*140	0.6	0.4*0.4*0.6	0.27*0.27*0.27	1550/251
3D FLAIR heavily T2W	3D	140*140	0.7	0.7*0.7*0.7	0.32*0.32*0.32	6000/385–1950
4D-TRAK	Coronal	240*240	3.0	1.3*1.3*3.0	1.0*1.0*1.5	2.9/1.29
2D TSE DWI	Coronal or axial	220*180	2.0	1.8*2.1*2.0	0.86*0.86*2.0	2702/59

Abbreviations: ACQ acquisition, *BB* black blood, *DWI* diffusion-weighted imaging, *FFE* fast field echo, *FLAIR* fluid-attenuated inversion recovery, *FOV* field of view, *REC* construction, *TE* echo time, *TI* inversion time, *TR* repetition time, *TRAK* time-resolved magnetic resonance angiography with K-space sharing, *TSE* turbo spin echo

[a] With possible spectral presaturation with inversion recovery (SPIR)

[b] With possible DIXON fat suppression

[c] With driven equilibrium radio-frequency reset pulse (DRIVE sequence)

Table 1.2 Scanning MR protocols of ear disorders

Chronic media otitis / cholesteatoma	External ear disorders	Inner ear disorders	Pulsatile tinnitus
Coronal TSE T1W	3D FFE T1W with fat suppression	Axial TSE T1W with fat suppression	3D FFE T1W with fat suppression
Coronal TSE T2W	Axial TSE T2W with and without fat suppression	3D FLAIR	Axial TSE T2W with and without fat suppression
Coronal TSE DWI[a]	Coronal TSE T2W with and without fat suppression		Coronal TSE T2W with and without fat suppression
3D TSE T2W	Coronal TSE DWI		3D TSE T2W
			3D TOF
	Intravenous contrast agent administration	*Intravenous contrast agent administration*	*Intravenous contrast agent administration*
	3D FFE T1W with fat suppression	3D TSE T2W[b]	4D-TRAK
		3D FLAIR	3D FFE T1W with fat suppression
		3D TSE T1W BB	
		After 4.5 h	
		3D FLAIR heavily T2W	

Abbreviations: *BB* black blood; *DWI* diffusion-weighted imaging, *FFE* fast field echo, *FLAIR* fluid attenuated inversion recovery, *TOF* time of flight, *TRAK* time-resolved MR angiography with K-space sharing, *TSE* turbo spin echo
[a]The acquisition on the axial plane is optional
[b]To cover part of the 10 min needed before the acquisition of postcontrast 3D FLAIR sequence, it is advantageous to inject a contrast agent before the acquisition of the 3D TSE T2W

and as a result, it is particularly useful in suspected labyrinthitis. In addition, it is highly sensitive in detecting post-contrast enhancement of the nerves within the internal auditory canal or of the facial nerve [7]. The heavily T2W 3D FLAIR sequence has been demonstrated to depict the membranous labyrinth. It is acquired 4.5 h after the intravenous contrast agent administration, because the contrast agent gradually accumulates in the perilymph but not in the endolymph, reaching its peak concentration at that time. The heavily T2W 3D FLAIR sequence allows to indirectly visualise the membranous labyrinth as a hypointense space surrounded by the enhanced perilymph. Although the intratympanic contrast agent administration has been reported to enhance the visualisation of the perilymph, the intravenous administration has several advantages: lesser invasiveness, bilateral examination in a single test session, and assessment of the blood-barrier permeability (while intratympanic administration uses the round window as delivery route in the labyrinthine compartment) [8, 9].

DWI Acquired with non-EPI technique, it has emerged as a pivotal tool in the diagnosis and management of cholesteatomas, providing a non-invasive and highly sensitive method for detecting these lesions. Cholesteatomas are characterised by their restricted diffusion, appearing hyperintense on DWI due to the dense keratin content and the lack of free water movement within the lesion. The utility of DWI extends to both primary and recurrent cholesteatomas, aiding in the early detection and precise localisation essential for surgical planning [5].

References

1. Conte G, Scola E, Calloni S, et al. Flat panel angiography in the cross-sectional imaging of the temporal bone: assessment of image quality and radiation dose compared with a 64-section multisection CT scanner. AJNR Am J Neuroradiol. 2017;38(10):1998–2002. https://doi.org/10.3174/ajnr.A5302.
2. Pyykkö I, Zou J, Gürkov R, Naganawa S, Nakashima T. Imaging of temporal bone. Adv Otorhinolaryngol. 2019;82:12–31. https://doi.org/10.1159/000490268.

3. Piergallini L, Scola E, Tuscano B, et al. Flat-panel CT versus 128-slice CT in temporal bone imaging: assessment of image quality and radiation dose. Eur J Radiol. 2018;106:106–13. https://doi.org/10.1016/j.ejrad.2018.07.013.
4. Juliano AF. Cross sectional imaging of the ear and temporal bone. Head Neck Pathol. 2018;12(3):302–20. https://doi.org/10.1007/s12105-018-0901-y.
5. Lingam RK, Connor SEJ, Casselman JW, Beale T. MRI in otology: applications in cholesteatoma and Meniere's disease. Clin Radiol. 2018;73(1):35–44. https://doi.org/10.1016/j.crad.2017.09.002. Epub 2017 Sep 29.
6. Veiga M, Kuhweide R, Demaerel V, De Pauw R, De Foer B, Casselman JW. Labyrinthine enhancement on 3D black blood MR images of the brain as an imaging biomarker for cisplatin ototoxicity in (lung) cancer patients. Neuroradiology. 2021;63(1):81–90. https://doi.org/10.1007/s00234-020-02504-x.
7. Conte G, Di Berardino F, Sina C, et al. MR imaging in sudden sensorineural hearing loss. Time to talk. AJNR Am J Neuroradiol. 2017;38(8):1475–9. https://doi.org/10.3174/ajnr.A5230.
8. Conte G, Caschera L, Tuscano B, et al. Three-tesla magnetic resonance imaging of the vestibular endolymphatic space: a systematic qualitative description in healthy ears. Eur J Radiol. 2018;109:77–82. https://doi.org/10.1016/j.ejrad.2018.10.023.
9. Zanetti D, Conte G, Scola E, Casale S, Lilli G, Di Berardino F. Advanced imaging of the vestibular endolymphatic space in Meniere's disease. Front Surg. 2021;8:700271. https://doi.org/10.3389/fsurg.2021.7002.

CT Imaging Anatomy

2

Francesco Maria Lo Russo, Giorgio Conte, Fabio Triulzi, Silvia Casale, and Elisa Scola

2.1 Introduction

The knowledge of middle and inner ear anatomy is essential for the diagnosis and presurgical planning of various pathological conditions. This chapter will describe in detail the anatomy of the bony structures of the middle and inner ear as shown by cone beam computed tomography (CBCT). CBCT provides three-dimensional high-resolution images.

2.2 The Middle Ear Space

The boundaries of the tympanic cavity are the scutum and tympanic membrane laterally, the tegmen tympani superiorly, the inner ear structures medially, and the jugular wall inferiorly. The tympanic cavity contains the ossicular chain and can be divided into three compartments: the epitympanum, the mesotympanum, and the hypotympanum. The epitympanum, or attic, is situated above the superior margin of the tympanic membrane and is in communication with the mastoid antrum through the aditus ad antrum; in the epitympanum are located the head of the malleus and the body and the short process of the incus. The mesotympanum is located between the level of the superior and inferior margin of the tympanic membrane, and it contains the majority of the ossicular chain as well as the tensor tympani and chorda tympani nerve. The hypotympanum lies below the inferior margin of the tympanic membrane and is in communication with the Eustachian tube [1, 2].

Important landmarks are present on the tympanic cavity walls. The medial wall hosts the facial nerve canal, oval window, cochlear promontory, and round window niche; in the posterior wall are located the facial nerve recess, the pyramidal eminence, sinus tympani, and round window niche, from lateral to medial. The Prussak's space is located in the lateral wall of tympanic cavity and is marginated by the pars flaccida and the scutum, a sharp spur of bone where the pars flaccida of tympanic membrane is inserted, and the neck of the malleus and the neck of the malleus medially [2, 3].

F. M. Lo Russo (✉) · S. Casale · E. Scola
Neuroradiology Unit, Fondazione IRCCS Ca' Granda Ospedale Maggiore Policlinico, Milan, Italy
e-mail: francesco.lorusso@policlinico.mi.it; silvia.casale@policlinico.mi.it; elisa.scola@policlinico.mi.it

G. Conte · F. Triulzi
Neuroradiology Unit, Fondazione IRCCS Ca' Granda Ospedale Maggiore Policlinico, Milan, Italy

Department of Pathophysiology and Transplantation, University of Milan, Milan, Italy
e-mail: giorgio.conte@policlinico.mi.it; fabio.triulzi@policlinico.mi.it

G. Conte et al. (eds.), *Atlas of Normal and Pathological Findings in Otoneuroradiology*,
https://doi.org/10.1007/978-3-032-08232-9_2

The Koerner septum is a bony structure that separates the mastoid air cells into medial and lateral compartments. It can be identified from the petrosquamous suture that extends posteriorly [4].

2.3 Ossicular Chain

The ossicular chain includes the malleus, the incus, and the stapes. The malleus is composed by the head, the neck, the anterior and lateral processes, and the manubrium. The manubrium is attached to the tympanic membrane, and the head forms the incudomalleolar joint together with the body of the incus. The incus has a "ice cream" shape on axial images and is composed by the body, the short and long processes, and the lenticular process. The lenticular process articulates with the head of the stapes. The stapes is composed by the head/capitellum, the anterior crus, the posterior crus, and the footplate which is located within the oval window [5].

These ossicles are held in place by various ligaments, joint capsules, and the tensor tympani and the stapedial muscles. The incus is the most susceptible to dislocation in case of trauma because it has few stabilizers. The footplate of the stapes is anchored to the oval window by the annular ligament. The mechanical energy of sounds is transformed into electrical energy thanks to the footplate that vibrates and displaces fluid in the inner ear's vestibule, stimulating the cochlea's hair cells [4, 5].

There are four ossicular ligaments: the superior malleal, the lateral malleal, the posterior malleal, and the posterior incudal ligaments.

The tensor tympani muscle emerges from the superior border of the cartilaginous part of the eustachian tube and then runs in the middle ear toward the cochleariform process where it turns laterally and attaches to the neck of the malleus. The stapedial tendon arises from the pyramidal eminence that is located in the posterior wall of the tympanic cavity and inserts into the capitellum of the stapes [6].

2.4 The Inner Ear

The inner ear is situated in the petrous portion of the temporal bone and consists in the osseous labyrinth, which includes the cochlea, the vestibule, and the semicircular canals. The cochlea has a spiral shape with two and a half turns around the modiolus. The cochlea contains the scala vestibuli, scala tympani, and scala media, which are three fluid-filled spaces; the interscalar septum separates the basal, the middle, and the apical turns. The osseous spiral lamina extends from the modiolus and divides the scala vestibuli from the scala tympani. The vestibular system comprises three semicircular canals (anterior, posterior, and lateral) that are ringlike structures with an enlarged end, the ampulla [4, 5] (Figs. 2.1, 2.2, 2.3, 2.4, 2.5, 2.6, 2.7, 2.8, 2.9, 2.10, 2.11, 2.12, 2.13, 2.14, 2.15, 2.16, 2.17, 2.18, 2.19, 2.20 and 2.21).

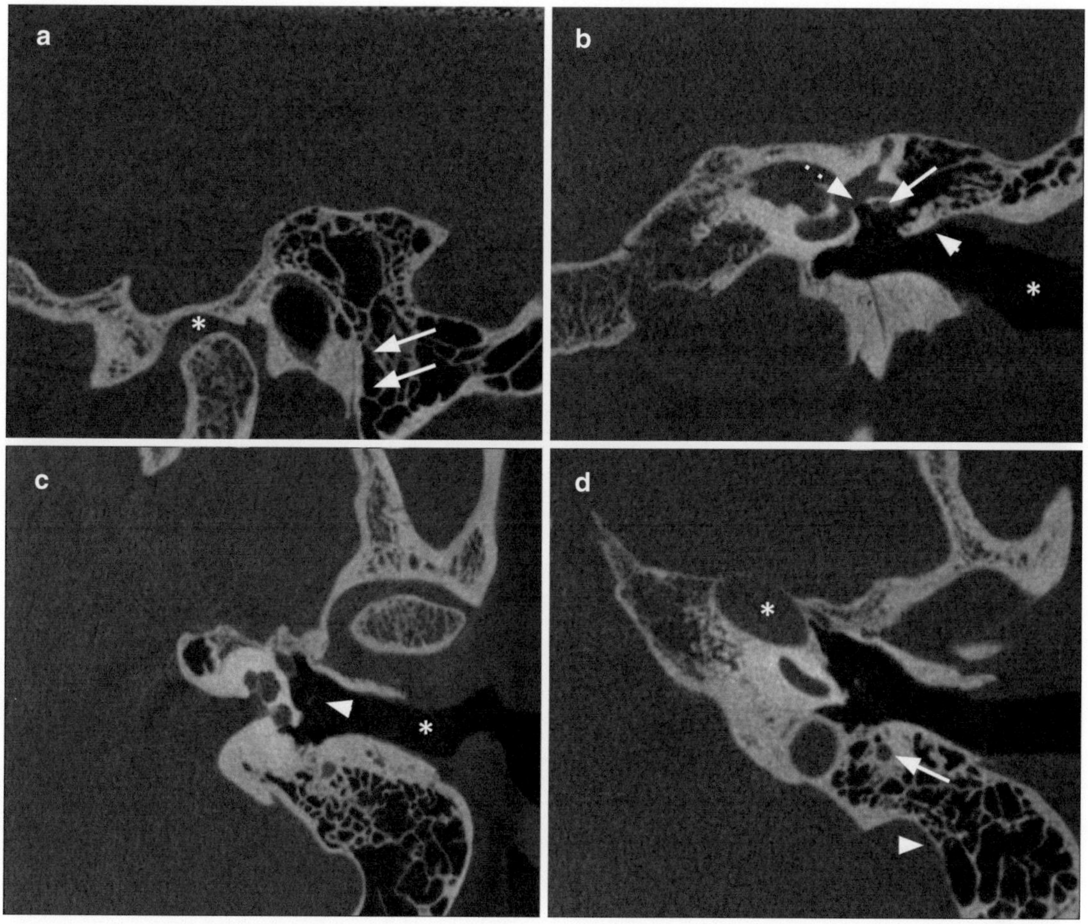

Fig. 2.1 External auditory canal. (**a**) Sagittal reformatted CBCT image shows the tympanic part of the temporal bone. The tympanic part forms the anterior wall, the floor, and part of the posterior wall of the external acoustic meatus, medially fuses with squamous part of the temporal bone and posteriorly is delimited from the mastoid by tympanomastoid fissure (arrows). Anteriorly it gives a contribution to the posterior wall of the mandibular fossa (asterisk). (**b**) Coronal reformatted CBCT image depicts the external auditory canal (EAC) as an S-shaped canal (asterisk). The medial margin of the EAC is the tympanic membrane which attaches inferiorly to the tympanic sulcus. Superiorly lies a bony crest, the scutum (short arrow). Medially it is possible to depict the niche of the oval window (dotted arrow). The tympanic part of the facial nerve (arrow) is seen adjacent to the fossa of the oval window. (**c**) Axial reformatted CBCT image passing through cochlear the middle turn of the cochlea depicts the EAC. The EAC (asterisk) is an S-shaped canal and extends from the concha, at the floor of the auricula, to the tympanic membrane (short arrow), which separates the external acoustic meatus from the middle ear. The external lateral third of EAC is cartilaginous, while the medial and proximal thirds are osseous and formed by the tympanic part and squamous part of the temporal bone. (**d**) Axial reformatted CBCT image passing through the cochlear basal turn depicts the normal cortex of the sigmoid sinus (arrowhead), which separates the sigmoid air cell from the sigmoid sinus. Laterally to the sigmoid sinus and anteriorly to the mastoid air cells, the mastoid segment of the VII cranial nerves (arrow) is shown. Anteriorly to the sigmoid sinus courses the petrous segment of the internal carotid artery (asterisk). *Abbreviations*: CBCT cone beam computed tomography, EAC external auditory canal

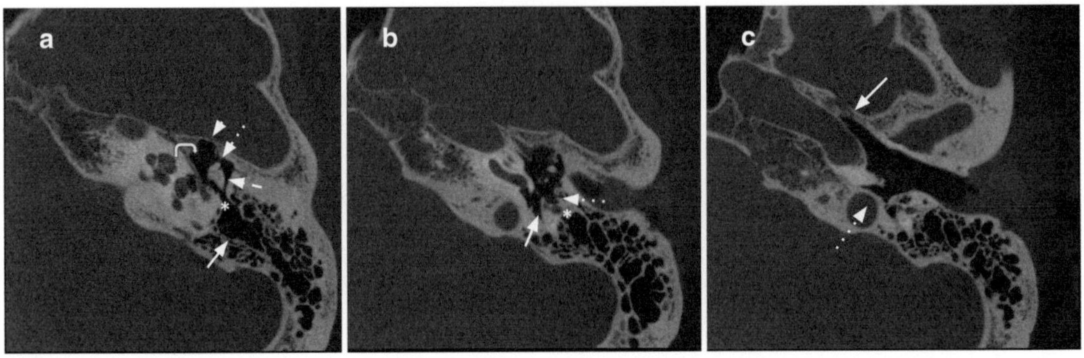

Fig. 2.2 Epitympanum, mesotympanum, and hypotympanum. (**a**) Axial reformatted CBCT image shows the epitympanum (short arrow), the most superior portion of the tympanic cavity. Posteriorly the epitympanum is in direct continuity with the mastoid antrum via the aditus ad antrum (asterisk) and thence the mastoid air cells. Its main contents are the head of the malleus (dotted arrow) and body and short process of the incus (dashed arrow). The normal appearance of these structures on axial CBCT gives rise to the "ice cream cone" sign. Anteriorly there is a discrete space, the anterior epitympanic recess, from which the rest of the epitympanum is separated by the cog (curved arrow). Laterally Prussak's space is located between the scutum and neck of the malleus. (**b**) A more caudal axial reformatted CBCT image shows the mesotympanic recess: the sinus tympani (arrow) is a small recess in the posterior wall medial to the pyramidal eminence and stapedius muscle origin. Lateral to the pyramidal eminence is the facial recess (dotted arrow). The upper mastoid portion of the facial nerve (asterisk) runs immediately posterior to the facial recess, giving it its name. The superior limit of the hypotympanum, the funiculus, is also shown extending from anterior pillar of round window niche toward jugular bulb along cochlear promontory. (**c**) A more caudal axial reformatted CBCT image depicts the hypotympanum. Anteriorly is the opening into the Eustachian tube (arrow) which passes anteromedially to the nasopharynx. The inferior limit is the funiculus and medially the jugular wall (dotted arrow) of the tympanic cavity. *Abbreviation*: CBCT cone beam computed tomography

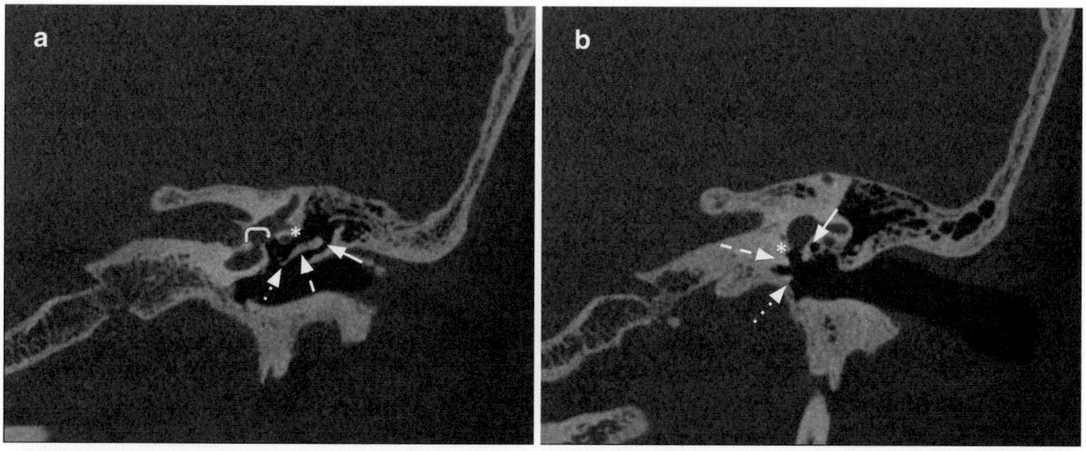

Fig. 2.3 Ossicular chain. (**a**) A coronal reformatted CBCT image shows the head of the malleus (arrow) articulating with the body of the incus (dashed arrow) in the epitympanum. The facet for articulation with the malleus is saddle shaped and forms nearly a right angle. The body of the incus continues infero-laterally in the mesotympanum and gives the attachment for superior ligament of the incus. Inferiorly, the long crus of the incus continues with the lentiform process (dotted arrow) which articulates with the head of the stapes. At this level it is possible to depict the tympanic part of the facial nerve (asterisk). The oval window niche is located in the medial wall of the posterior part of the mesotympanum and harbors the stapes. It is bounded superiorly by the tympanic portion of the facial nerve and inferiorly by the promontory. Medially lies the oval window (curved arrow), a kidney-shaped aperture in the medial wall of the mesotympanum. The footplate of the stapes is attached to the oval window by the annular ligament. (**b**) A coronal reformatted CBCT image shows the round window niche (asterisk) which is situated below the oval window, separated by a posterior extension of the promontory, the subiculum (arrow). More medially it is possible to depict the posterior pillar of the round window (dashed arrow) and inferiorly the pyramidal eminence (dotted arrow). *Abbreviation*: CBCT cone beam computed tomography

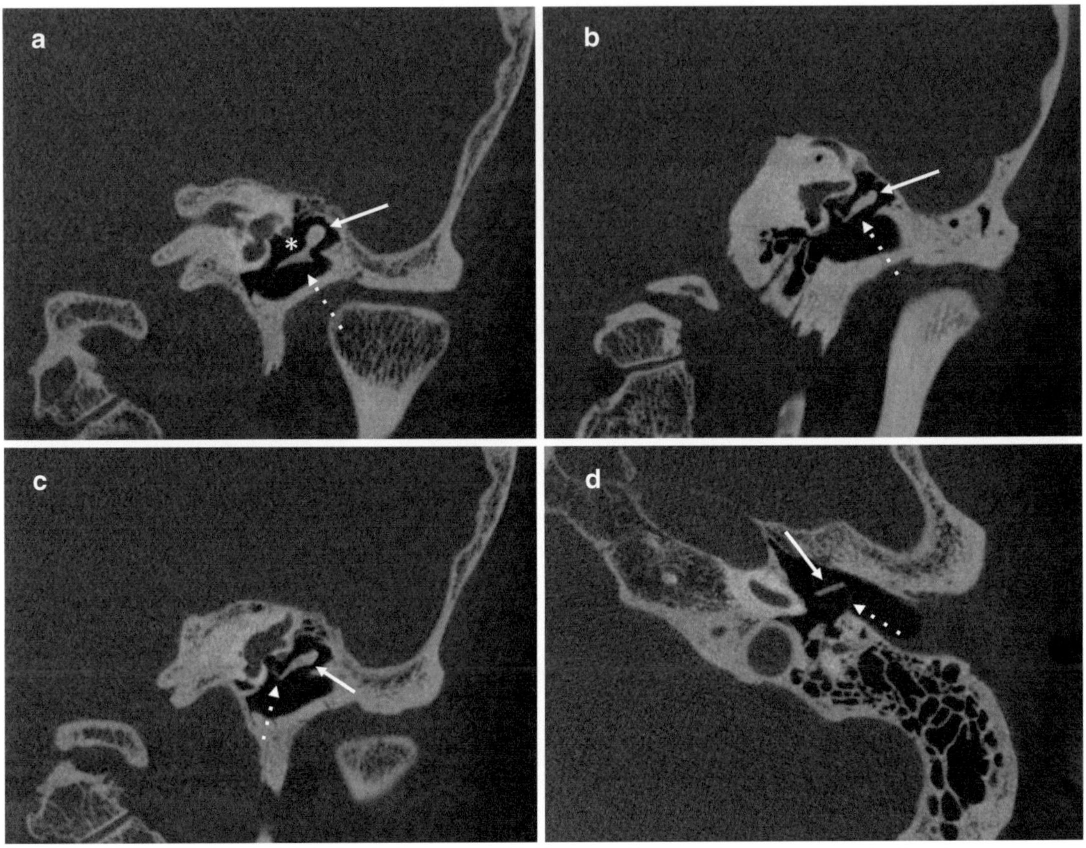

Fig. 2.4 **Malleus and incus.** (**a**) A coronal reformatted CBCT image shows the head of the malleus (arrow) in the epitympanum, just beneath the neck (asterisk) of the malleus which continues with the manubrium (dotted arrow), directed downward, medially, and backward in the mesotympanum. The lateral margin of the malleus is connected with the tympanic membrane. (**b**) A coronal reformatted CBCT image shows the head of the malleus (arrow) articulating with the body of the incus (dotted arrow) in the epitympanum, with a saddle-shaped articulation. (**c**) A coronal reformatted CBCT image shows the long process of the incus (arrow) continuing with the lenticular process (dotted arrow) which articulates the head of the stapes. The stapes lies in the oval window niche and consists of the crura and the footplate which is attached thanks to the annular ligament to the oval window. (**d**) An axial reformatted CBCT image shows the manubrium (arrow) of the malleus projecting toward the tympanic membrane (dotted arrow). *Abbreviation*: CBCT cone beam computed tomography

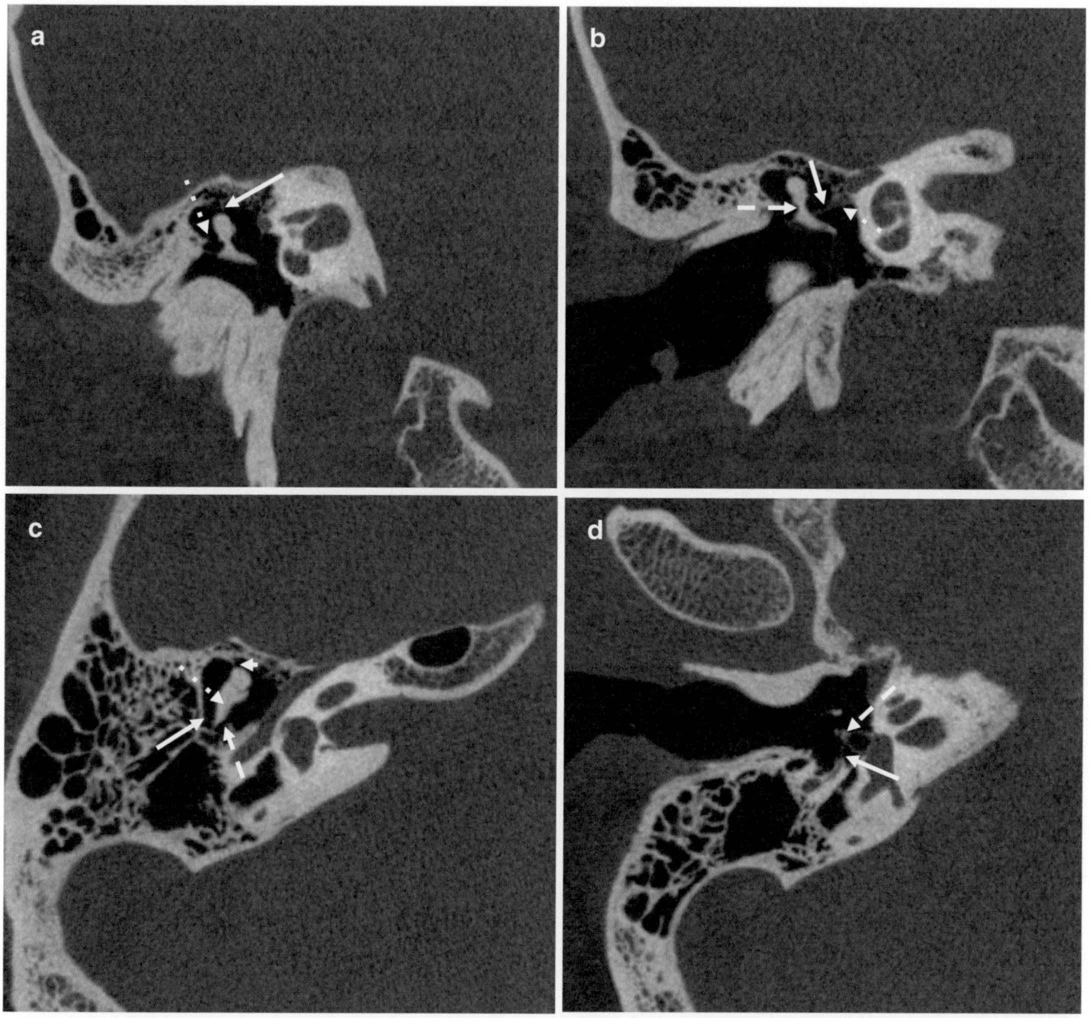

Fig. 2.5 **Ossicular chain**. (**a**) A coronal reformatted CBCT image depicts the superior malleolar ligament (arrow) that cores from the epitympanum to the head of the malleus, the lateral malleolar ligament (dotted arrow) arising from the bony margin of the tympanic notch to the neck of the malleus. (**b**) A coronal reformatted CBCT image depicts the tendon of the tensor tympani muscle (arrow) which arises from the cochleariform process (dotted arrow) and attaches to the neck of the malleus (dashed arrow). (**c**) An axial CBCT depicts the posterior incudal ligament, which is divided in the lateral (arrow) and medial part (dashed arrow), arising from the incudal fossa and inserting in the short process of the incus (dotted arrow), and the anterior malleolar ligament (short arrow) that cores from the anterior epytimpanic wall and inserts to the head of the malleus. (**d**) An axial reformatted CBCT image depicts the tendon of the stapedius muscle which arises from the apex of the pyramidal eminence (arrow) and inserts onto the posterior surface of the neck of the stapes (dashed arrow). *Abbreviation*: CBCT cone beam computed tomography

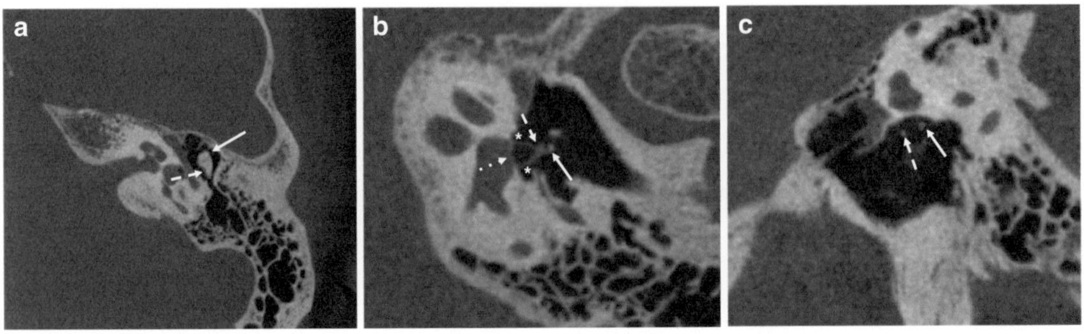

Fig. 2.6 **Ossicular chain.** (**a**) Axial reformatted CBCT image shows the head of the malleus (arrow) articulating with the body of the incus (dashed arrow) in the epitympanum. The facet for articulation with the malleus is saddle shaped and forms nearly a right angle. The body of the incus continues infero-laterally in the mesotympanum. Inferiorly, the long crus of the incus continues with the lentiform process which articulates with the head of the stapes. (**b**) Axial reformatted CBCT image shows the stapes that consists of the head (dashed arrow), which articulates with the lenticular process of the incus (arrow). The anterior and posterior crura (asterisks) continue with the footplate (dotted arrow), which attaches to the oval window thanks to the annular ligaments. (**c**) Coronal reformatted CBCT image depicts the anterior (dashed arrow) and posterior crura (arrow) of the stapes lining in the oval window niche. *Abbreviation*: CBCT cone beam computed tomography

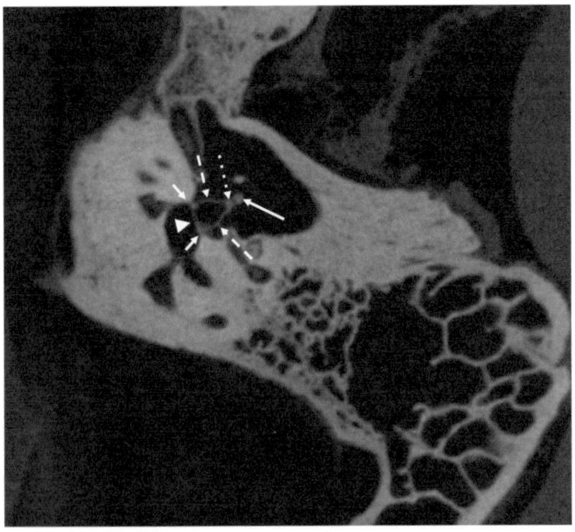

Fig. 2.7 **The stapes.** An axial reformatted postmortem CBCT image shows the stapes. The stapes consists of a head-neck (dotted arrow) articulating with the lenticular process of the incus (arrow). The neck of the stapes connects the head and the crura (dashed arrows) and offers the attachment for the stapedius muscle. The stapes continues with the footplate (arrowhead), which is attached thanks to the annular ligament (short arrows) to the oval window and lies in the oval window niche. *Abbreviation*: CBCT cone beam computed tomography

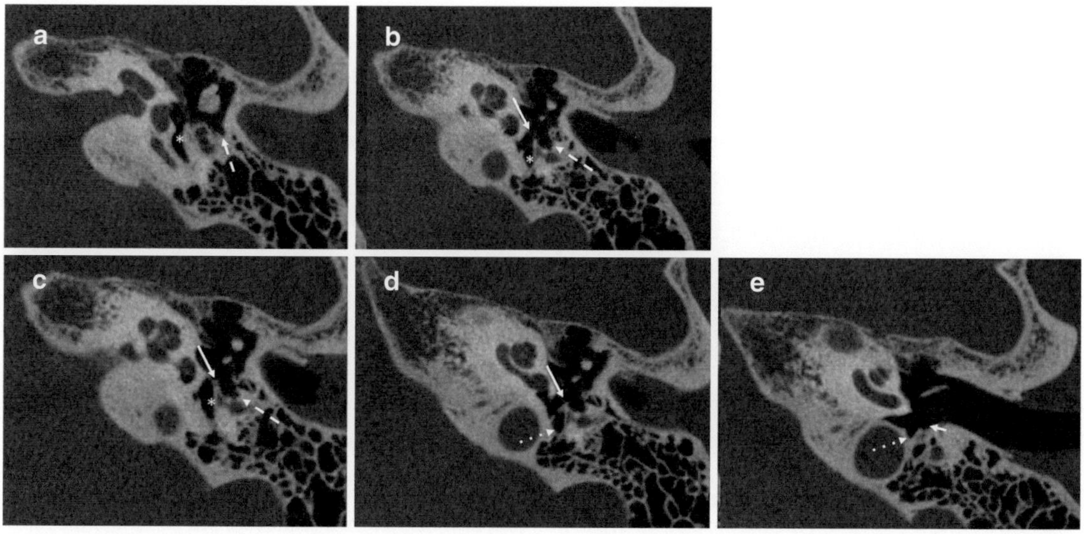

Fig. 2.8 **The retrotympanic spaces.** (**a**) The retrotympanum is divided in four spaces, the pyramidal eminence (arrow in **b**) is its main landmark that divide the medial and lateral compartiments. From the pyramidal eminence arise the chordal ridge, which goes laterally and transversally to the chordal eminence, and the ponticulus, which goes medially and transversally toward the cochlear promontory. In the medial retrotympanum two spaces can be defined: the sinus tympani (dotted arrow in **d** and **e**) inferiorly to the ponticulus and the posterior tympanic sinus (asterisk in **a**, **b**, and **c**) superiorly to the ponticulus. In the lateral retrotympanum two spaces can be defined: the lateral tympanic sinus (short arrow in **e**) inferiorly to the chordal ridge and the facial recess (dashed arrow in **a**, **b** and **c**) superiorly to the chordal ridge. *Abbreviation*: CBCT cone beam computed tomography

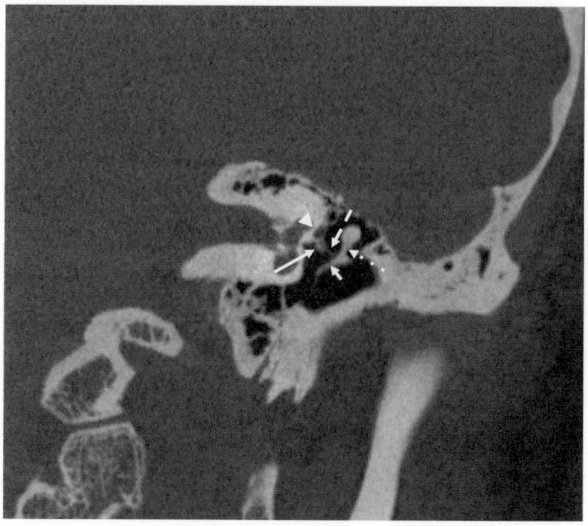

Fig. 2.9 **Tensor tympani muscle.** A coronal reformatted CBCT image shows the tensor tympani muscle which arises from the cartilaginous portion of the auditory tube and then reflects at the cochleariform process (arrow). The belly (arrowhead) attaches thanks to a tendon (dashed arrow) to the neck of the malleus (dotted arrow). It is possible to depict the manubrium of the malleus (short arrow) which attaches to the tympanic membrane. *Abbreviation*: CBCT cone beam computed tomography

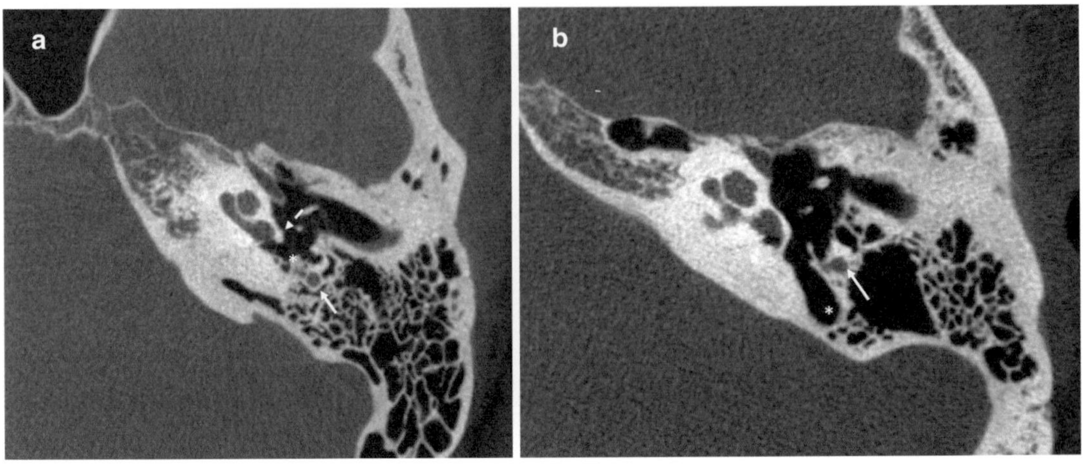

Fig. 2.10 **Sinus tympani morphology.** (**a**) An axial CBCT depicts a sinus tympani type A. In type A, the sinus tympany (asterisk) is shallow and doesn't extend medially and posteriorly beyond the mastoid portion of the facial nerve (arrow). Dashed arrow points to cochlear promontory. (**b**) An axial CBCT depicts a deep sinus tympani type C which is deep with posterior extension (asterisk) beyond to the mastoid portion of the facial nerve (arrow). In these cases, the sinus tympani is very large, and these patients usually have a well-pneumatized mastoid. *Abbreviation*: CBCT cone beam computed tomography

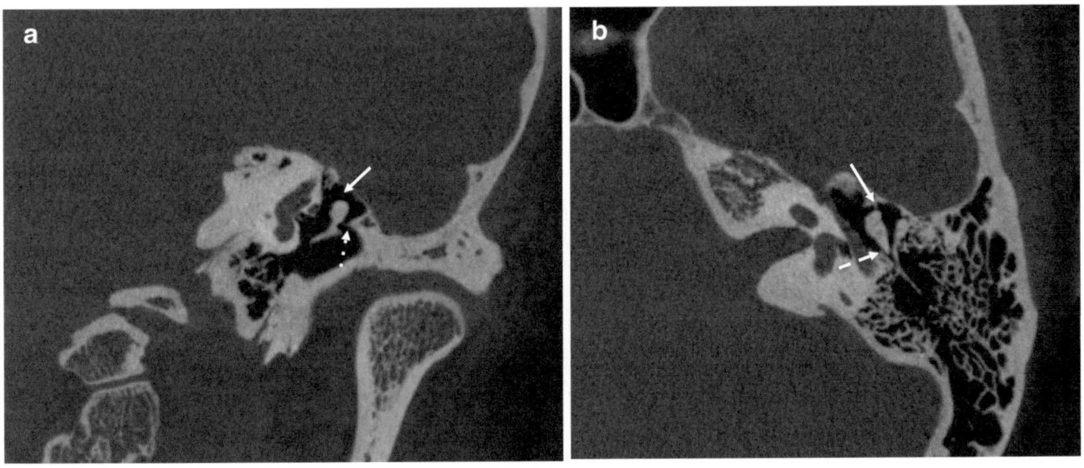

Fig. 2.11 **Ossicular ligaments.** (**a**) A coronal reformatted CBCT image depicts the ligaments of the malleus. The superior ligament (arrow) descends from the epitympanum to the head of the malleus. The lateral (dotted arrow) arises from the bony margin of tympanic notch and attaches to the neck of the malleus. (**b**) An axial reformatted CBCT image shows the anterior ligament of the malleus (arrow) originating from anterior epitympanic wall and attaching to head of the malleus and the posterior incudal ligament (dashed arrow) originating from the short process of the incus and attaching to the fossa incudis. *Abbreviation*: CBCT cone beam computed tomography

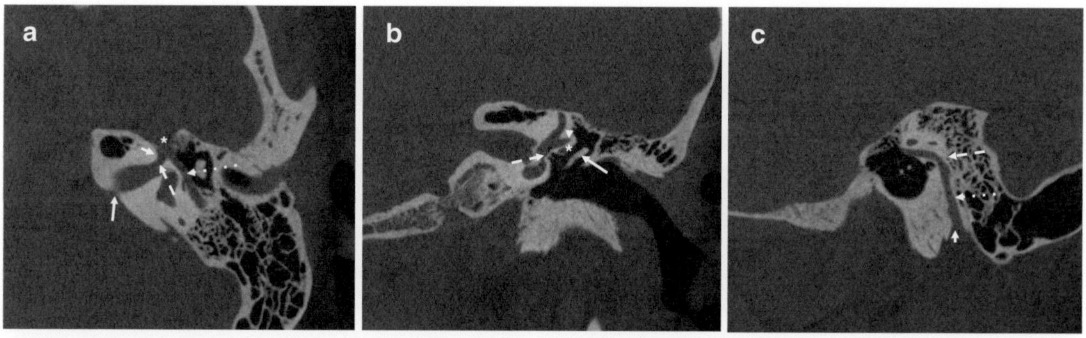

Fig. 2.12 Bony canal of the facial nerve. (**a**) Axial reformatted CBCT image indicates the intracanalicular segment of the facial nerve, which courses from the internal porus acusticus (arrow) through the internal auditory canal to the fundus (dashed arrow). The shortest segment of the facial nerve is the labyrinthine segment (short arrow) which travels anterior-laterally from the fundus and superior to the cochlea until it reaches the geniculate ganglion. The geniculate ganglion lies in geniculate fossa (asterisk). At the geniculate ganglion, the facial nerve makes a 75 degree turn posteriorly to become the tympanic segment (dotted arrow). (**b**) Coronal reformatted CBCT image depicts the tympanic segment (asterisk) of the facial nerve. The segment runs from the geniculate ganglion to the second (or posterior) genu. Within the tympanic cavity, the facial nerve passes medial to the incus (arrow). It runs posterior-superior to the cochleariform process (not shown), superior and lateral to the oval window (dashed arrow), and then inferior to the lateral semicircular canal (arrowhead). (**c**) At the pyramidal process, the tympanic segment turns inferiorly at a 95–125° angle at the second genu (dashed arrow) to become the mastoid or vertical segment (dotte arrow). The mastoid segment of the facial nerve runs posteromedially along the external auditory canal to its exit from the temporal bone at the stylomastoid foramen (short arrow). Two branches arise from the mastoid segment: the nerve to the stapedius and the chorda tympani. The nerve exits the temporal bone at the stylomastoid foramen, entering the substance of the parotid gland. *Abbreviation*: CBCT cone beam computed tomography

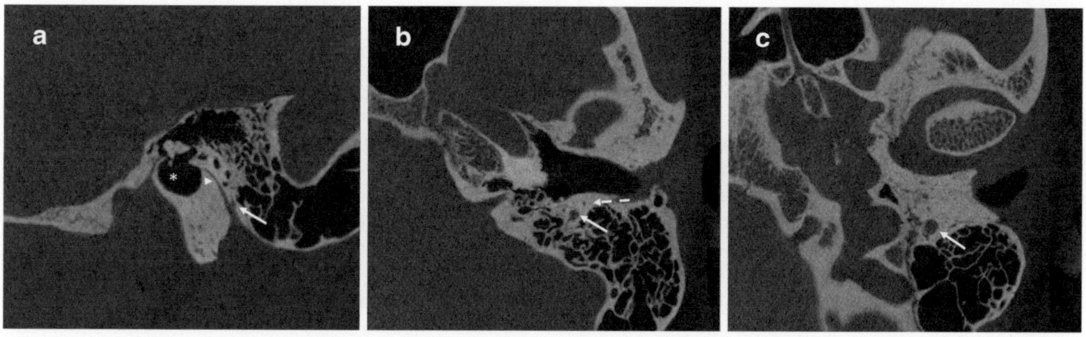

Fig. 2.13 Chorda tympani bony canal. (**a**) A coronal reformatted CBCT image shows the posterior canaliculus (arrowhead) of the facial nerve. Chorda tympani aescends vertically within the posterior canaliculus in the anterior and lateral aspect of the mastoid bone, just posterior to the EAC (asterisk). The chorda tympani carries afferent taste fibers from the two anterior thirds of the tongue and joins the mastoid segment of the facial nerve just before exiting the stylomastoid foramen (arrow). (**b**) An axial reformatted CBCT image shows the mastoid portion of facial nerve (arrow) and the accompanying posterior canaliculus (dashed arrow). (**c**) Axial CBCT shows the stylomastoid foramen (arrow) as a rounded opening at the inferior end of the facial canal. It is located on the inferior surface of the petrous temporal bone, between the base of the styloid process and the mastoid process of the temporal bone. It transmits the facial nerve and stylomastoid artery (branch of posterior auricular artery or, sometimes, occipital artery). *Abbreviation*: CBCT cone beam computed tomography

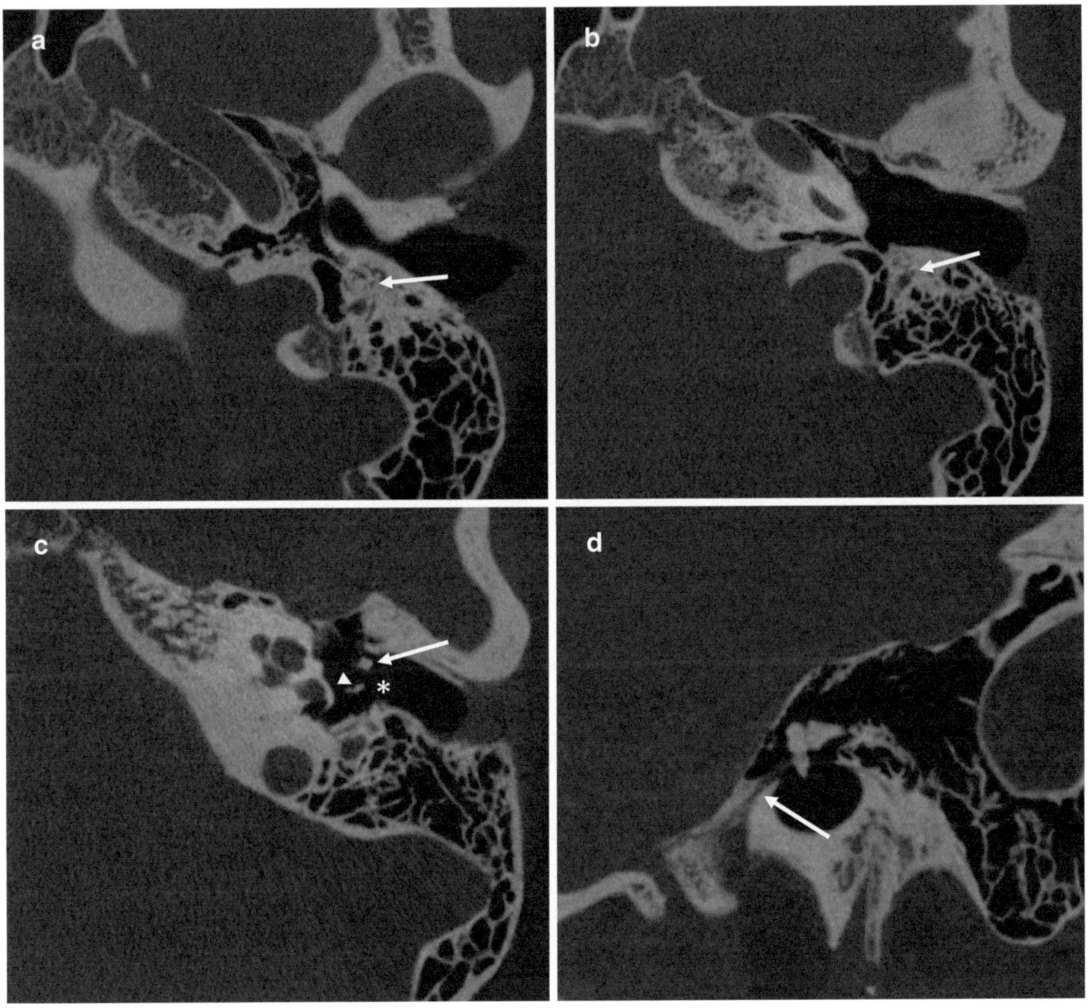

Fig. 2.14 Chorda tympany bony canal. (**a**) An axial reformatted CBCT image shows the origin of the chorda tympani (arrow) at the level of the distal mastoid segment of the facial nerve. Here, the chorda tympani leaves the facial nerve and courses in the posterior canaliculus which is antero-lateral to the course of the facial canal. (**b**) An axial reformatted CBCT image passing through the external auditory canal shows the posterior canaliculus coursing antero-lateral to the facial canal (arrow), approaching the middle ear. (**c**) The chorda tympani leaves the posterior canaliculus at the level of the tympanic annulus and enters in the middle ear. Here, the chorda tympani passes immediately medial to the tympanic membrane (asterisk), between the malleus (arrow) and incus (arrowhead), to reach the anterior canaliculus. (**d**) A sagittal CBCT shows the anterior canaliculus (arrow) passing medial to the glenoid fossa, along the petrotympanic fissure to exit the skull base. It trasmits the chorda tympani along with the anterior tympanic artery (branch of the external carotid artery). *Abbreviation*: CBCT cone beam computed tomography

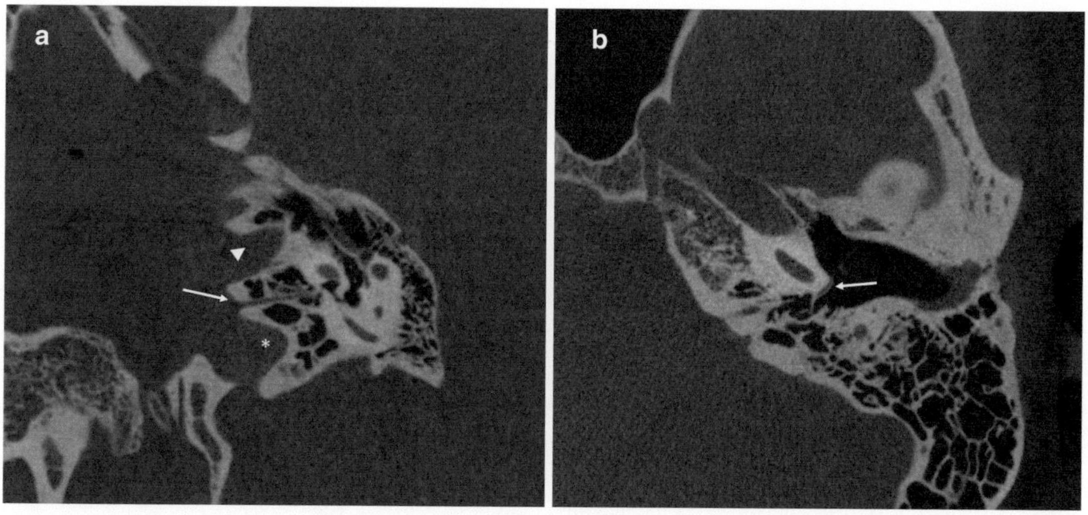

Fig. 2.15 **Inferior tympanic canaliculus.** (**a**) A reformatted CBCT image passing through the jugular foramen depicts the inferior tympanic canaliculus (arrow), a bony canal that separates the opening of the carotid canal (arrowhead) anteromedially from the jugular foramen (asterisk) posterolaterally. It is located medially to the styloid foramen and the styloid process of the temporal bone. Inside the inferior tympanic canaliculus lies the inferior tympanic artery (branch of the ascending pharyngeal artery) in addition to the tympanic branch of the glossopharyngeal nerve (Jacobson nerve). (**b**) An axial CBCT depicts the tympanic nerve (arrow) emerging on the promontory of the middle ear, on its medial wall and anterior to the round window. It exits through the internal aperture of the tympanic canaliculus which lies anterior to the inferior half of the round window. *Abbreviation*: CBCT cone beam computed tomography

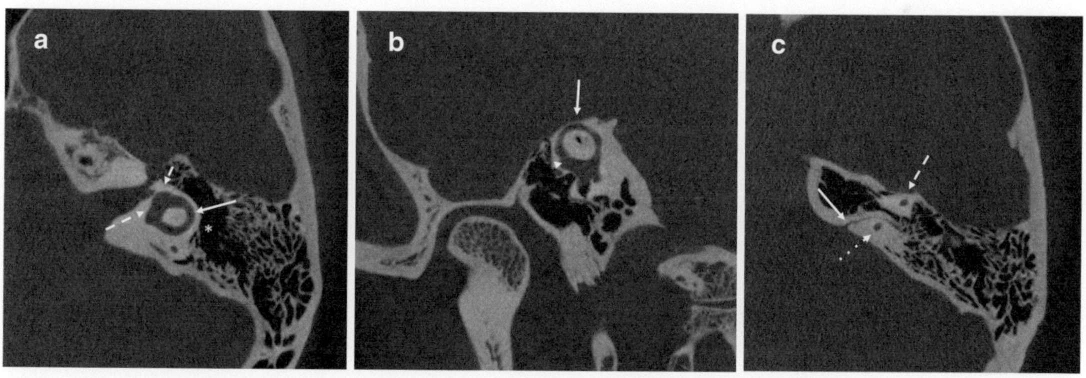

Fig. 2.16 **Semicircular canals and subarcuate canal.** (**a**) An axial reformatted CBCT image depicts the lateral semicircular (arrow) which slightly protrudes into the epitympanum (asterisk). It is in close contact with the midtympanic portion of the facial nerve, which passes along the undersurface of the lateral semicircular canal. Each semicircular canal has an enlargement at one end, forming a bony ampulla (short arrow) that contains the cristae with the vestibular sensory epithelium and that opens in the vestibule (dashed arrow). The non-ampullary end of the semicircular canal joins the vestibule as well. (**b**) A coronal CBCT depicts the superior semicircular canal. The upper bony margin of the superior semicircular canal forms a convexity in the petrous roof, the arcuate eminence (arrow). The non-ampullary end of the superior semicircular canal opens in the vestibule and joins with the posterior semicircular canals to form a common crus (arrowhead). (**c**) An axial reformatted CBCT image depicts the subarcuate canal (arrow). It is a thin canal coursing between the anterior (dashed arrow) and posterior part (dotted arrow) of the superior semicircular canal which joins the mastoid antrum to the posterior cranial fossa. It contains the subarcuate artery and vein. *Abbreviation*: CBCT cone beam computed tomography

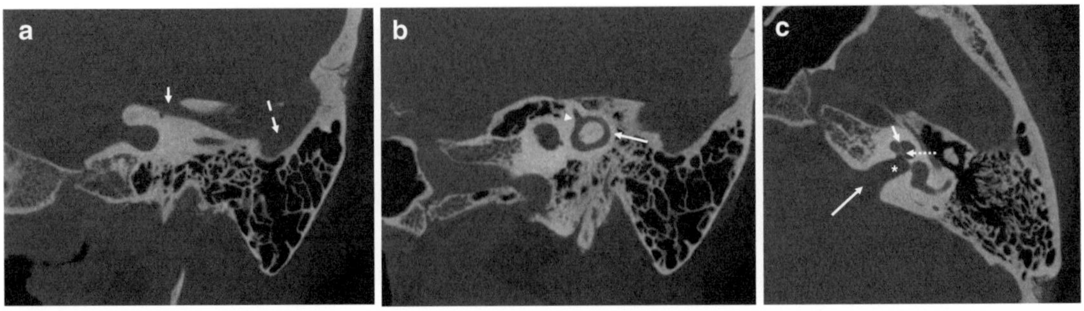

Fig. 2.17 Superior petrosal sinus, semicircular canals, and internal auditory canal. (**a**) A parasagittal reformatted CBCT image depicts the superior petrosal sinus (arrow) which drains in the cavernous sinus. It courses posterolaterally, along the superior aspect of the petrous temporal bone, to drain into the sigmoid sinus (dashed arrow). The superior petrosal sinus receives the labyrinthine vein, hence participating in the draining of the inner ear structures. (**b**) A sagittal reformatted CBCT image depicts the posterior semicircular (arrow). The non-ampullary portion of the posterior semicircular joins the non-ampullary portion of the superior semicircular canal forming a common crus (arrowhead) which opens in the vestibule. (**c**) An axial CBCT reformat depicts the IAC. The porus acusticus (arrow) of the IAC opens in the ponto-cerebellar-cistern angle. The IAC courses anterolaterally to the fundus (asterisk), a thin cribriform plate separates the IAC from the cochlea and the vestibule. The fundus is divided in a superior and inferior segments by the transverse crest (also called falciform crest). The superior half is further divided into anterior and inferior segments by Bill's bar. The base of the cochlea connects with the IAC at the fundus. The cochlea is a snail-shaped structure which makes approximately two and a half turns around a central axis, the modiolus (dotted arrow), which contains the Rosenthal's canal housing the cohlear nerve. It is divided in thee turns (basal, middle, apical) by thin bony plate, the interscalar septum (short arrow). The basal turn of the cochlea has two openings in the tympanic cavity, the round window and the oval window, and the latter is in contact with the footplate of the stapes thanks to the annular ligament. *Abbreviations*: CBCT cone beam computed tomography, IAC internal audditory canal

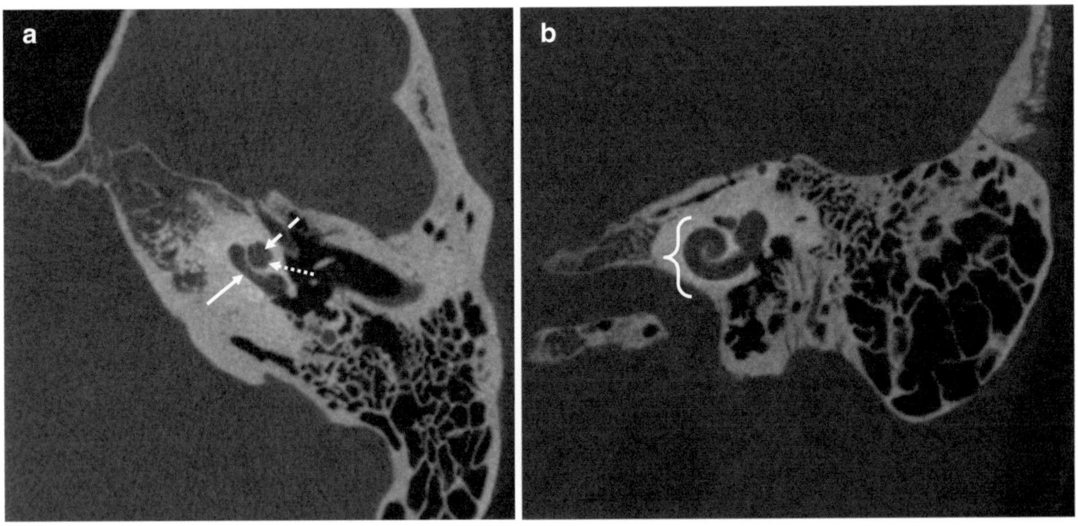

Fig. 2.18 Cochlea. (**a**) An axial reformatted CBCT image depicts the cochlea. The cochlea is a spiral-shaped structure and consists of three turns (precisely 2.5 turns) separated by the interscalar septum: the basal (arrow), middle (dotted arrow), and apical turn (dashed arrow). Each turn is subdivided into three compartments or scalae: the scala vestibuli, which lies superior to the cochlear duct and abuts the oval window, and the scala tympani, which lies inferior to the cochlear duct and terminates at the round window. Scala vestibuli and scala timpani contain perilymph. The scala media contains endolymph, and the potential difference of the endolymph and the perilymph is essential for the activity of the stereocilia of the hairy cells of the organ of Corti. (**b**) A double oblique reformatted CBCT image shows the entire length of the cochlea (bracket) in a single slice. The double oblique reformat is performed setting the reconstruction plane parallel to the basal turn in the axial and coronal plane. *Abbreviation*: CBCT cone beam computed tomography

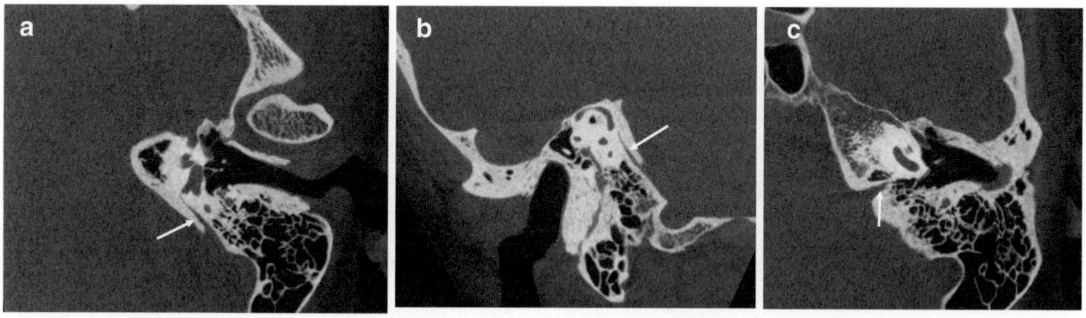

Fig. 2.19 Vestibular and cochlear aqueduct. (**a**) An axial reformatted CBCT image depicts the vestibular aqueduct (arrow). The vestibular aqueduct is a bony canal connecting the vestibule and the posterior surface of the petrous bone. It harbors the endolymphatic duct, which ends with the endolymphatic sac, a blind pouch between the layers of the dura mater within the cranial cavity. (**b**) A parasagittal reformatted CBCT image along the Poschl's plane of the petrous bone shows the vertical course of the vestibular aqueduct (arrow). (**c**) An axial reformatted CBCT image depicts the cochlear aqueduct (arrow). The cochlear aqueduct extends from the scala tympani of the basal turn of the cochlea and runs parallel and posteriorly to the internal auditory canal. It opens lateral to the jugular foramen in the inferior surface of the petrous part of the temporal bone. Contrary to the vestibular aqueducts, it is a patent communication between the subarachnoid cavity and the membranous labyrinth. *Abbreviation*: CBCT cone beam computed tomography

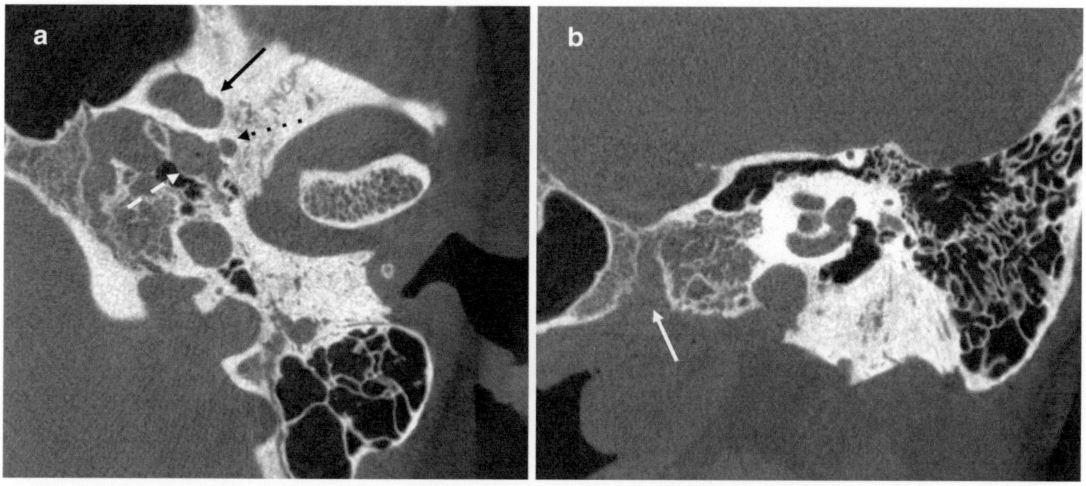

Fig. 2.20 Foramina in the middle cranial fossa. (**a**) An axial CBCT depicts the anatomy of the foramina in the middle cranial fossa. The foramen ovale (black arrow) is an oval-shaped opening in the posterior base of the greater wing of the sphenoid bone. The mandibular division of the trigeminal nerve (CN V3), accessory meningeal artery, emissary veins between the cavernous sinuses and pterygoid plexus, otic ganglion, and occasionally the nervus spinosus and lesser petrosal nerve pass through the oval foramen. Posteriorly and laterally it is possible to recognize the foramen spinosum (black dotted arrow); it connects the middle cranial fossa with the infratemporal fossa. It transmits the middle meningeal artery, middle meningeal vein, and the nervus spinosus. Medially there is the foramen lacerum (dashed arrow), at the continuation of the petrosphenoidal and petroclival fissures. The foramen transmits the small meningeal branches of the ascending pharyngeal artery and emissary veins from the cavernous sinus to the pterygoid venous plexus. The greater petrosal nerve enters to join with the deep petrosal nerve and leaves anteriorly as the nerve of the pterygoid canal. (**b**) A sagittal CBCT shows the foramen ovale (arrow) which offers a communication between the middle cranial fossa and the infratemporal fossa. *Abbreviation*: CBCT cone beam computed tomography

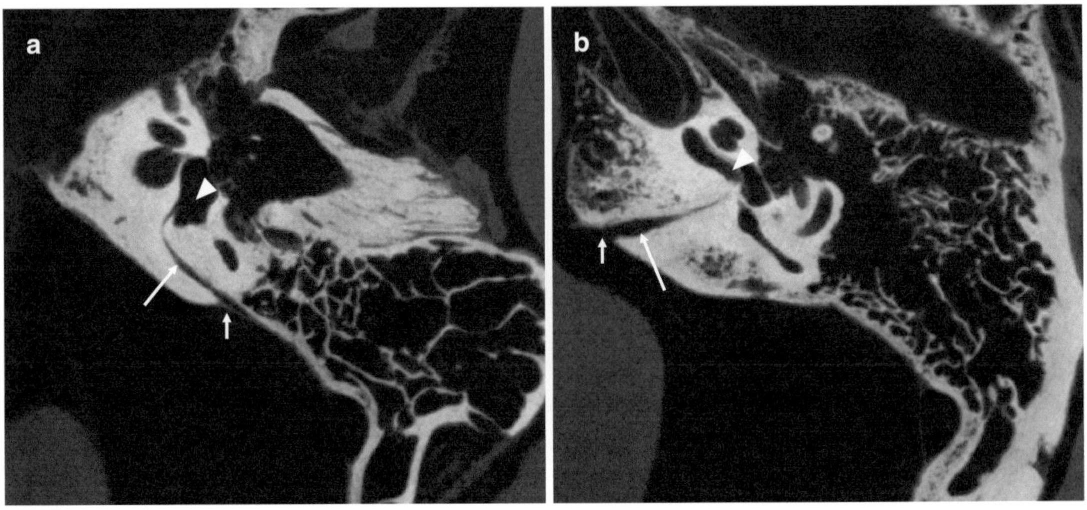

Fig. 2.21 **Vestibular and cochlear aqueducts.** (**a**) An axial reformatted CBCT image obtained postmortem depicts the vestibular aqueduct (arrow), connecting the vestibule (arrowhead) and the posterior surface of the petrous bone. Note that the dura mater (short arrow) covers the vestibular acqueduct thus the endolymphatic sac is extradural. (**b**) An axial reformatted CBCT image depicts the cochlear aqueduct (arrow). The cochlear aqueduct extends from the scala tympani of the basal turn (arrowhead) of the cochlea and runs parallel and posteriorly to the internal auditory canal. It is a patent communication between the subarachnoid space and the scala tympani because the dura mater does not cover its ostium (short arrow), for this reason the composition of the cerebrospinal fluid and the perlymph in the basal turn are similar. *Abbreviation*: CBCT cone beam computed tomography

References

1. Marchioni D, Molteni G, Presutti L. Endoscopic anatomy of the middle ear. Indian. J Otolaryngol Head Neck Surg. 2011;63(2):101–13. https://doi.org/10.1007/s12070-011-0159-0. Epub 2011 Feb 23. PMID: 22468244; PMCID: PMC3102170.
2. Nogueira JF, Mattioli F, Presutti L, Marchioni D. Endoscopic anatomy of the retrotympanum. Otolaryngol Clin N Am. 2013;46(2):179–88. https://doi.org/10.1016/j.otc.2012.10.003. Epub 2013 Jan 5. PMID: 23566904.
3. Marchioni D, Piccinini A, Alicandri-Ciufelli M, Presutti L. Endoscopic anatomy and ventilation of the epitympanum. Otolaryngol Clin N Am. 2013;46(2):165–78. https://doi.org/10.1016/j.otc.2012.10.002. Epub 2012 Nov 27.
4. Juliano AF, Ginat DT, Moonis G. Imaging review of the temporal bone: part I. Anatomy and inflammatory and neoplastic processes. Radiology. 2013;269(1):17–33. https://doi.org/10.1148/radiol.13120733.
5. Lane JI, Lindell EP, Witte RJ, DeLone DR, Driscoll CL. Middle and inner ear: improved depiction with multiplanar reconstruction of volumetric CT data. Radiographics. 2006;26(1):115–24. https://doi.org/10.1148/rg.261055703.
6. Lemmerling MM, Stambuk HE, Mancuso AA, Antonelli PJ, Kubilis PS. CT of the normal suspensory ligaments of the ossicles in the middle ear. AJNR Am J Neuroradiol. 1997;18(3):471–7. PMID: 9090405; PMCID: PMC8338412.

MRI of the Internal Auditory Canal, Labyrinth, and Middle Ear

3

Guido Del Vecchio, Andrea Fontana,
Giorgio Conte, Francesco Maria Lo Russo,
Luca Caschera, Fabio Triulzi,
Antonia Valentina Genovese, and Elisa Scola

The MRI examination of the temporal bone employs high-resolution T2-weighted sequences to investigate the anatomy of the cerebellopontine angle and inner ear. The high-resolution T2-weighted images have different techniques and names according to the MR scan vendor. It provides detailed imaging of the inner ear and its nerves, serving as a valuable complement to CT scans, particularly in assessing surgical candidates. This is especially crucial in pediatric cochlear implantation cases, where abnormalities in the labyrinth may be associated with facial and cochlear nerve malformations. Advancements in imaging technology, such as the development of contrast-enhanced heavily T2-weighted 3D FLAIR on a 3 Tesla scanner, now allow the visualization of the membranous labyrinth and the evaluation of pathological conditions affecting the labyrinth itself. See Chap. 9, for a detailed description of the anatomy of membranous labyrinth.

3.1 Anatomy of the Internal Acoustic Canal

The internal auditory canal (IAC) contains the facial nerve, vestibulocochlear nerve, nervus intermedius, and labyrinthine artery. Emerging just posterosuperior to the facial nerve, the vestibulocochlear nerve initially appears as a single large nerve before branching into the cochlear, superior, and inferior vestibular nerves near the porus acusticus. In the majority of cases, 3-T imaging reveals the nervus intermedius, which exits the brainstem laterally to the motor root of the facial nerve and follows a path along the posterior aspect of cranial nerve VII. It ultimately joins the facial nerve just proximal to the meatal foramen at the fundus of the IAC. Additionally, in 20–40% of individuals, there is an entry of the anterior inferior cerebellar artery (AICA) into the IAC, typically without clinical significance (Figs. 3.1, 3.2, 3.3, and 3.4).

G. Del Vecchio · F. M. Lo Russo · L. Caschera
A. V. Genovese · E. Scola (✉)
Neuroradiology Unit, Fondazione IRCCS Ca' Granda Ospedale Maggiore Policlinico, Milan, Italy
e-mail: guido.delvecchio@policlinico.mi.it; francesco.lorusso@policlinico.mi.it; luca.caschera@policlinico.mi.it; valentina.genovese@policlinico.mi.it; elisa.scola@policlinico.mi.it

A. Fontana
School in Radiodiagnostics, Università degli Studi di Milano, Milan, Italy

G. Conte · F. Triulzi
Neuroradiology Unit, Fondazione IRCCS Ca' Granda Ospedale Maggiore Policlinico, Milan, Italy

Department of Pathophysiology and Transplantation, University of Milan, Milan, Italy
e-mail: giorgio.conte@policlinico.mi.it; fabio.triulzi@policlinico.mi.it

G. Conte et al. (eds.), *Atlas of Normal and Pathological Findings in Otoneuroradiology*,
https://doi.org/10.1007/978-3-032-08232-9_3

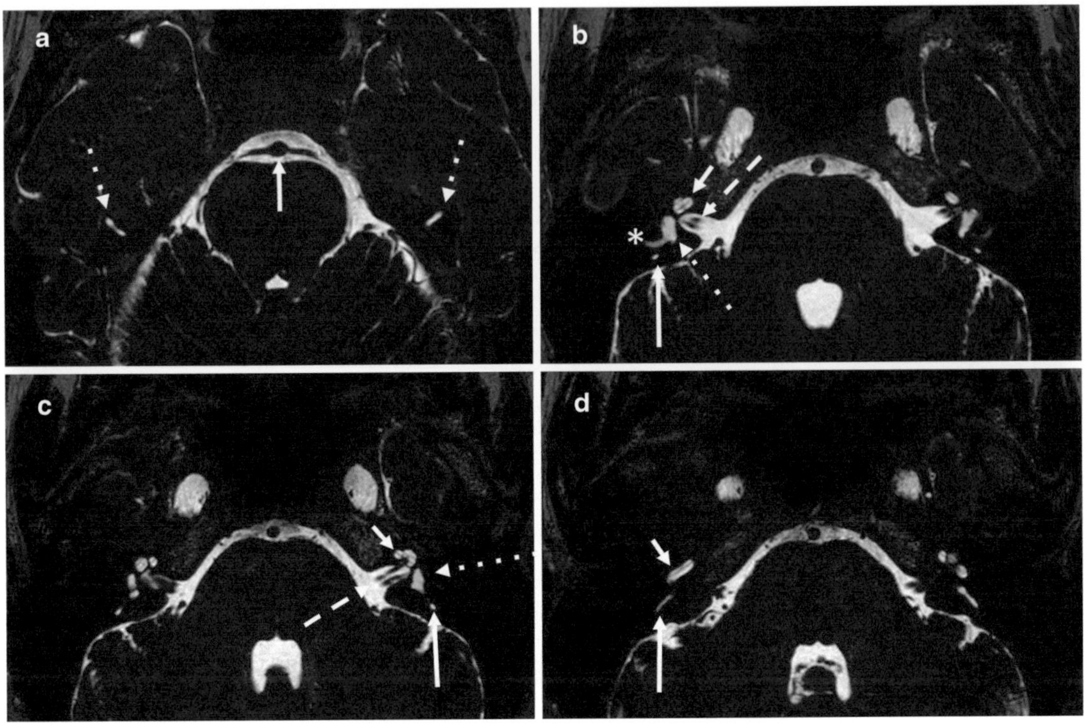

Fig. 3.1 Internal acoustic canal, axial plane. (**a**) Axial 3D TSE-T2W image passing cranial to the plane of IAC shows the superior semicircular canal (dotted arrows) and the basilar artery (arrow). (**b**, **c**) Axial 3D TSE-T2W image passing through the upper portion of IAC. Intracanalicular segment of facial and vestibular nerves, anteriorly and posteriorly, respectively, in the IAC (dashed arrow). Some inner ear structures are shown: vestibule (dotted arrows), posterior semicircular canal (arrow), lateral semicircular canal (asterisk), apical and medial turns of the cochlea (short arrows). (**d**) Axial 3D TSE-T2W image passing just below the IAC plane; posterior semicircular canal (arrow) is better seen, basal turn of the cochlea (short arrow). *Abbreviations: IAC* = internal auditory canal, *TSE* = turbo spin echo

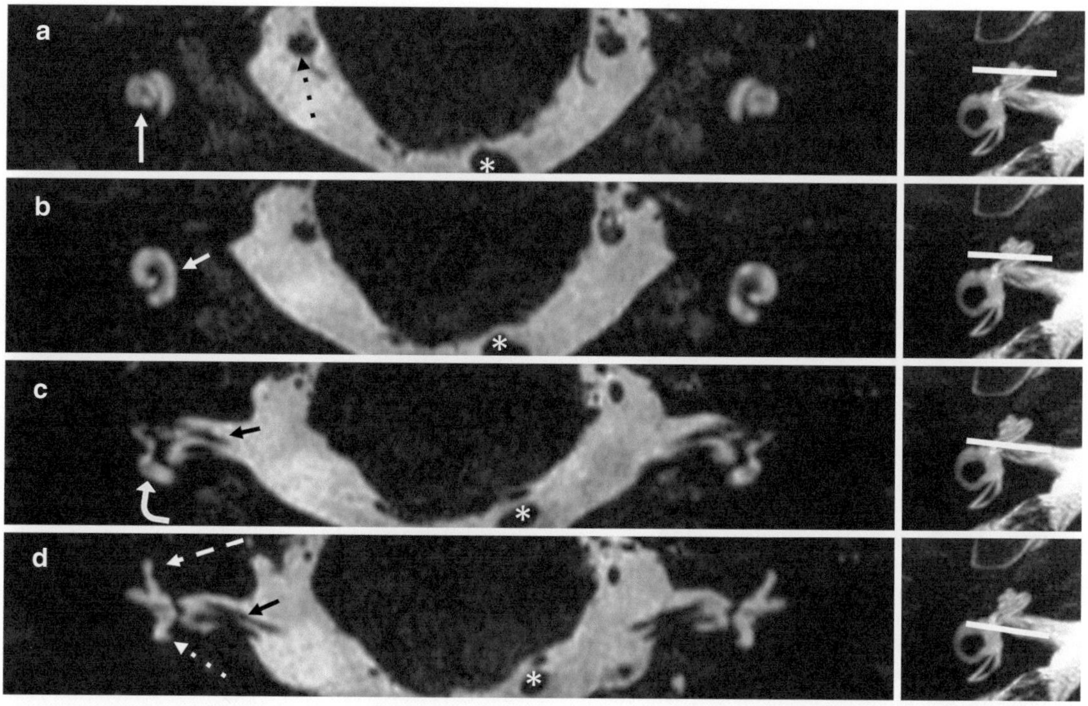

Fig. 3.2 Internal acoustic canal, coronal plane. (**a**–**d**) coronal MIP reconstructed 3D TSE-T2W anterior to posterior planes show apical (arrow in **a**) and medial (short arrow in **b**) turns of the cochlea, the vestibule (curved arrow in **c**), the superior semicircular canal (dashed arrow in **d**) and the posterior semicircular canal (dotted arrow in **d**). Figures (**c**) and (**d**) show the intracanalicular segment of the facial nerve and statoacoustic nerve bundle (black short arrow). Note the basilar artery (asterisks) and right 5th cranial nerve (black dotted arrow in **a**). *Abbreviations: TSE* = turbo spin echo, *IAC* = internal auditory canal, *MIP* = maximum intensity projection

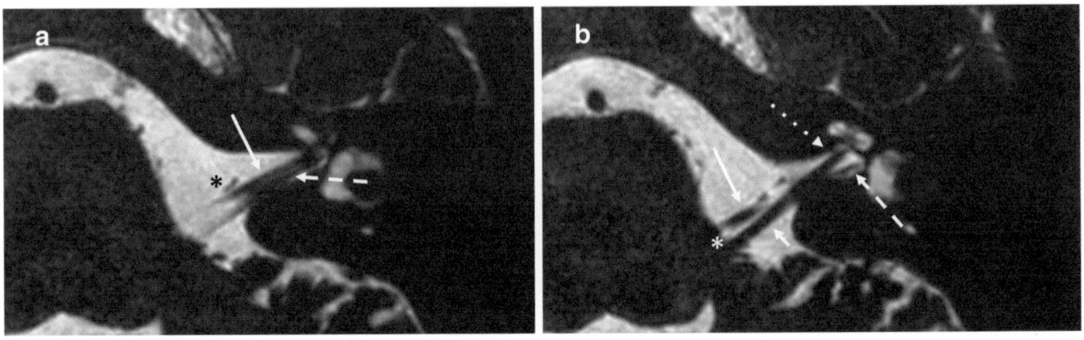

Fig. 3.3 Internal acoustic canal and VII and VIII nerve anatomy. The IAC is a bony canal within the petrous part of the temporal bone, coated with dura mater and arachnoid meninges and filled with CSF. The opening is called porus acusticus, the lateral boundary is the fundus, where the canal splits into three distinct openings. The facial nerve (arrow in **a** and **b**) originates from the retro-olivary groove at the bulbopontine sulcus (white asterisk in **b**) , located medially to the cochleo-vestibular nerve (short arrow in **b**). The facial nerve courses upwards and laterally in the cistern, above the VIII nerve, reaching and traversing the anterosuperior quadrant of the cerebellopontine angle, and remains superior to the cochlear nerve up to the facial canal. The cochleovestibular nerve keeps its two components closely associated until the IAC. At the middle third of IAC, it divides into three components: the cochlear nerve anteriorly (dotted arrow in **b**) and the vestibular nerve inferiorly. The vestibular nerve, immediately after the division, shows a swelling (the vestibular ganglion). Distal to the ganglion, the vestibular nerve divides into a superior branch, the superior vestibular nerve (dashed arrow in **a**), and an inferior branch, the inferior vestibular nerve (dashed arrow in **b**). The cochleovestibular nerve is typically 1.5 to 2 times larger in diameter than the facial nerve. (**a, b**) axial 3D TSE-T2W images in the plane passing through the IAC in cranial-caudal direction. (**a**) axial TSE-T2W shows facial nerve (arrow) and superior vestibular nerve (dotted arrow). Note the anterior-inferior cerebellar artery (AICA) looping into the proximal portion of the IAC (black asterisk). (**b**) axial TSE-T2W shows cisternal segment of facial (arrow) and vestibulocochlear (short arrow) nerves. Note also the vestibulocochlear nerve split in the IAC in cochlear nerve (dotted arrow) which runs through the Rosenthal canal and inferior vestibular nerve (dashed arrow). *Abbreviations: IAC* = internal acoustic canal, *CSF* = cerebrospinal fluid, *TSE* = turbo spin echo

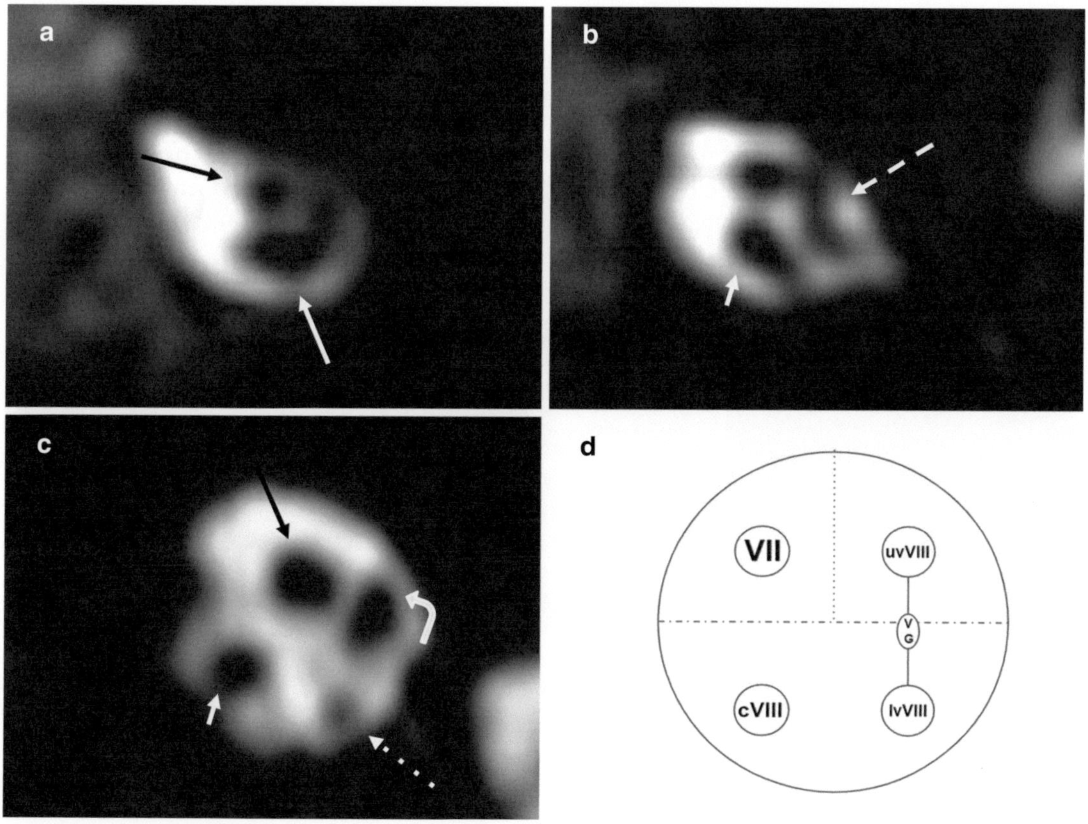

Fig. 3.4 Internal acoustic canal and VII e VIII nerve anatomy (continues from Fig. 3.3). (**a**) proximal IAC para-sagittal 3D TSE-T2W image shows two nerves, the facial nerve superiorly (black arrow) and the vestibulo-cochlear nerve inferiorly (arrow) (**b**) third middle IAC para-sagittal 3D TSE-T2W shows the statoacoustic bundle division into the cochlear nerve inferiorly (short arrow) and the vestibular nerve (dashed arrow). (**c**) distal IAC parasagittal 3D TSE-T2W shows four nerves: the facial nerve superior-anterior (black arrow), the cochlear nerve anterior-inferior (short arrow), the superior vestibular nerve posterior-superior (curved arrow), and the inferior vestibular nerve posterior-inferior (dotted arrow). (**d**) schematic representation of figure (**c**) also showing Bill's barr (dotted line) and falciform crest (dotted and dashed line), two bony ridges not appreciable on standard 3D TSE-T2W MRI sequence. *Abbreviations*: *TSE* = turbo spin echo, *IAC* = internal acoustic canal, *VII* = facial nerve; *cVIII* = cochlear branch of the eighth cranial nerve, *uvVIII* = upper vestibular component of the eighth cranial nerve, *lvVIII* = lower vestibular component of the eighth cranial nerve

3.2 Anatomy of the Labyrinth

The labyrinth comprises a bony labyrinth and a membranous labyrinth, with the former being divided into semicircular canals, vestibule, and cochlea, best assessed using CBCT. MRI depicts the fluid content of the labyrinth (Figs. 3.5, 3.6, 3.7, 3.8, 3.9, 3.10, and 3.11). Within the bony labyrinth lies the membranous labyrinth, consisting of ducts and sacs containing endolymph, separated from the bone by perilymphatic fluid (Figs. 3.9, 3.10, and 3.11). In the osseous vestibule, the utricle, adjacent to the semicircular canals and innervated by the superior vestibular nerve, detects horizontal acceleration. The saccule, near the cochlea and innervated by the saccular branch of the inferior vestibular nerve, detects vertical linear acceleration. The semicircular canals house the semicircular ducts; the superior and lateral are innervated by the superior vestibular nerve, while the posterior is innervated by the inferior vestibular nerve. The ducts have focal dilations called ampullae, each containing a crista ampullaris, detectable on high-resolution T2-weighted images. The cochlea consists of the scala media, bordered by perilymphatic channels called the scala tympani and scala vestibuli. The scala vestibuli transmits fluid waves from the oval window, and the scala tympani allows pressure decompression by propagating waves to the round window;the two scalae met togheter at the helicotrema in the cochlea apex. The spiral lamina along the inner wall of the cochlea is visible on heavily T2-weighted images, acting as a landmark between the scala vestibuli and tympani. The scala media, between these structures, is bordered by the Reissner membrane ventrally, basilar membrane dorsally, and spiral ligament and otic capsule laterally.

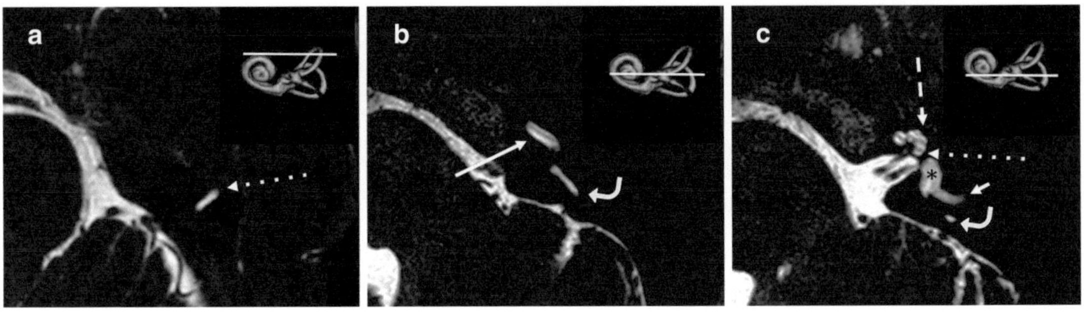

Fig. 3.5 Petrous labyrinth, axial plane. The labyrinth comprises the semicircular canals, the vestibule, and the cochlea. The cochlea, a shell-shaped spiral, makes between two-and-a-half and two-and-three-quarters turns around the modiolus, which contain the spiral ganglion. The vestibular system comprises the vestibule and three semicircular canals (anterior, posterior, and lateral), that are ringlike structures with an enlarged end, the ampulla. (**a–c**) Axial 3D TSE-T2W image shows the basal (arrow in **b**), the middle (dotted arrow in **c**), and the apical turns (dashed arrow in **c**) of the cochlea. Note also the vestibule (black asterisk in **c**), the superior semicircular canal (dotted arrow in **a**), the posterior semicircular canal (curved arrow in **c**), and the lateral semicircular canal (short arrow in **c**). *Abbreviation: TSE* = turbo spin echo

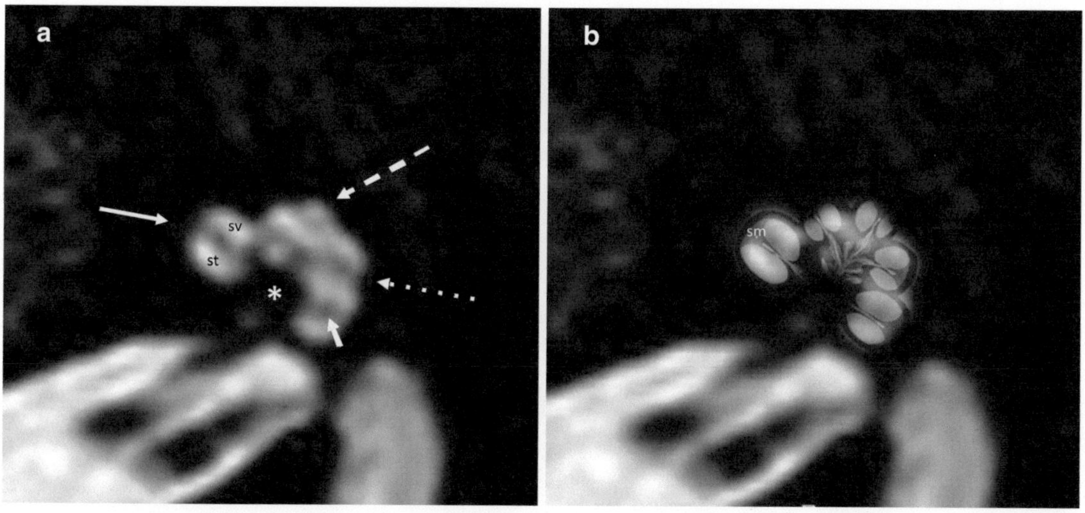

Fig. 3.6 The cochlea, axial plane. The cochlea consists of the scala media, bordered by two perilymphatic channels called the scala tympani and the scala vestibuli. The scala vestibuli transmits fluid waves from the oval window, whilst the scala tympani allows pressure decompression by propagating waves to the round window; the two scalae met together at the helicotrema in the cochlea apex. The spiral lamina along the inner wall of the cochlea is visible on heavily T2-weighted sequences, and works as a landmark between the scala vestibuli and tympani. The scala media, between these structures, is bordered by the Reissner membrane ventrally, basilar membrane dorsally, and spiral ligament and otic capsule laterally. (**a**) axial 3D TSE-T2W image shows the the middle (arrow), and the apical (dashed and dotted arrows) turns of the cochlea, the modiolus (asterisk), and the spiral lamina (short arrow) which divides the scala tympani (st) and the scala vestibuli (sv). (**b**) Schematic representation of (**a**) showing the scala media (sm), bordered by the Reissner membrane (not visible on MR imaging). *Abbreviation: TSE* = turbo spin echo

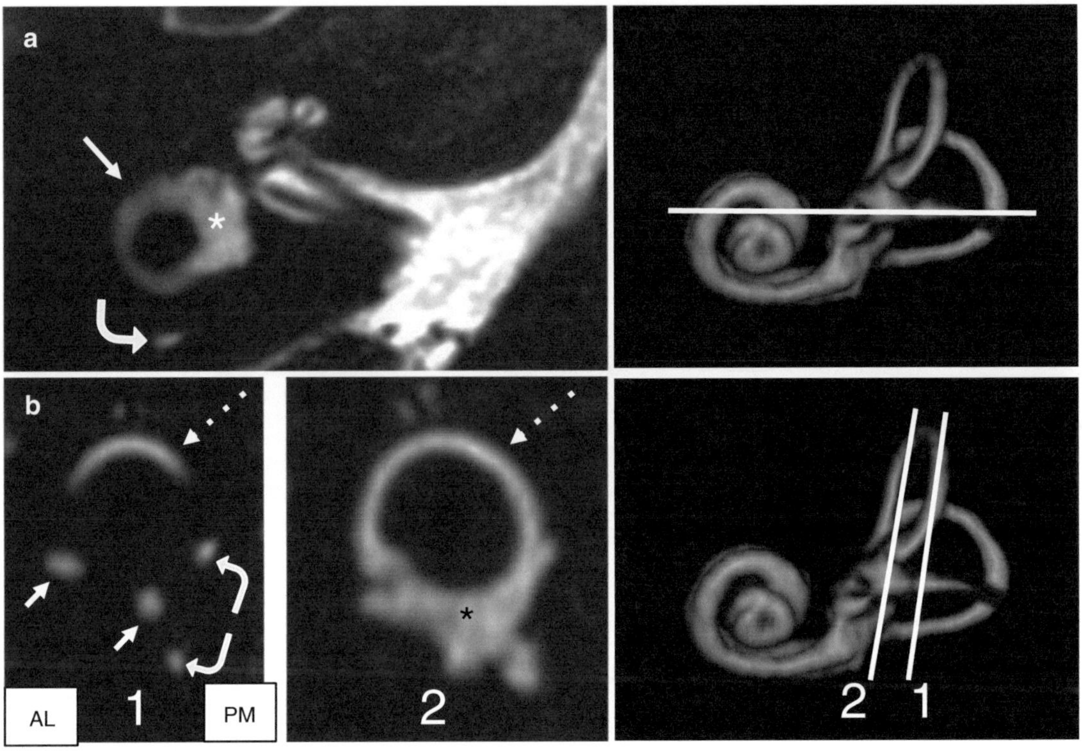

Fig. 3.7 Semicircular canals. The semicircular canals are part of the vestibular system and bony labyrinth and house the semicircular ducts. The superior and lateral semicircular ducts are innervated by the superior vestibular nerve, while the posterior semicircular duct is innervated by the inferior vestibular nerve. (**a**) Axial 3D TSE-T2WE: lateral semicircular canal (arrow), posterior semicircular canal (curved arrow), and vestibule (asterisk). (**b**, **1-2**) 3D TSE-T2W image in the Pöschl plane, perpendicular to the long axis of temporal bone and parallel to superior semicircular canal (dotted arrows); in the image we can also see theposterior semicircular canal (curved arrows), the lateral semicircular canal (short arrows), and the common crus (black asterisk).*Abbreviations: TSE* = turbo spin echo, *AL* = anterior lateral side, *PM* = posterior medial side

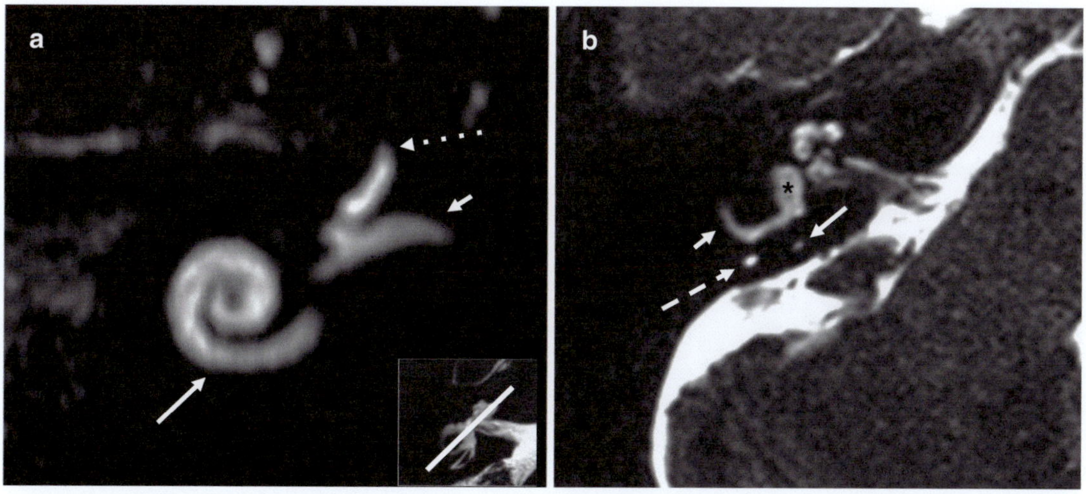

Fig. 3.8 Stenvers view and vestibular aqueduct. (**a**) 3D TSE-T2W oblique reformat image parallel to the petrous portion of the temporal bone (Stenvers view) shows the two-and-a-half turns of the cochlea (arrow), the superior semicircular canal (dotted arrow), the lateral semicircular canal (short arrow). (**b**) axial TSE-T2W image shows the vestibular aqueduct (arrow): when not enlarged the vestibular aqueduct is barely recognizable on standard MRI, the lateral semicircular canal (short arrow), the posterior semicircular canal (dashed arrow), and the vestibule (black asterisk). *Abbreviations: TSE* = turbo spin echo, *MRI* = magnetic resonance image

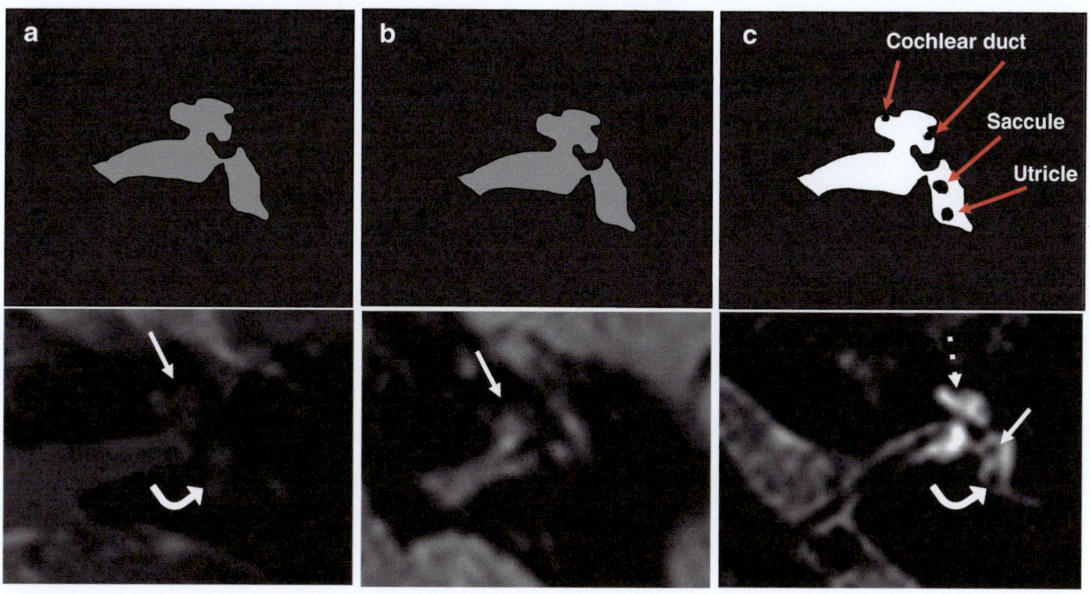

Fig. 3.9 MR imaging of the membranous labyrinth. (**a**) pre-contrast axial TSE-T1-weighted image and (**b**) axial 3D FLAIR image acquired 10 minutes after the contrast medium intravenous injection show the cochlea (arrows) and the vestibule (curved arrow in **a**); normally these structures are barely visible in these sequences. (**c**) axial 3D FLAIR image acquired 4 hours after the contrast medium intravenous shows the membranous labyrinth: the contrast medium diffuses into the perilymph but not in the endolymph giving a perilymph positive image and a negative endolymph image allowing the depiction of membranous labyrinth as dark structures (as displayed in the upper row diagram). Note that only the delayed FLAIR acquisition allows the depiction of membranous labyrinth: in fact, in the lower row image, we can clearly see the saccule (arrow) and the utricle (curved arrow); normally the scala media is not or barely visible as a round flow voids in the scala vestibuli (dotted arrow). *Abbreviations: TSE* = turbo spin echo, *FLAIR* = fluid-attenuated inversion recovery

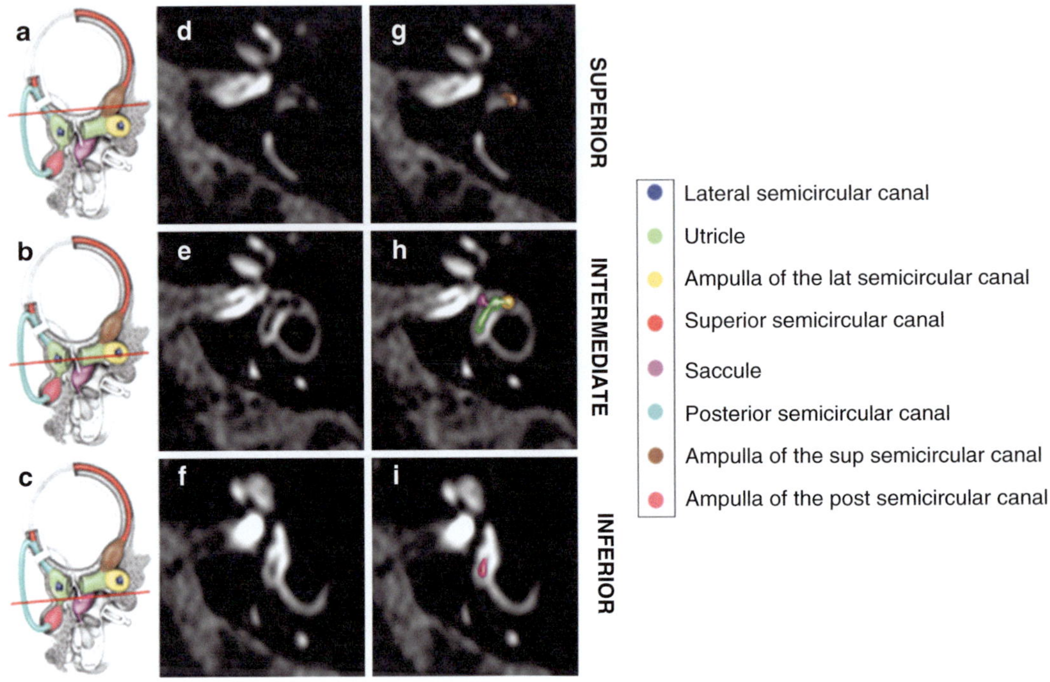

Fig. 3.10 MRI schematization of the membranous labyrinth. On the left (**a**–**c**) is a schematic representation of the membranous labyrinth in the sagittal plane, parallel to the SSC (modified under free concession from Max Brödel; Three unpublished drawings of the anatomy of the human ear, W.B. Saunders Company 1946). On the axial intermediate plane, the membranous labyrinth components show a Y-shaped arrangement with the long arm represented by the utricle and the short arm represented by the saccule and the LSC ampulla (**e**, **h**). On a more cranial plane the ampulla of the SCC is shown (**d, g**). On the axial plane, the saccule presents a round shape only on the intermediate section (**e**, **h**). This is confirmed on the axial inferior plane, where the vestibule is almost entirely represented by the perilymph, with only the most caudal portion of the PSC ampulla visible (**f**, **i**). *Abbreviations: MRI* = magnetic resonance imaging, *SSC* = superior semicircular canal, *LSC* = lateral semicircular canal, *PSC* = posterior semicircular canal. The images are modified from Conte et al. [4]

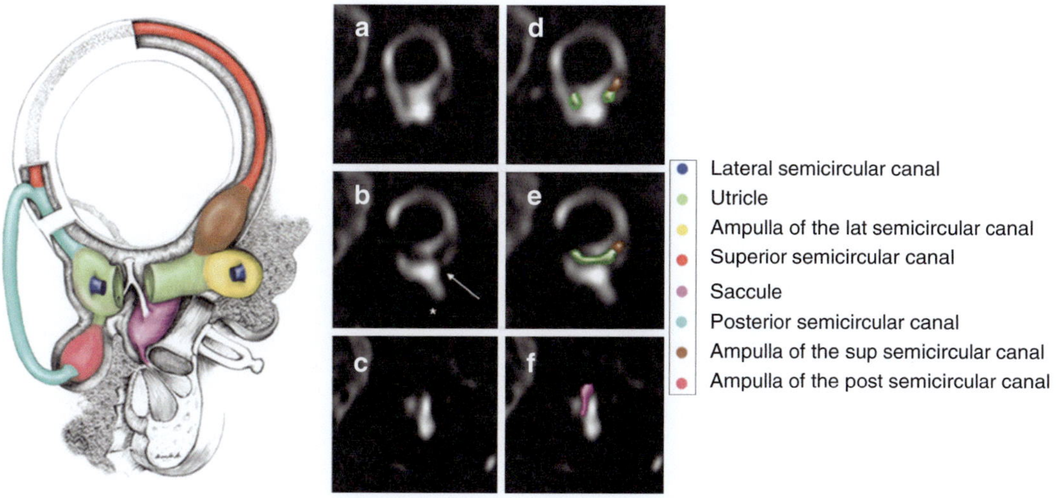

Fig. 3.11 MRI schematization of the membranous labyrinth (continues from Fig. 3.10). On the left is a schematic representation of the membranous labyrinth in the sagittal plane, parallel to the SSC (modified under free concession from Max Brödel; Three unpublished drawings of the anatomy of the human ear, W.B. Saunders Company 1946). On the right are reformatted oblique sagittal MRI, (**a**, lateral sagittal plane; **b**, intermediate sagittal plane; **c**, medial sagittal plane) with the corresponding colored representational images (**d–f**). Arrow: oval window; asterisk: round window. *Abbreviations: MRI* = magnetic resonance imaging, *SSC* = superior semicircular canal. The images are modified from Conte et al. [4]

References

1. Tien RD, Felsberg GJ, Macfall J. Fast spin-echo high-resolution MR imaging of the inner ear. Am J Roentgenol. 1992;159:395–8. https://doi.org/10.2214/ajr.159.2.1632364.
2. Naganawa S, Koshikawa T, Fukatsu H, Ishigaki T, Aoki I, Ninomiya A. Fast recovery 3D fast spin-echo MR imaging of the inner ear at 3 T. AJNR Am J Neuroradiol. 2002;23(2):299–302. PMID: 11847059; PMCID: PMC7975244.
3. Nakashima K, Morikawa M, Ishimaru H, Ochi M, Kabasawa H, Hayashi K. Three-dimensional fast recovery fast spin-echo imaging of the inner ear and the vestibulocochlear nerve. Eur Radiol. 2002;12(11):2776–80. https://doi.org/10.1007/s00330-002-1493-0. Epub 2002 Jun 21. PMID: 12386773.
4. Conte G, Caschera L, Tuscano B, Piergallini L, Barozzi S, Di Berardino F, Zanetti D, Scuffi C, Scola E, Sina C, Triulzi F. Three-Tesla magnetic resonance imaging of the vestibular endolymphatic space: a systematic qualitative description in healthy ears. Eur J Radiol. 2018;109:77–82. https://doi.org/10.1016/j.ejrad.2018.10.023. Epub 2018 Oct 24.

4 Ear Malformations

Giorgio Conte, Antonia Valentina Genovese, Guido Del Vecchio, Federica Di Berardino, Diego Zanetti, Silvia Casale, Elisa Scola, and Fabio Triulzi

4.1 Introduction

Congenital malformations of the ear occur in approximately 1 in 3800 live births [1]. The etiology may be genetic (isolated or syndromic) or secondary to factors such as congenital infection, chemical agents, malnutrition, irradiation, Rh incompatibility, hypoxia, and drug exposure. Considering the differences in the embryogenesis of the outer/middle ear (first and second branchial arches) and the inner ear (otic placode), malformations can affect the outer and/or middle ear without involving the inner ear and vice versa.

Herein, we briefly describe and provide a pictorial essay on the malformations of the external auditory canal (EAC), middle ear, and inner ear. Reference linear measurements useful for assessing suspected ear malformations are reported in Table 4.1 and illustrated in Figs. 4.1 and 4.2.

G. Conte (✉) · F. Triulzi
Neuroradiology Unit, Fondazione IRCCS Ca' Granda Ospedale Maggiore Policlinico, Milan, Italy

Department of Pathophysiology and Transplantation, University of Milan, Milan, Italy
e-mail: giorgio.conte@policlinico.mi.it; fabio.triulzi@policlinico.mi.it

A. V. Genovese · G. Del Vecchio · S. Casale · E. Scola
Neuroradiology Unit, Fondazione IRCCS Ca' Granda Ospedale Maggiore Policlinico, Milan, Italy
e-mail: valentina.genovese@policlinico.mi.it; guido.delvecchio@policlinico.mi.it; silvia.casale@policlinico.mi.it; elisa.scola@policlinico.mi.it

F. Di Berardino · D. Zanetti
Audiology Unit, Fondazione IRCCS Ca' Granda Ospedale Maggiore Policlinico, Milan, Italy

Department of Clinical Sciences and Community Health, Università degli Studi di Milano, Milan, Italy
e-mail: federica.diberardino@policlinico.mi.it; diego.zanetti@policlinico.mi.it

G. Conte et al. (eds.), *Atlas of Normal and Pathological Findings in Otoneuroradiology*,
https://doi.org/10.1007/978-3-032-08232-9_4

Table 4.1 Reference linear measurements

Measurement	Reference values	Measurement technique
EAC width	>4 mm	EAC diameter measured on axial plane [2] (Fig. 4.1a)
Tympanic cavity width	>3 mm	Measured from promontory to atretic plate/tympanic membrane in coronal plane [2] (Fig. 4.1b)
Oval window width	>2 mm (>1.5 mm in children)	Diameter is measured on coronal plane where the oval window enters the vestibule [3] (Fig. 4.1c)
Round window width	>1.5 mm	Width is measured between the bony edges of the RW opening on coronal plane [4] (Fig. 4.1c)
Vestibular aqueduct	>1.5 mm	Midpoint between the external aperture and the common crus [5] (Fig. 4.1d)
Cochlear width	> 4.5 mm	Maximum diameter measured in an axial plane tangentially to the two inferior extremities of modiolus [6] (Fig. 4.2a)
Cochlear nerve canal width	>2 mm (1.5 mm in children)	Measurements of the canal were performed tangentially to the two inferior extremities of the modiolus [6] (Fig. 4.2a)
Cochlear length	> 8.10 mm and < 9.59 mm	Largest distance from the round window, through the modiolar axis measured in an oblique plane parallel to cochlea basal turn [7] (Fig. 4.2b)
Cochlear height	> 4.3 mm	Maximal height measured on a coronal plane perpendicular to oval window [8] (Fig. 4.2c)
Lateral SCC bony island	> 3 mm	Measurement of bony island perpendicular to long axis of vestibule [9] (Fig. 4.2d)

Abbreviations: *EAC* external auditory canal, *RW* round window, *SCC* semicircular canal

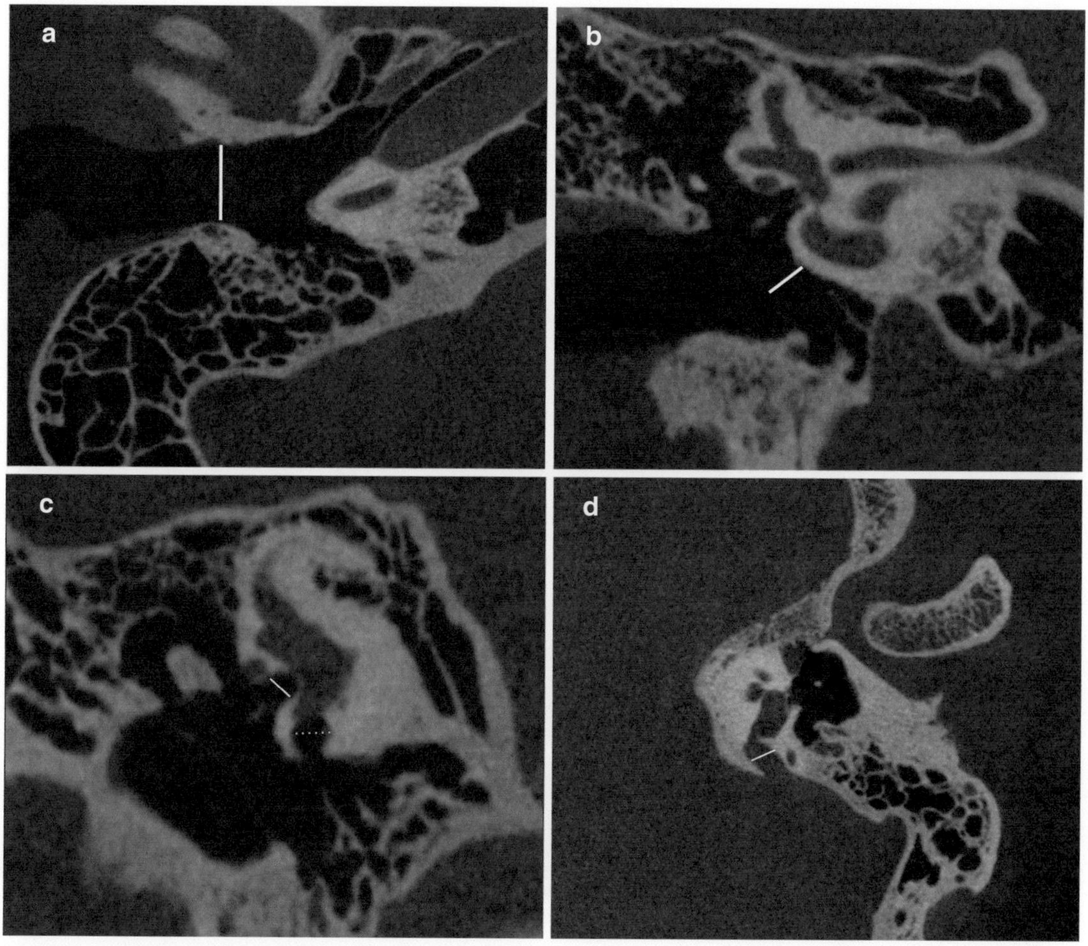

Fig. 4.1 Reference measurements of normal the ear anatomy. (**a**) Axial CBCT image shows the diameter (white line) of the EAC; (**b**) Coronal CBCT image shows the width of the tympanic cavity (white line), measured from promontory to tympanic membrane; (**c**) coronal oblique CBCT image shows the diameters of the oval (white line) and round (dotted line) windows; (**d**) axial oblique CBCT image parallel to the stapes shows the vestibule aqueduct width (white line), measured between the external aperture and the common crus. *Abbreviations*: CBCT = cone-beam computed tomography, EAC = external auditory canal

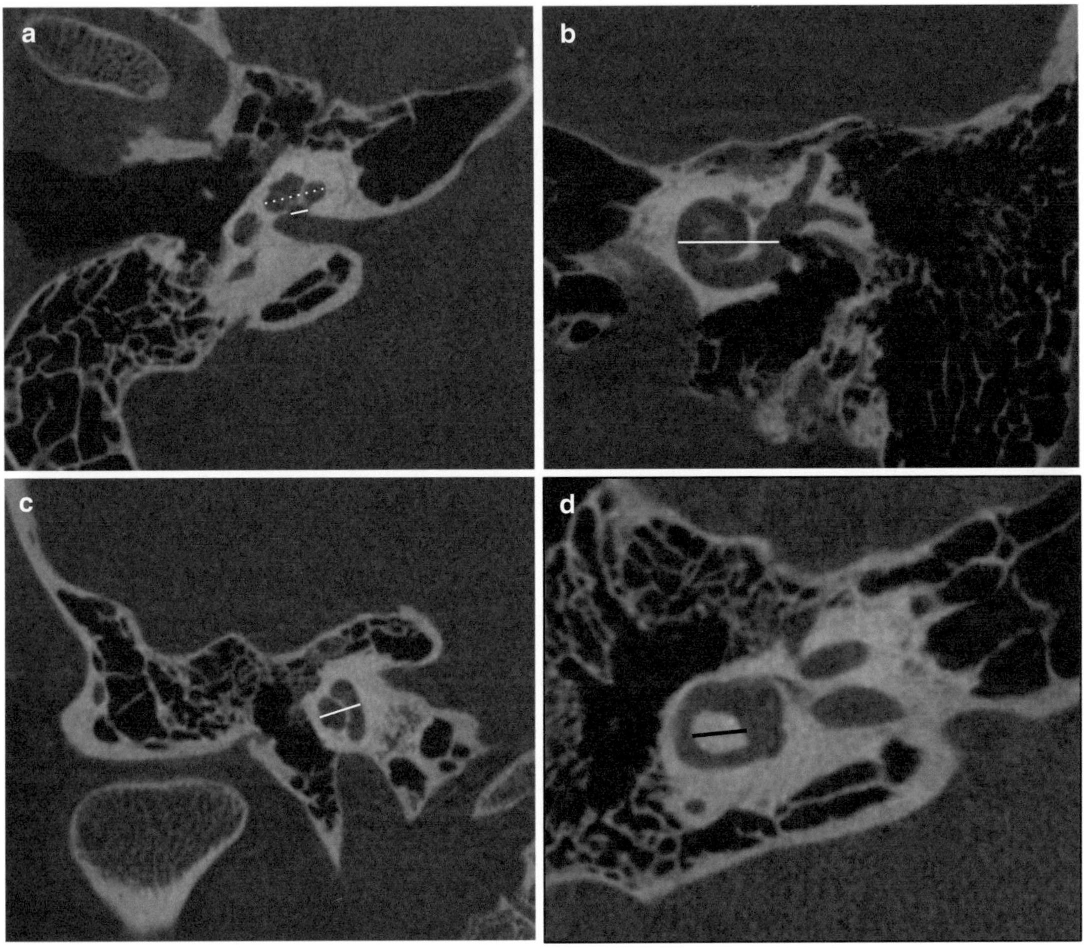

Fig. 4.2 **Reference measurements of the ear anatomy**. (**a**) Axial oblique CBCT image parallel to the short modiolar axis shows the width of the cochlea (dotted line) and the cochlear nerve canal (white line); (**b**) oblique CBCT parallel to cochlea basal turn shows the cochlear length measurement (white line); (**c**) coronal oblique CBCT perpendicular to oval window shows the cochlear height (white line); (**d**) axial oblique CBCT shows the lateral SCC bony island (black line). *Abbreviations*: CBCT = cone-beam computed tomography, SCC = semicircular canal

4.2 EAC Malformation

EAC malformations (Figs. 4.3, 4.4, 4.5, 4.6, 4.7, 4.8, 4.9, 4.10 and 4.11) can be summarized into three types:

- *Shortness and/or marked angulation of the cartilaginous canal*
- *Stenosis of the cartilaginous and/or bony canal*
- *Partial or complete EAC atresia*, which may be membranous or bony, where the tympanic membrane is replaced by a fibrous or bony atretic plate, respectively.

EAC stenosis has an increased predisposition for cholesteatoma formation. EAC atresia is more frequently associated with middle ear malformations than EAC stenosis. Various classification systems have been proposed to assess the severity of EAC deformities. The Weerda classification is simpler and commonly used for clinical assessment; it categorizes EAC abnormalities based on the extent and severity of stenosis or atresia [1].

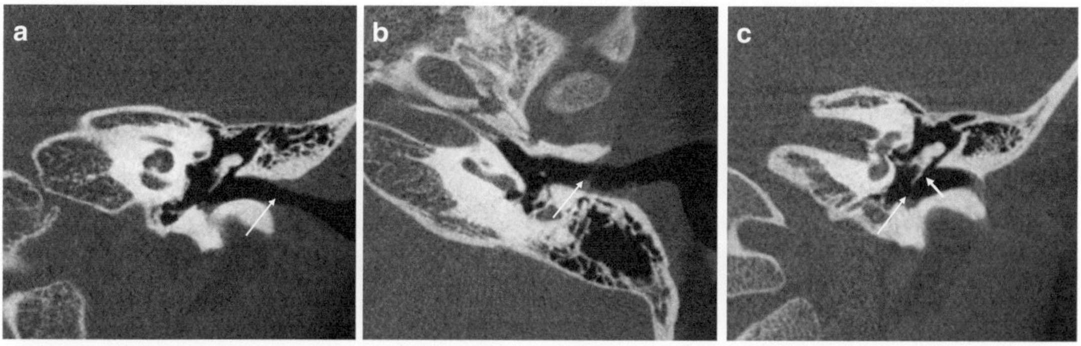

Fig. 4.3 **EAC stenosis type A according to Weerda's classification.** (**a, b**) Coronal and axial CBCT images show horizontalized and narrowed EAC (arrow); (**c**) on coronal oblique CBCT the tympanic cavity (long arrow) and the manubrium of the malleus (short arrow) are hypoplasic. *Abbreviations*: CBCT = cone-beam computed tomography, EAC = external auditory canal

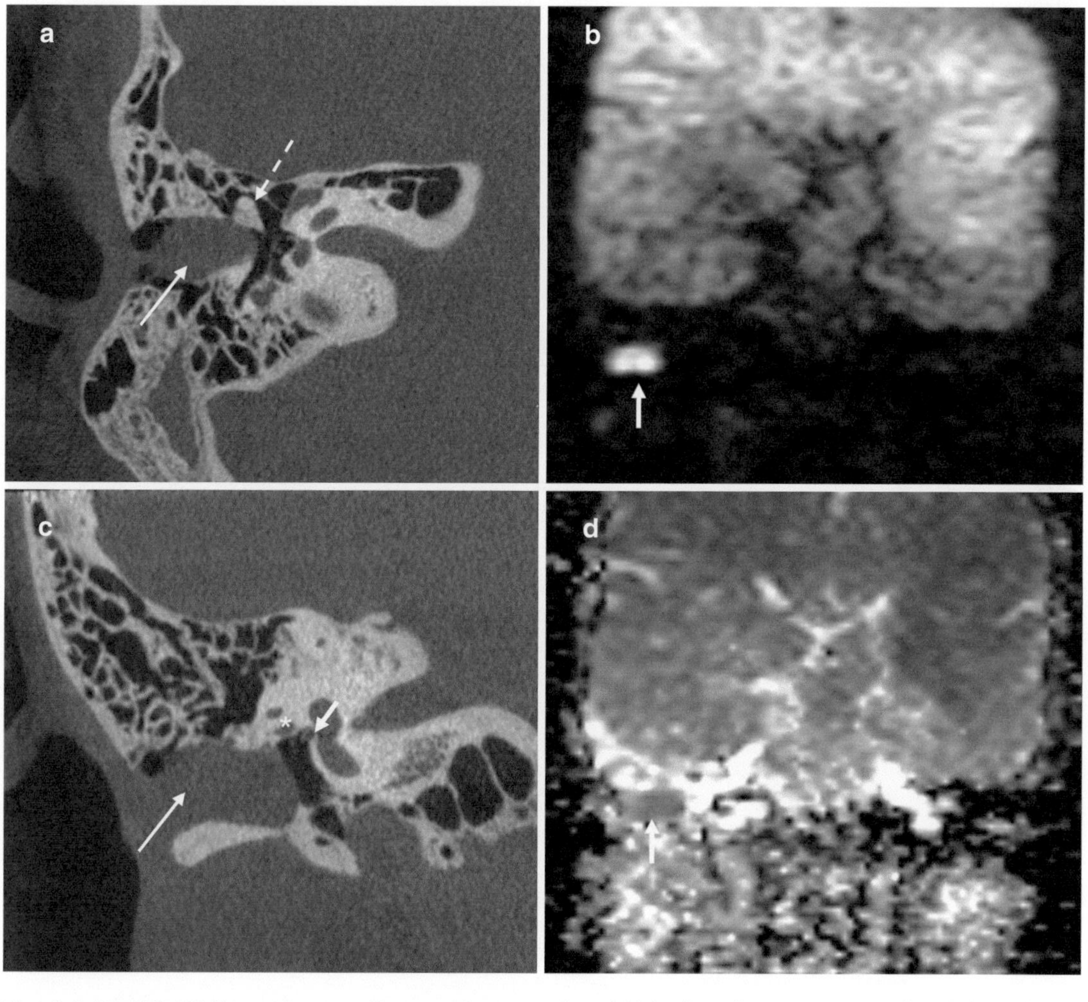

Fig. 4.4 **Partial EAC atresia type B according to Weerda's classification, after surgical canaloplasty**. (**a, c**) Axial and coronal CBCT images show a soft tissue mass (long arrow) within the reconstructed EAC, which causes bone scalloping. The tympanic cavity is mildly hypoplastic, the ossicular chain is displaced anteriorly (dashed arrow), the tympanic tract of the facial nerve (asterisk) is along the tegmen tympani, and the oval window is narrow (short arrow). (**b, d**) Coronal DWI and ADC map show restricted diffusion of the mass within the EAC, suggesting for cholesteatoma. *Abbreviations*: ADC = apparent diffusion coefficient, CBCT = cone-beam computed tomography, DWI = diffusion weighted-imaging, EAC = external auditory canal

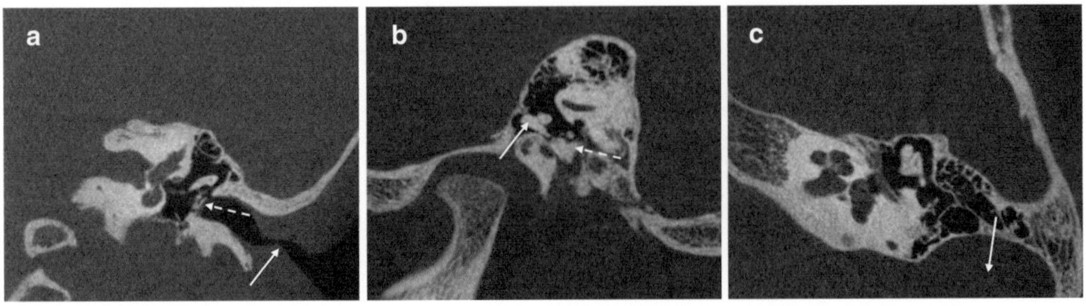

Fig. 4.5 Partial EAC atresia type B according to Weerda's classification. (**a**) Coronal CBCT image shows stenosis (arrow) of the cartilaginous part of the EAC and a bony medial atretic plate (dashed arrow); (**b**) sagittal oblique CBCT image shows dysmorphism of the malleus (arrow) close to the atretic plate (dashed arrow); (**c**) axial CBCT image shows procidence of the sigmoid sinus (arrow) into the mastoid. *Abbreviations*: CBCT = cone-beam computed tomography, EAC = external auditory canal

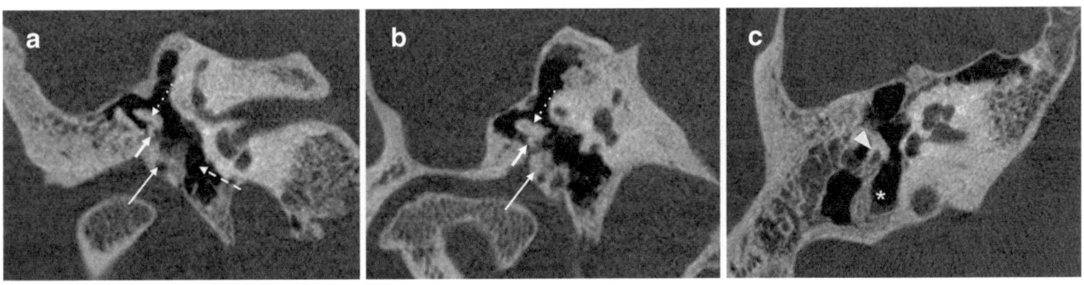

Fig. 4.6 Complete bony EAC atresia type C according to Weerda's classification. (**a**, **b**) Coronal oblique CBCT images show absence of the EAC with bony atretic plate (long arrow), hypoplastic tympanic cavity (dashed arrow), rudimental malleus (short arrow), and dysmorphism of the incus (dotted arrow) with absence of long process. (**c**) axial CBCT image shows lateralization the mastoid segment of the facial nerve (arrowhead) and deep sinus tympani (asterisk). *Abbreviations*: CBCT = cone-beam computed tomography, EAC = external auditory canal

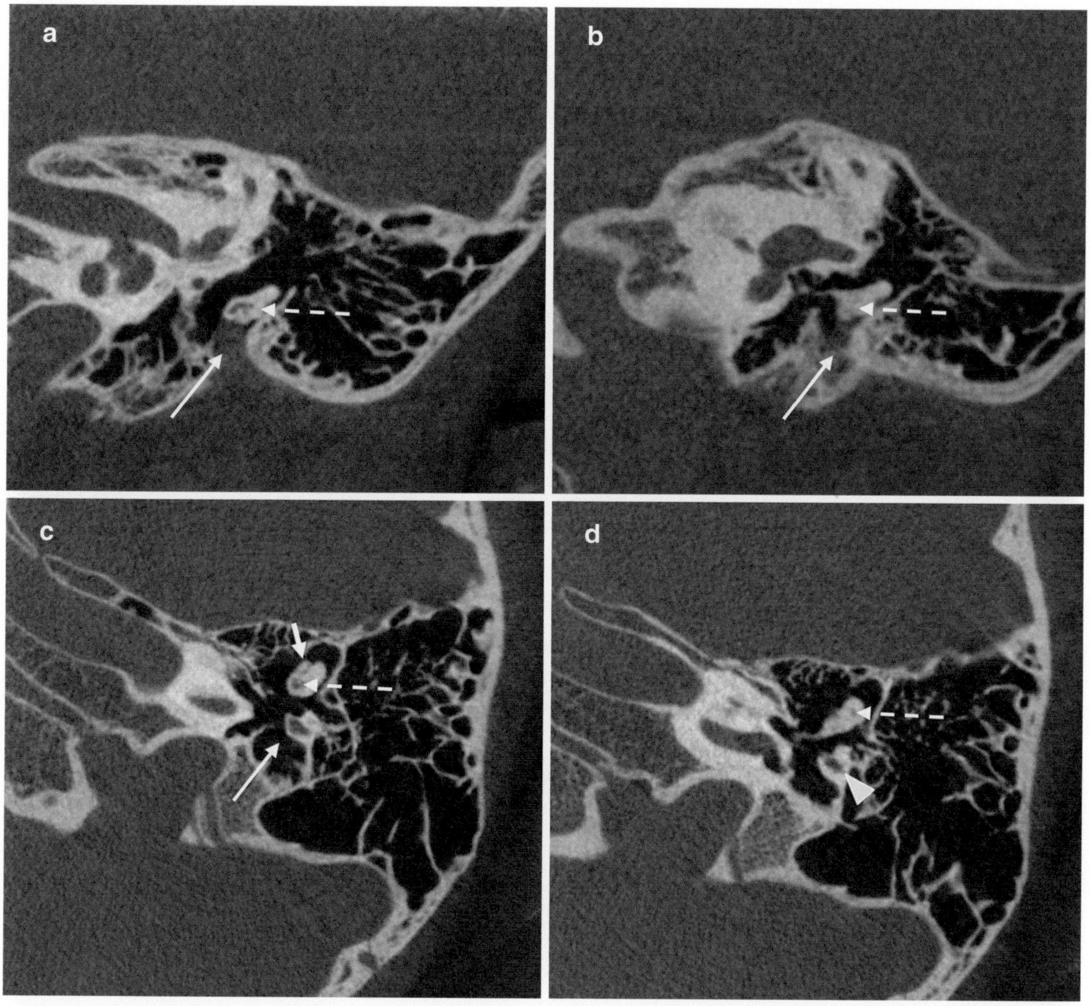

Fig. 4.7 Complete cartilaginous EAC atresia type C according to Weerda's classification. (**a**, **b**) Coronal oblique CBCT images show absence of the EAC and a membranous atretic plate (arrow), marked dysmorphism of the incus (dashed arrow) which is fused with the atretic plate and shows a large body and thin horizontalized long process; (**c**, **d**) axial CBCT images show small rudimental head of the malleus (short arrow) with partially fusion of the joint with the incus (dashed arrow), lateralization the mastoid segment of the facial nerve (arrowhead). *Abbreviations*: CBCT = cone-beam computed tomography, EAC = external auditory canal

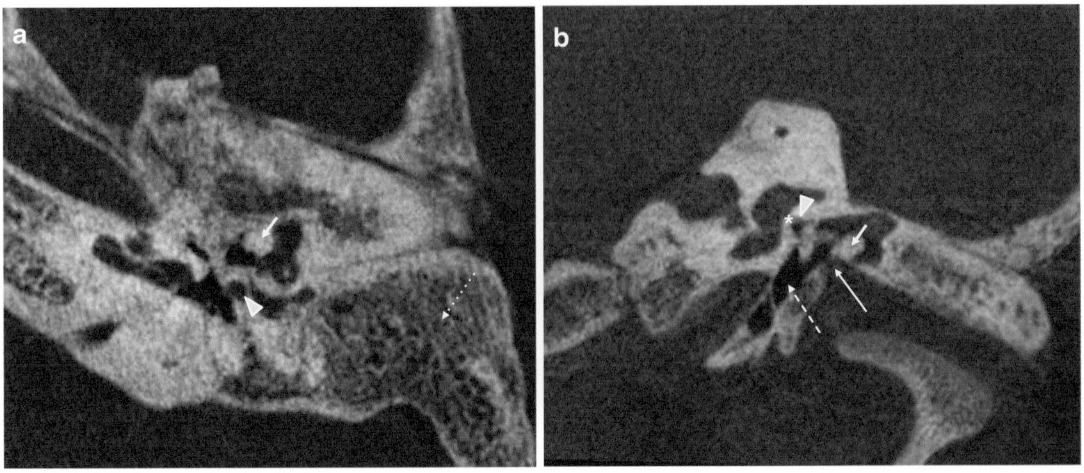

Fig. 4.8 Complete cartilaginous EAC atresia type C according to Weerda's classification. (**a**) Axial and (**b**) coronal CBCT images show absence of the EAC and a membranous atretic plate (arrow), hypoplastic tympanic cavity (dashed arrow), deformation of the malleus (short arrow) and its fixation to the epitympanic recess, absent stapes and incus, oval window stenosis (asterisk), abnormal facial nerve course (arrowhead), and hypopneumatized mastoid (dotted arrow). *Abbreviations*: CBCT = cone-beam computed tomography, EAC = external auditory canal

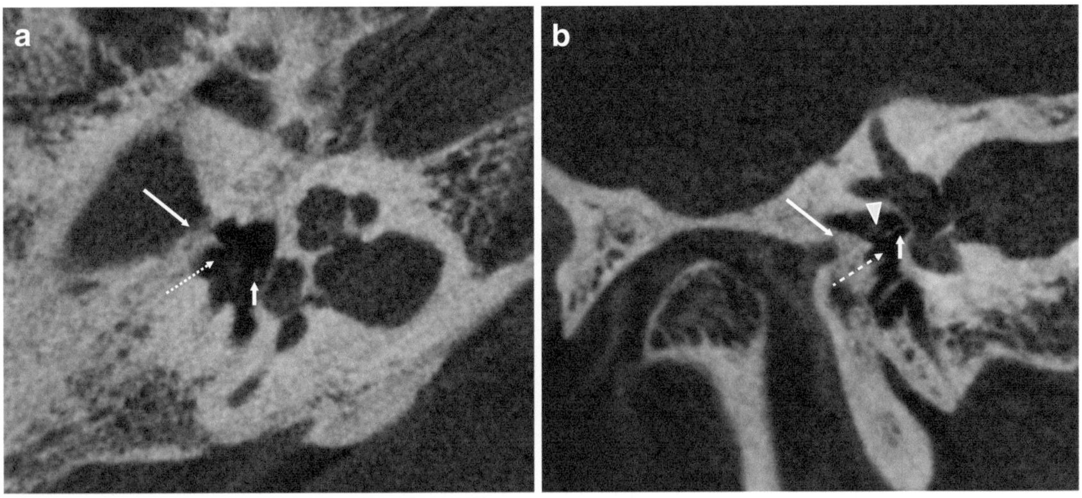

Fig. 4.9 Complete bony EAC atresia type C according to Weerda's classification. (**a**) Axial and (**b**) coronal CBCT images show absence of the EAC and a bony atretic plate (arrow), hypoplastic tympanic cavity (dashed arrow), absence of the malleus and incus, monopod stapes (short arrow), and dehiscence of the tympanic segment of the facial nerve along the tegmen tympany (arrowhead). *Abbreviations*: CBCT = cone-beam computed tomography, EAC = external auditory canal

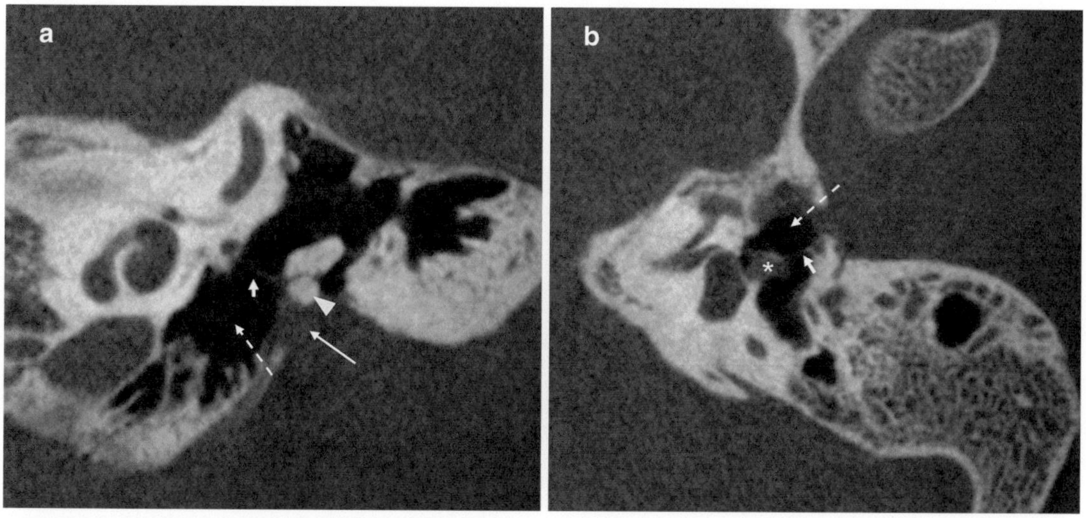

Fig. 4.10 **Complete cartilaginous EAC atresia type C according to Weerda's classification.** (**a**) Coronal and (**b**) axial CBCT images show absence of the EAC and a membranous atretic plate (long arrow), hypoplastic tympanic cavity (dashed arrow), rudimental head of the malleus (arrowhead), thin and fibrous long process of the incus (short arrow), and soft tissue replacing the stapes at the oval window (asterisk). *Abbreviations*: CBCT = cone-beam computed tomography, EAC = external auditory canal

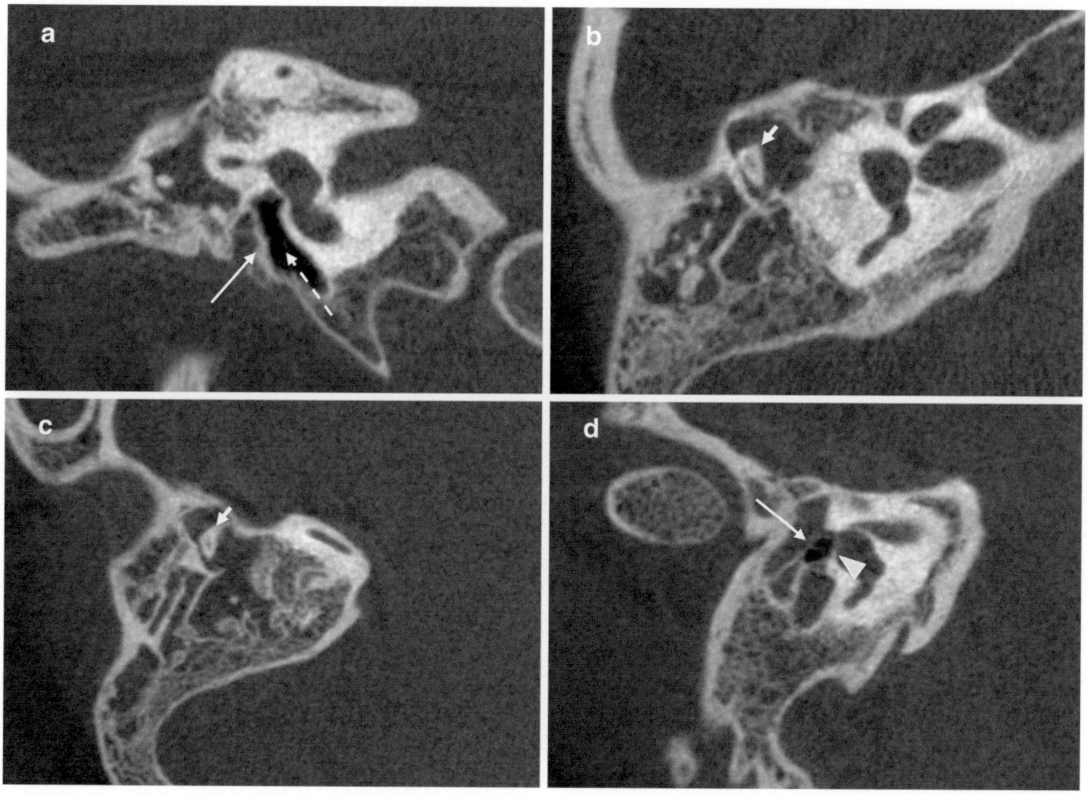

Fig. 4.11 **Complete bony EAC atresia type C according to Weerda's classification**. (**a**) Coronal and (**b–d**) axial CBCT images show absence of the EAC with bony atretic plate (long arrow), hypoplastic tympanic cavity (dashed arrow), absence of malleus and small dysmorphic incus (short arrow) which is displaced anteriorly into epitympanic recess, and small stapes (arrowhead) articulated with the atretic plate (arrow). *Abbreviations*: CBCT = cone-beam computed tomography, EAC = external auditory canal

Table 4.2 Jahrsdoerfer's grading system

Structures	Configuration	Points
EAC	Normal Fibrotic atresia Bony atresia	2 1 0
Aeration of mastoid	Distinct Moderate Absent	2 1 0
Size of tympanic cavity	Large Moderate Eburnated	2 1 0
Aeration of tympanic cavity	Distinct Moderate Absent	2 1 0
Facial nerve	Normal Slightly aberrant Strongly aberrant	4 2 0
Course of arteries and veins	Normal Slightly aberrant Strongly aberrant	2 1 0
Malleus and incus	Normal Dysplastic Absent	2 1 0
Stapes	Normal Dysplastic Absent	4 2 0
Oval window	Open Closed	4 0
Round window	Open Closed	4 0
	Maximum score	28

Abbreviations: *EAC* external auditory canal

The most commonly used scoring system developed to predict postoperative hearing outcomes in these patients is Jahrsdoerfer's grading system (Table 4.2) [10].

4.3 Middle Ear Malformation

Middle ear malformations (Figs. 4.12, 4.13, 4.14, 4.15, 4.16, 4.17, 4.18, 4.19, 4.20, 4.21, 4.22, 4.23, 4.24 and 4.25) include malformations of the tympanic cavity, which may or may not be combined with ossicular malformations. The tympanic cavity is considered normal when the distance from the tympanic membrane/atretic plate to the promontory is >3 mm on coronal imaging [2]. In moderate malformations, there is hypoplasia of the tympanic cavity with rudimentary or aplastic ossicles. In severe malformations, the tympanic cavity may be aplastic or cleft-like.

Ossicular malformations can involve the entire ossicular chain or isolated bones. Malformations of the malleus and incus are more common than those of the stapes. Below are the most frequent ossicular malformations:

- *Malleus* (Figs. 4.14, 4.17, 4.18, 4.19 and 4.20):
  - Hypoplasia/dysplasia of the head and manubrium
  - Fixation within the epitympanic recess
  - Aplasia
- *Incus* (Figs. 4.12, 4.15, 4.20 and 4.24):
  - Absence or hypoplasia of the long process
  - Variations in the position of the long process (e.g., horizontal rotation and fixation)
  - Complete incus aplasia
- *Incudomalleolar joint*:
  - Malleo-incudal fusion (boomerang appearance)
  - Malleo-incudal malalignment
  - Malleo-incudal disarticulation
- *Incudostapedial joint*:
  - Bony/fibrous fusion
  - Malalignment/widening/disarticulation of the incudostapedial joint.
- *Stapes* (Figs. 4.12, 4.14, 4.20, 4.21, 4.22, 4.23, and 4.24):
  - Complete absence of the stapes, associated with oval window atresia
  - Monopodal stapes (single crus)
  - Crural fusion, where the anterior and posterior crura of the stapes are fused, forming a ring
  - Double stapes, with additional linear hyperdensity from the footplate to the anterior/posterior crura or head
  - Hypo/aplasia
  - Ossification of the stapes
  - Displaced superstructure, which may be morphologically normal but disconnected from the footplate
  - Fixation of the stapes superstructure to the pyramidal eminence, facial canal, or promontory

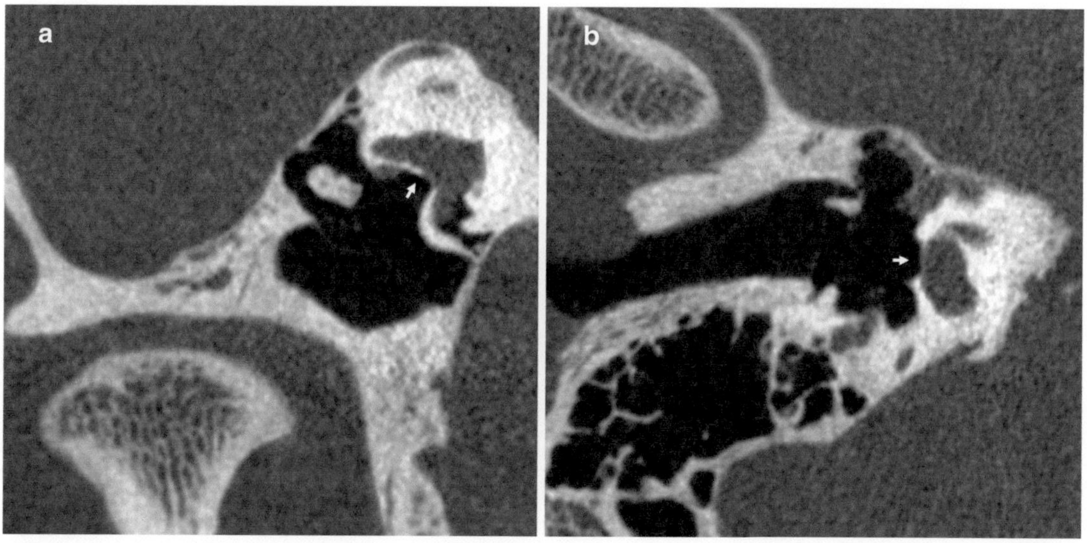

Fig. 4.12 Malformation of the incus and stapes. (**a**) Coronal and (**b**) axial CBCT images show absence of the long process of the incus and of the stapes at the level of the oval window (short arrow). *Abbreviation*: CBCT = cone-beam computed tomography

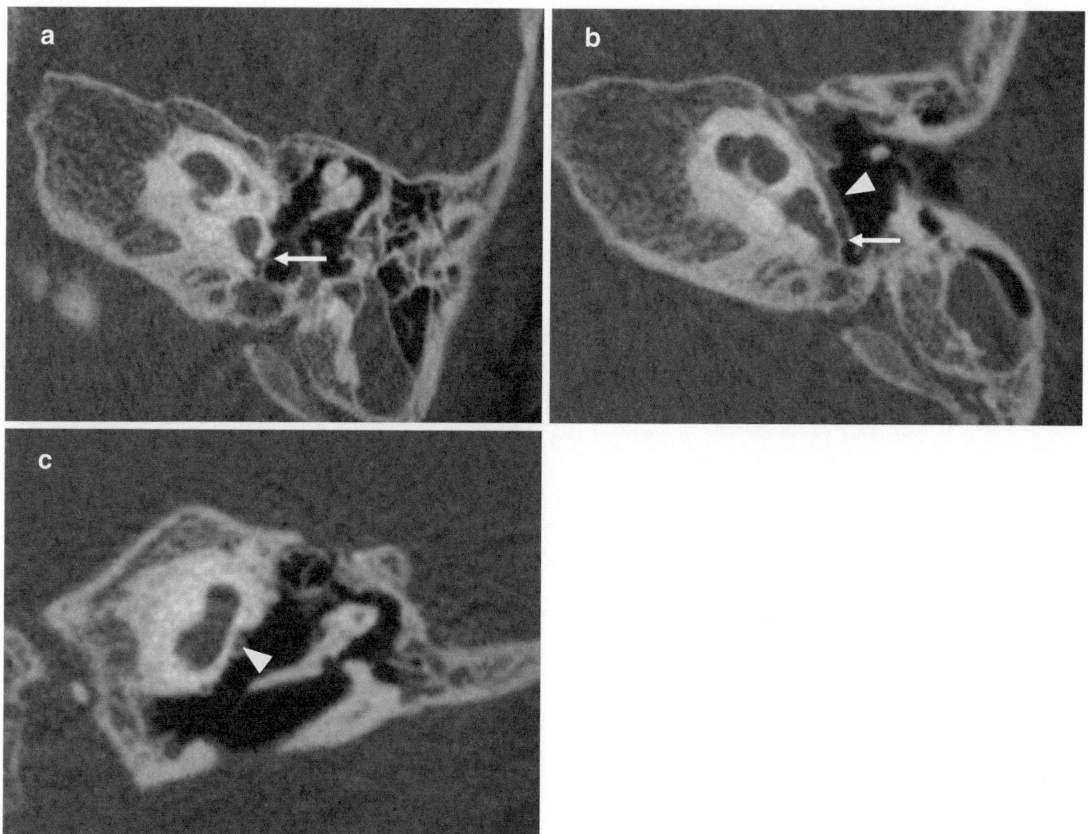

Fig. 4.13 Middle ear malformations in Goldenhar syndrome. (**a**, **b**) Axial and (**c**) coronal CBCT images show hypoplastic tympanic cavity, oval window atresia with displaced facial nerve canal (arrowhead), absent stapes, and round window stenosis (arrow). *Abbreviation*: CBCT = cone-beam computed tomography

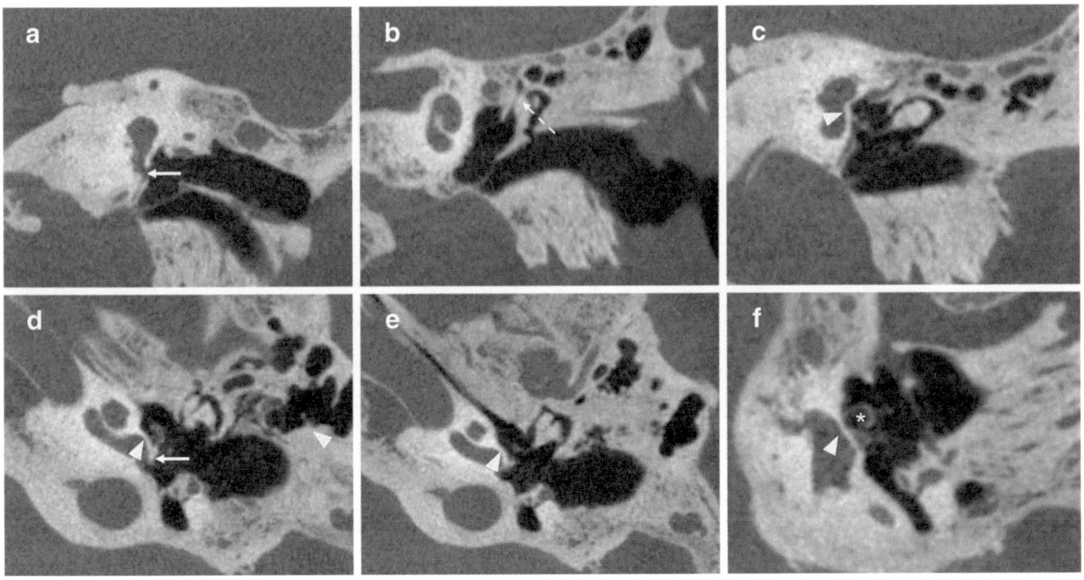

Fig. 4.14 **Ossicular chain and window malformation in a patient treated for cholesteatoma.** (**a**–**c**) Coronal and (**d**–**f**) axial CBCT images show round window stenosis (arrow), oval window atresia (arrowhead), dysmorphic stapes (asterisk) which is attached more caudally, and fusion of the malleolar head (dashed arrow) with the tegmen. *Abbreviation*: CBCT = cone-beam computed tomography

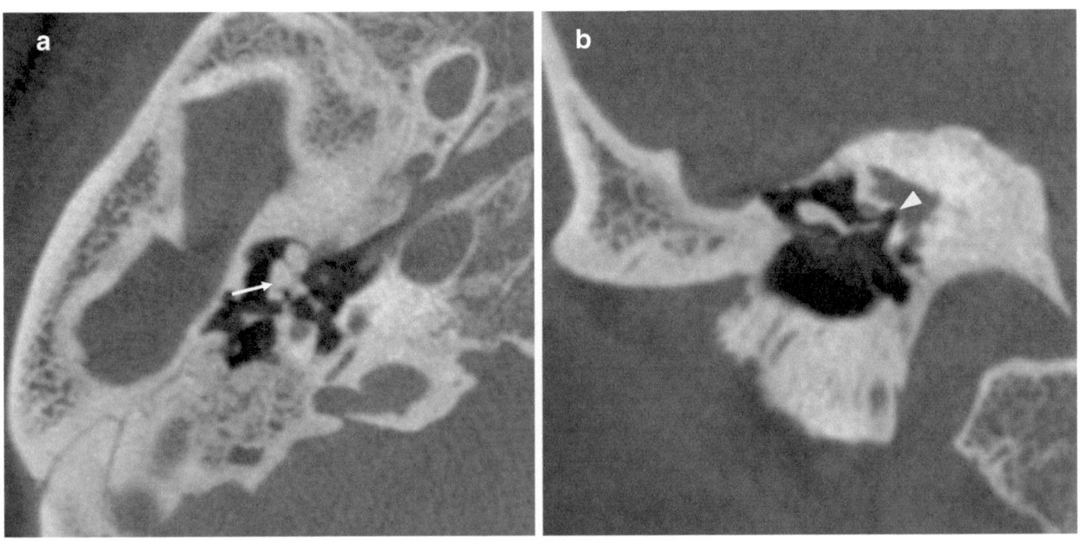

Fig. 4.15 **Incus and oval window malformations.** (**a**) Axial and (**b**) coronal CBCT images show the "boomerang" shape of the incus (arrow) and oval window stenosis (arrowhead). *Abbreviation*: CBCT = cone-beam computed tomography

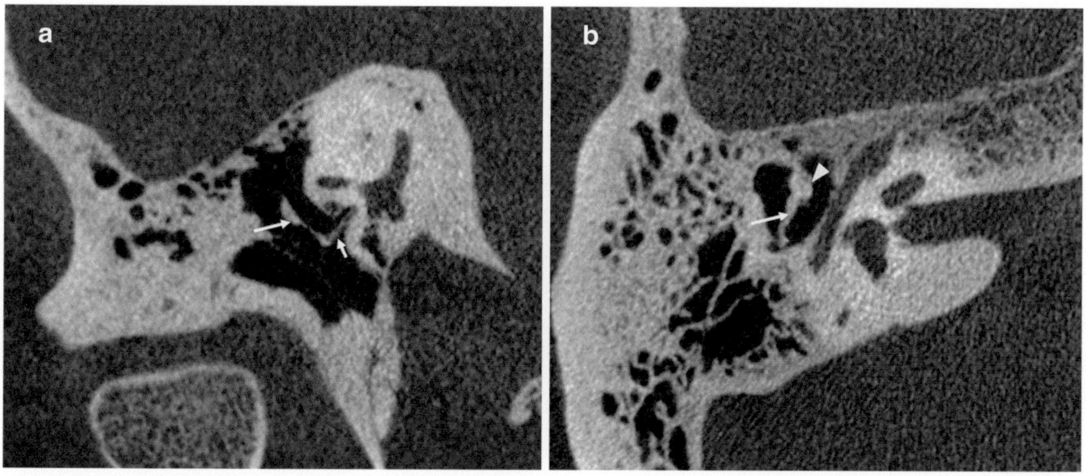

Fig. 4.16 Incus malformation. (**a**) Coronal and (**b**) axial CBCT images show "ribbonlike" incus (arrow) articulated with the malleus (arrowhead) and the stapes (short arrow). *Abbreviation*: CBCT = cone-beam computed tomography, EAC

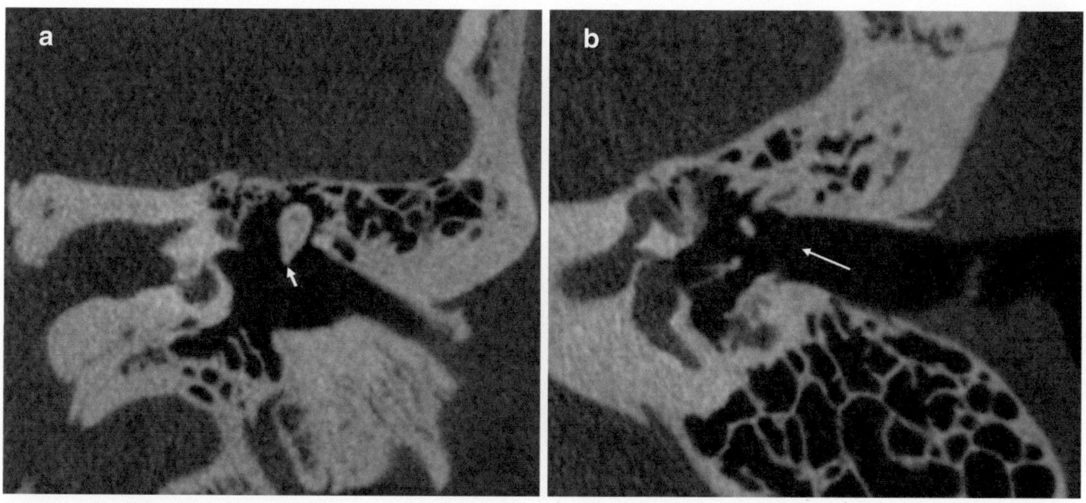

Fig. 4.17 Malleus malformation. (**a**) Coronal and (**b**) axial CBCT images show mild stenosis of the mesial portion of the EAC (long arrow) and absence of the malleolar manubrium (short arrow). *Abbreviations*: CBCT = cone-beam computed tomography, EAC = external auditory canal

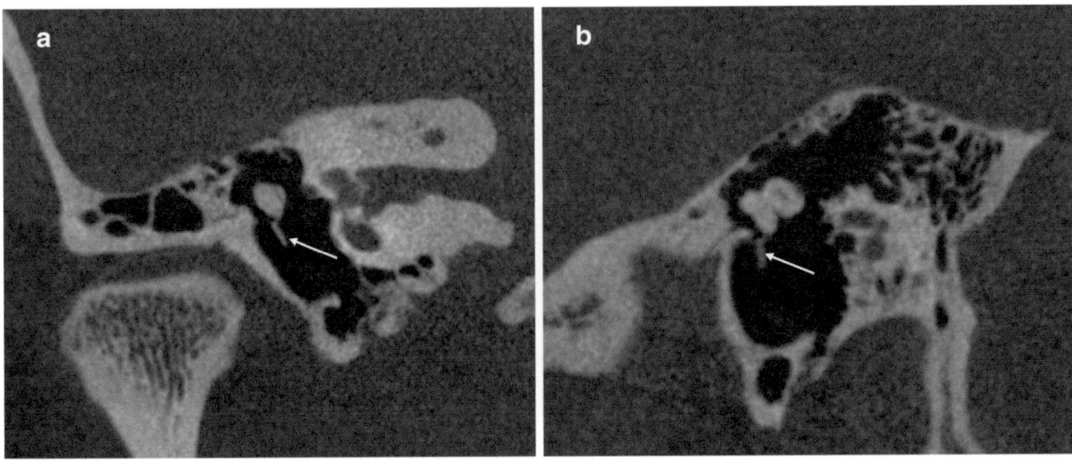

Fig. 4.18 **Malleolar manubrium hypoplasia.** (**a**) Coronal and (**b**) sagittal CBCT images show hypoplasia of the manubrium (arrow). *Abbreviation*: CBCT = cone-beam computed tomography

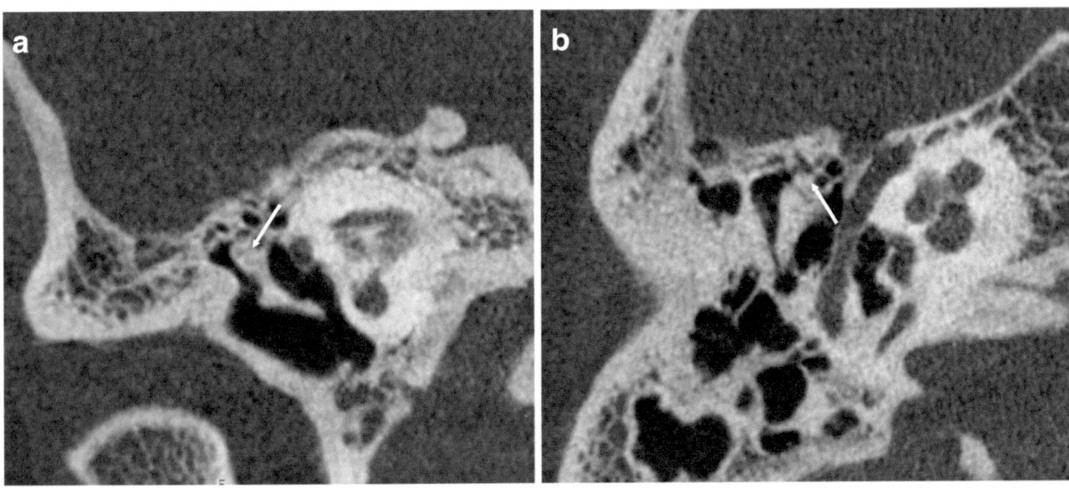

Fig. 4.19 **Malleus fixation.** (**a**) Coronal and (**b**) axial CBCT images show the fusion of the malleus head (arrow) with the tegmen. *Abbreviation*: CBCT = cone-beam computed tomography

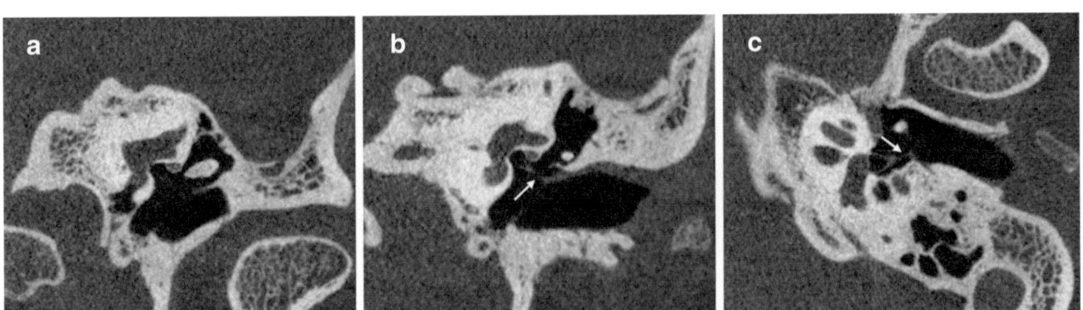

Fig. 4.20 **Ossicular chain malformation in Kniest syndrome**. (**a**, **b**) Coronal and (**c**) axial CBCT images show absence of the long process of the incus; the stapes head is connected to the tympanic membrane through a fibrous shoot (arrow). *Abbreviation*: CBCT = cone-beam computed tomography

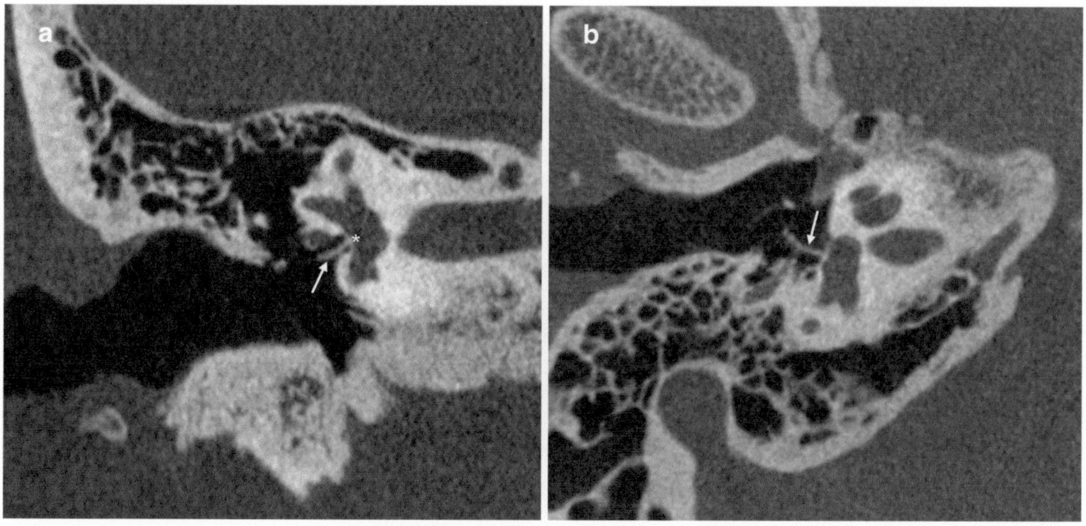

Fig. 4.21 **Stapes and oval window malformation**. (**a**) Coronal and (**b**) axial CBCT images show monopod stapes (arrow) and oval window stenosis (asterisk). *Abbreviation*: CBCT = cone-beam computed tomography

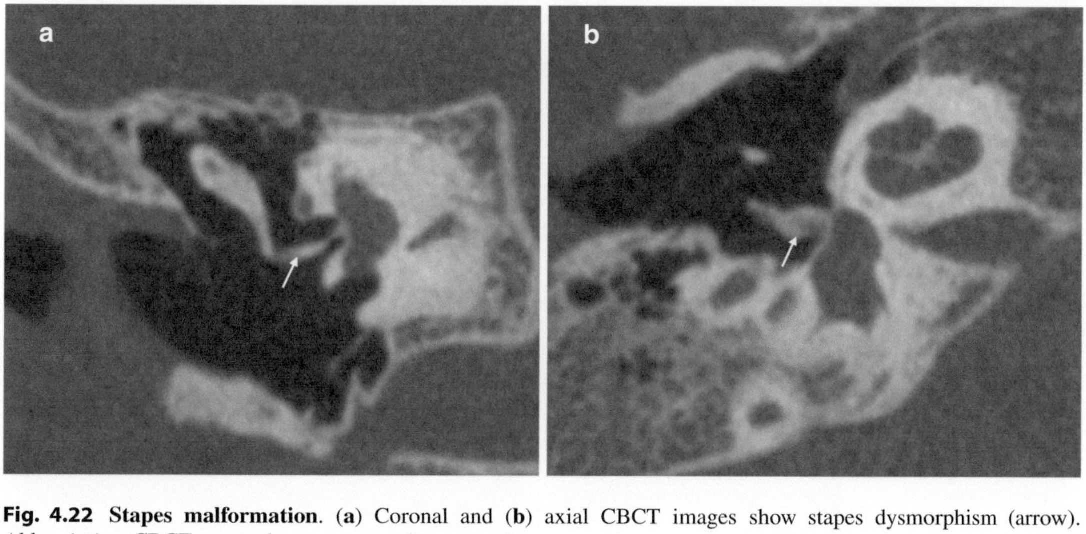

Fig. 4.22 **Stapes malformation**. (**a**) Coronal and (**b**) axial CBCT images show stapes dysmorphism (arrow). *Abbreviation*: CBCT = cone-beam computed tomography

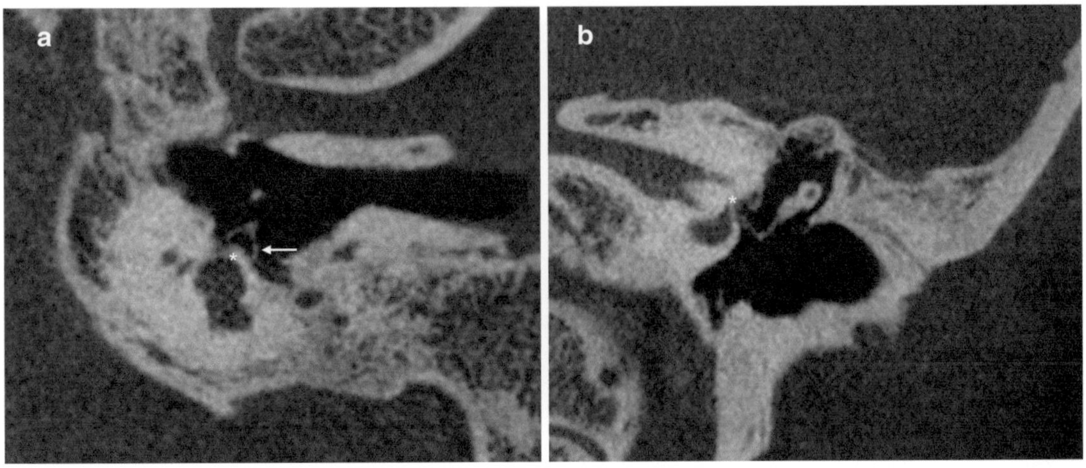

Fig. 4.23 **Stapes malformation.** (**a**) Axial and (**b**) coronal CBCT images show oval window stenosis and partial ossification (asterisk), slender appearance of the stapes crus (arrow). *Abbreviation*: CBCT = cone-beam computed tomography

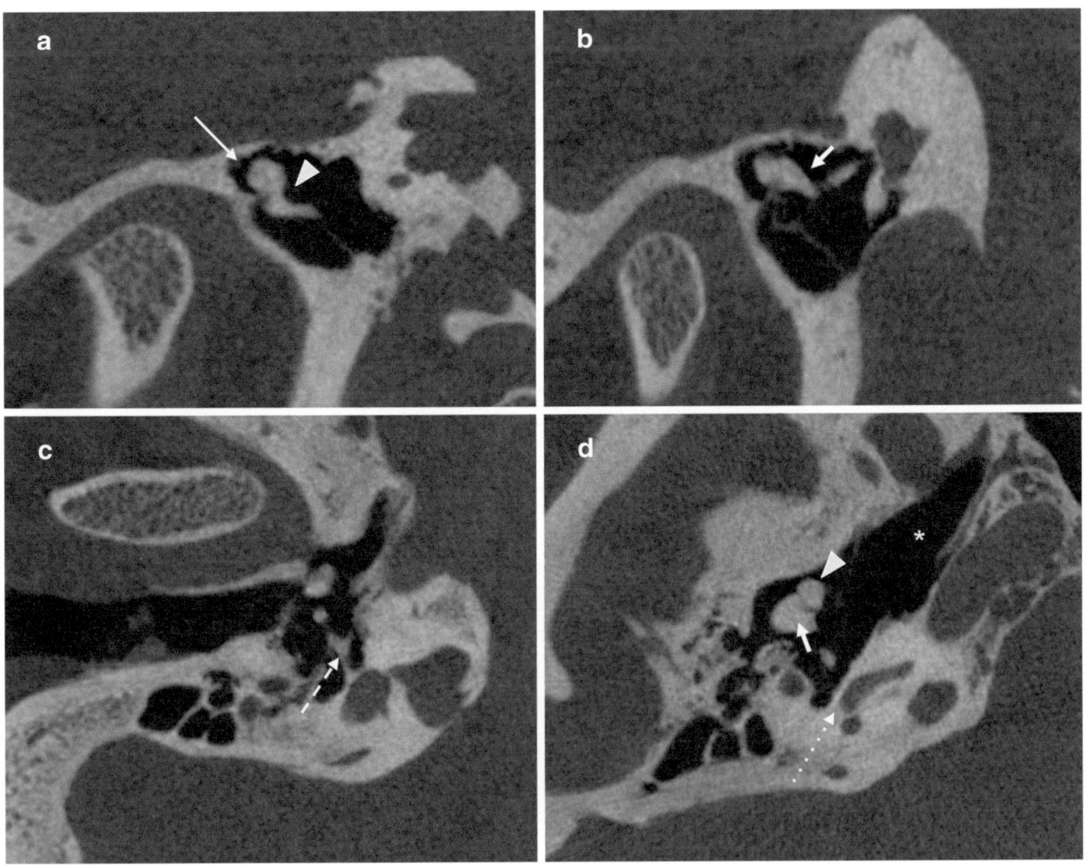

Fig. 4.24 **Middle ear malformation**. (**a**, **b**) Coronal and (**c**, **d**) axial CBCT images show hypoplasic epitympanum (arrow), enlarged protympanum (asterisk), short malleus (arrowhead) and incus (short arrow), dysmorphism of the stapes (dashed arrow), and round window atresia (dotted arrow). *Abbreviation*: CBCT = cone-beam computed tomography

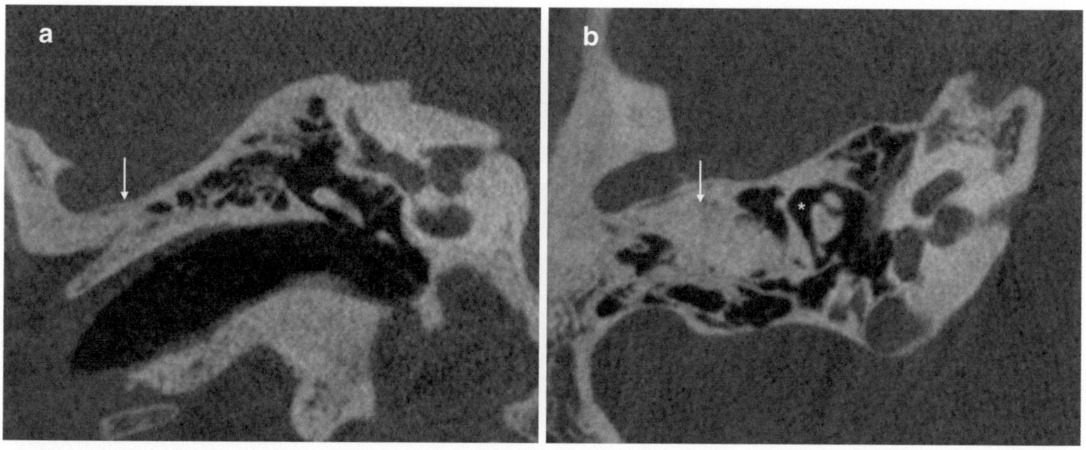

Fig. 4.25 **Hypoplasia of the tympanic cavity and mastoid**. (**a**) Coronal and (**b**) axial CBCT images show hypoplasic tympanic cavity (asterisk) and mastoid (arrow). *Abbreviation*: CBCT = cone-beam computed tomography

- Footplate fixation, with thickening of the interface between the vestibule and oval window niche
- Hypoplasia/aplasia of the footplate

Aberrant facial nerves are frequently encountered, including dehiscence of the fallopian canal, inferior displacement of the tympanic segment, and aberrant courses of the facial nerve and/or chorda tympani. The facial nerve canal may exhibit anomalies in position, caliber, number, course, and bony integrity, affecting one or more segments (Figs. 4.6, 4.7, 4.8, 4.9, 4.13 and 4.26).

Oval window anomalies are often associated with stapes and tympanic segment anomalies of the facial nerve due to their close embryological development. The oval window is considered stenotic when it measures ≤1 mm on the coronal plane. In cases of atresia, there is complete obliteration of the oval window by a thick bony plate (Figs. 4.8, 4.13, 4.14, 4.15, 4.21, 4.23 and 4.27).

Round window stenosis occurs when its diameter is less than 1.5 mm and is atretic when it is obliterated by a bony plate of the otic capsule at the interface of the middle ear and scala tympani (Figs. 4.13, 4.14, 4.24, 4.27, 4.29 and 4.30).

4.4 Inner Ear Malformation

Inner ear malformations (Figs. 4.26, 4.27, 4.28, 4.29, 4.30, 4.31, 4.32, 4.33, 4.34, 4.35, 4.36, 4.37, 4.38, 4.39, 4.40 and 4.41) are classified according to Sennaroglu's classification [11]. We also provide a flow chart of an imaging algorithm useful for radiologists in defining malformations.

Complete labyrinthine aplasia (CLA), also known as Michel aplasia, is an extremely rare condition caused by developmental arrest of the otic placode during the third gestational week [12]. It is characterized by the complete absence of inner ear structures and can be divided into (a) CLA with absent petrous bone, (b) CLA without otic capsule, and (c) CLA with otic capsule.

Rudimentary otocyst is a rare condition caused by an insult occurring likely at the beginning of the formation of the otocyst (3rd–4th week). There is a millimetric inner ear structure with an oval or round shape without the internal auditory canal (IAC).

Cochlear aplasia (CA) is defined as the absence of the cochlear duct, while vestibular and endolymphatic structures may develop normally

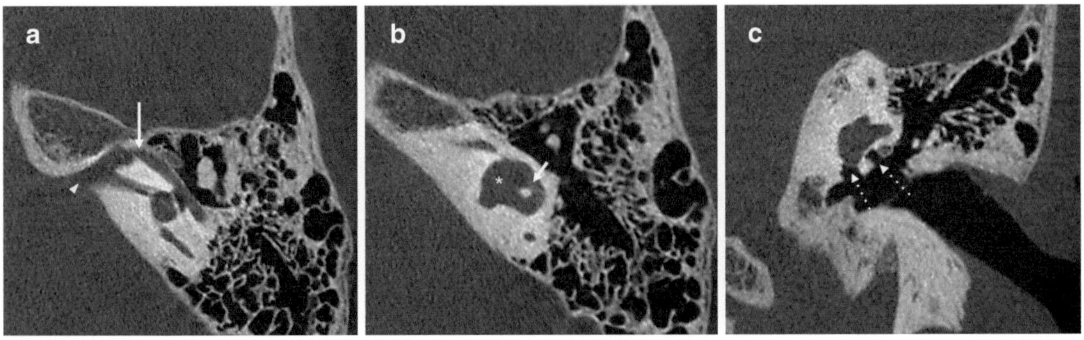

Fig. 4.26 Cochlear aplasia with dilated vestibule (CADV). (**a**, **b**) Axial and (**c**) coronal CBCT images show hypoplasic IAC (arrowhead) and complete absence of the cochlea; the labyrinthine segment of the facial nerve is anteriorly dislocated in the usual location of the cochlea (long arrow); the vestibule (asterisk) and lateral semicircular canal (short arrow) are short and dilated. Round and oval window are normal (dotted arrows). *Abbreviations*: CBCT = cone-beam computed tomography, IAC = internal auditory canal

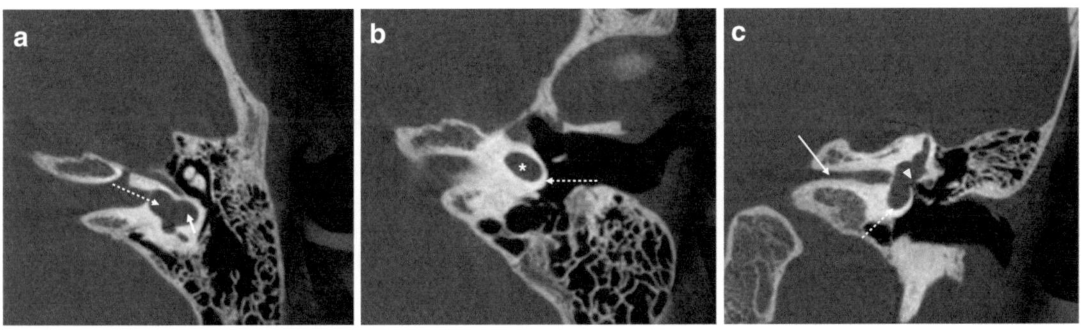

Fig. 4.27 Cochlear hypoplasia type I with dilated vestibule. (**a**, **b**) Axial and (**c**) coronal CBCT images show stenosis of the IAC (long arrow), cochlea has an ovoid shape without internal architecture (asterisk), the vestibule (dotted arrow) is dysmorphic with agenesia of the lateral SCC (short arrow), the oval window (arrowhead) is narrow, and the round window (dashed arrow) is absent. *Abbreviations*: CBCT = cone-beam computed tomography, IAC = internal auditory canal, SCC = semicircular canal

but can also exhibit abnormalities (cochlear aplasia with dilated vestibule, CADV). The insult typically occurs around the 5th week. Dense otic bone is present at the site where the cochlea would normally be. It is crucial to distinguish this anomaly from labyrinthitis ossificans, where normal-sized bone is present anterior to the IAC, with the cochlear promontory bulging formed by the basal turn of the cochlea. These characteristics are absent in cases of CA (Figs. 4.26 and 4.27).

Common cavity (CC) results from developmental arrest between the 4th and 5th weeks before there is clear differentiation into cochlea and vestibule. CC is a round or ovoid structure containing cochlear and vestibular neural elements, with the IAC opening into the center. Semicircular canals (SCC) are frequently malformed but may occasionally appear normal. It is important to differentiate CC from CADV because cochlear implantation may provide hearing in a CC, whereas in CADV, no functional stimulation will occur with cochlear implantation. In CADV, the dilated vestibule and SCC are located in the posterolateral part of the IAC fundus, which is usually normal in morphology, while in CC, the IAC is typically deformed, is angled posteriorly, and enters the cavity usually at its center.

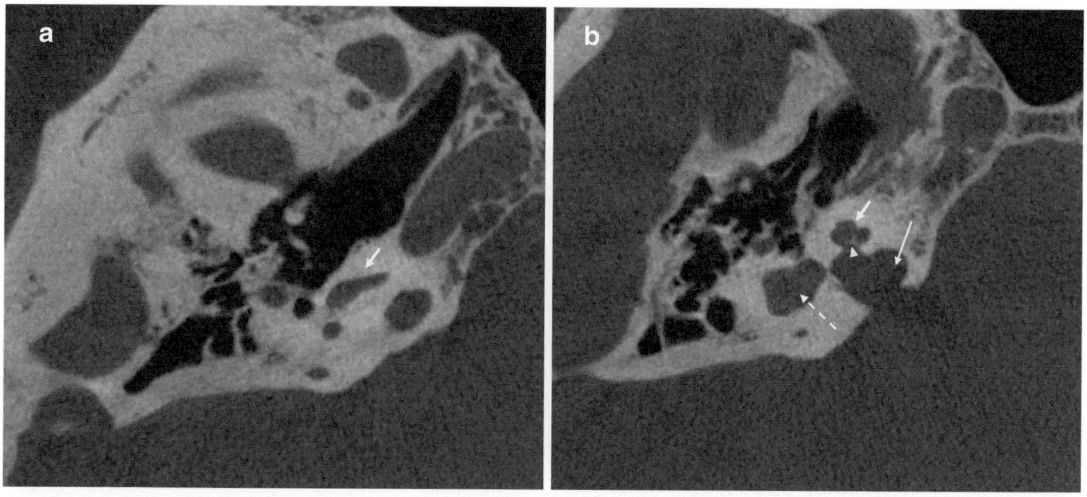

Fig. 4.28 Cochlear hypoplasia type II. (**a**, **b**) Axial CBCT images show dysmorphic IAC with a large diverticulum on its anterior wall (arrow), the cochlea is small (short arrow), and its internal architecture is partially defective: the modiolus (arrowhead) is short and there is no clear ISS between apical and middle turns. The vestibule is irregularly dilated (dashed arrow) along with agenesia of the lateral SCC. *Abbreviations*: CBCT = cone-beam computed tomography, IAC = internal auditory canal, ISS = interscalar septum, SCC = semicircular canal

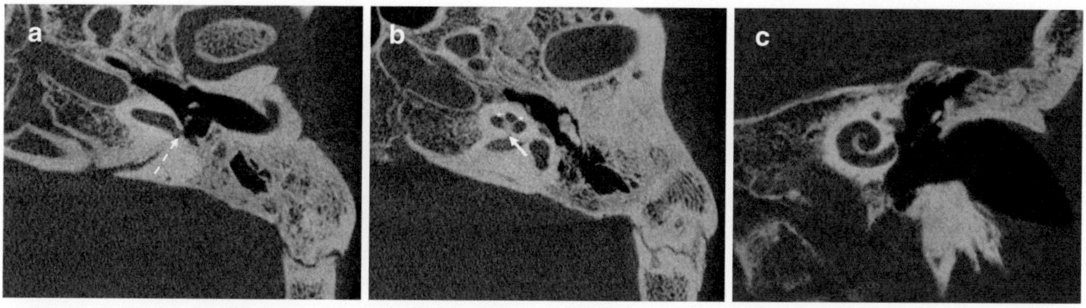

Fig. 4.29 Cochlear hypoplasia type III in CHARGE syndrome. On (**a**, **b**) axial CBCT the cochlea is smaller than usual, the ISS is normal (asterisks), the cochlear canal is stenotic (arrow), and the round window is narrow (dashed arrow); (**c**) oblique coronal reconstruction CBCT shows 1.5 turns of the cochlea. *Abbreviations*: CBCT = cone-beam computed tomography, ISS = interscalar septum

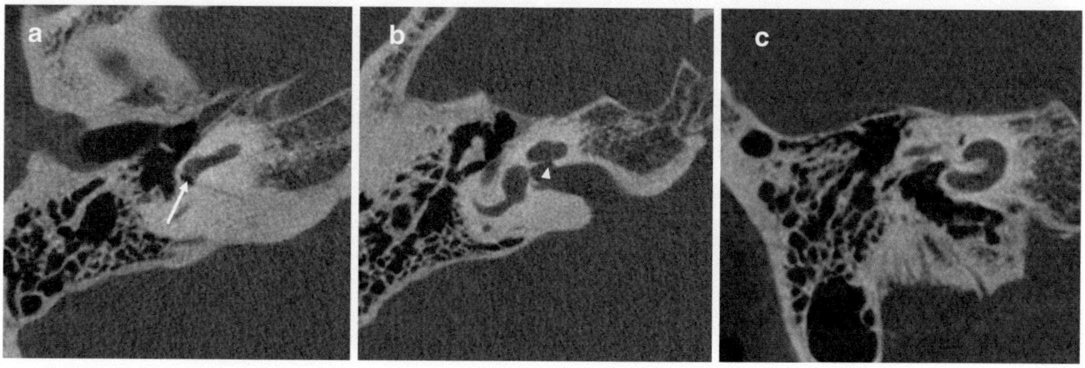

Fig. 4.30 Cochlear hypoplasia type III. (**a**, **b**) Axial CBCT images show small cochlea, the cochlear canal (arrowhead) is defective at the fundus of IAC, and the round window is narrow (arrow); (**c**) oblique coronal reconstruction CBCT shows less than 1.5 turns of the cochlea. *Abbreviations*: CBCT = cone-beam computed tomography, IAC = internal auditory canal

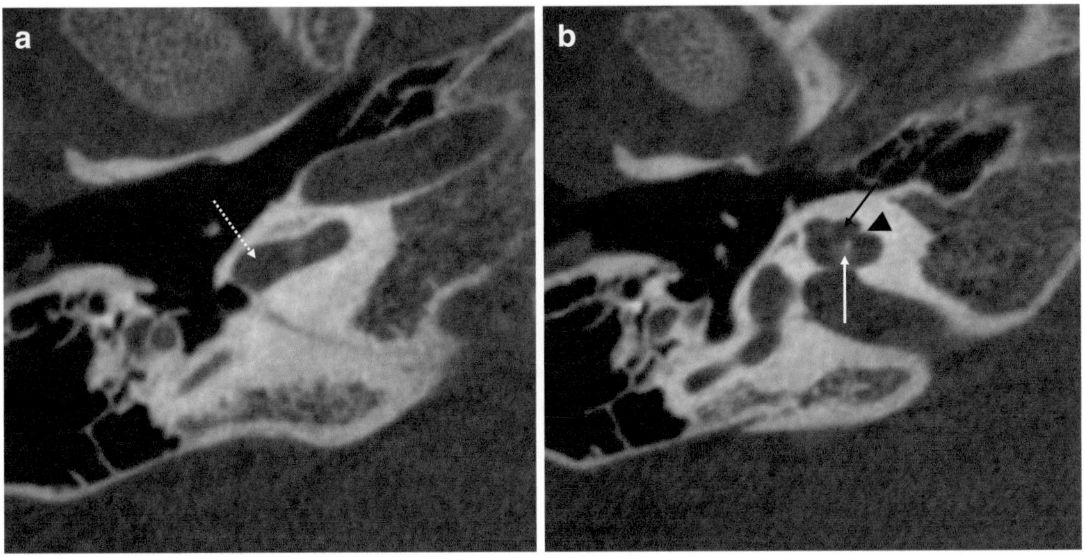

Fig. 4.31 **Cochlear hypoplasia Type IV**. (**a**, **b**) Axial CBCT images show small cochlea, the modiolus (arrow) and the ISS (balck arrowhead) are normal, the upper turns (black arrow) are small while the basal turn is normal (dotted arrow). *Abbreviations*: CBCT = cone-beam computed tomography, ISS = interscalar septum

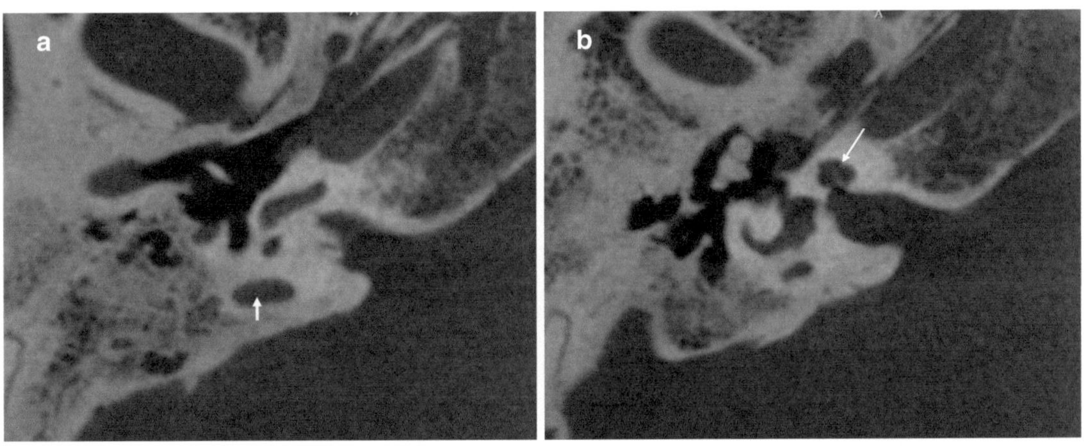

Fig. 4.32 **Not classifiable cochlear hypoplasia**. (**a**, **b**) Axial CBCT images show a small cochlea (arrow), with 2.5 turns, the modiolus and ISS are preserved, and the vestibular aqueduct is enlarged (short arrow). *Abbreviations*: CBCT = cone-beam computed tomography, ISS = interscalar septum

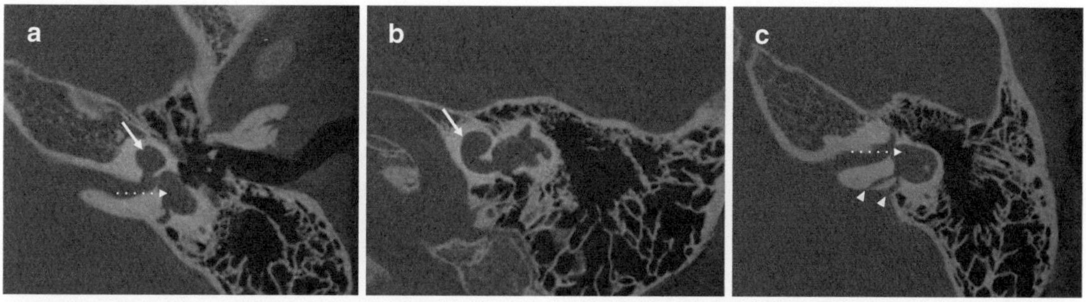

Fig. 4.33 Incomplete partition type I. (**a**, **c**) Axial and (**b**) oblique coronal CBCT images show cochlea with normal external dimension, with a cystic-like appearance lacking the entire modiolus and ISS, and the vestibule (dotted arrow) is enlarged along with dysplastic SCCs; on (**c**) axial CBCT two thin canals (arrowheads) extending from the medial wall of the vestibule (dotted arrow): one could be a small vestibular aqueduct, the second one an aberrant nervous canal. *Abbreviations*: CBCT = cone-beam computed tomography, ISS = interscalar septum, SCC = semicircular canal

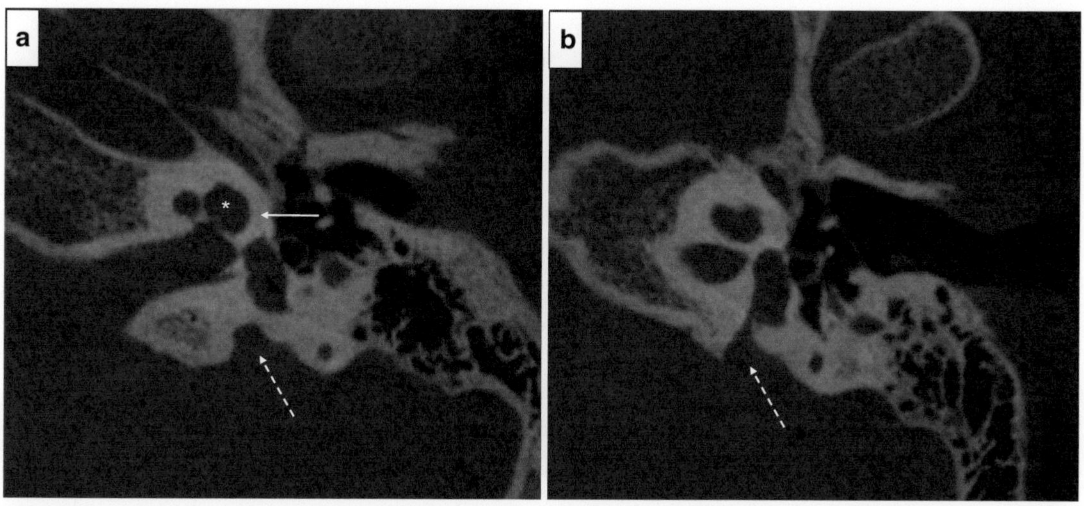

Fig. 4.34 Incomplete partition type II with EVA. (**a**, **b**) Axial CBCT images show a defective modiolus and ISS in the apical part of the cochlea, with a cystic-like middle and apical turns (asterisk) and smooth lateral cochlear contour (arrow), and the EVA (dashed arrow). *Abbreviations*: CBCT = cone-beam computed tomography, EVA = enlarged vestibular acqueduct, ISS = interscalar septum

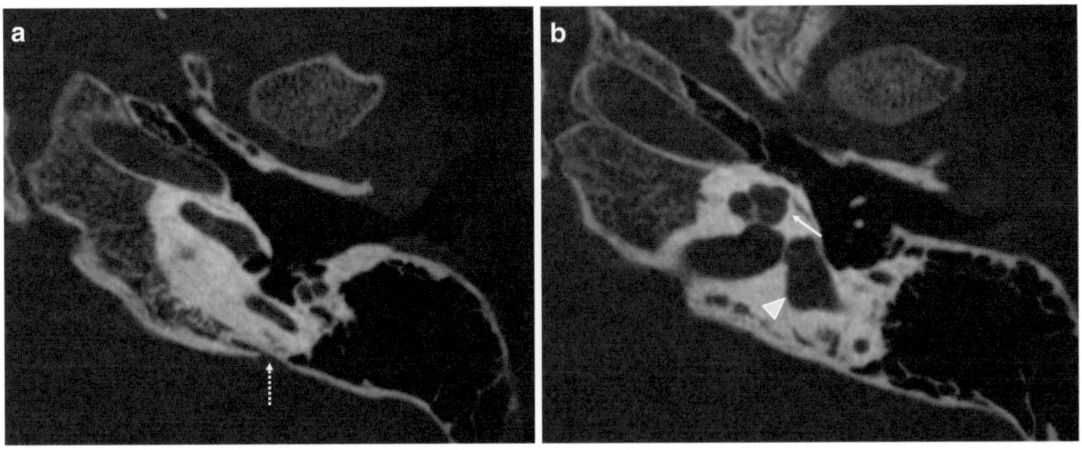

Fig. 4.35 **Incomplete partition type II without EVA**. (**a**, **b**) Axial CBCT images show a cystic cochlear apex with a smooth lateral contour of the apical and middle turns (arrow), the vestibule is enlarged (arrowhead), and the vestibular aqueduct is normal (dashed arrow). *Abbreviations*: CBCT = cone-beam computed tomography, ISS = interscalar septum

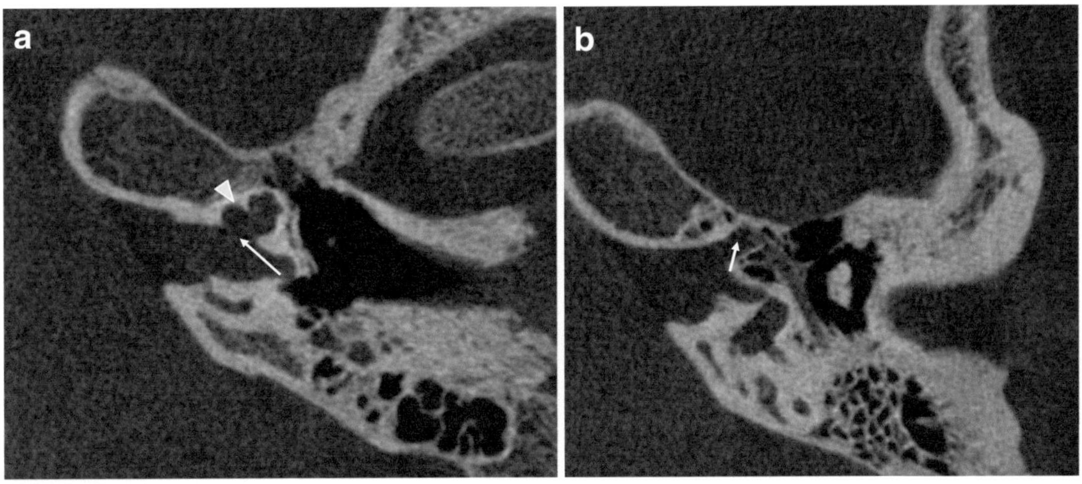

Fig. 4.36 **Incomplete partition type III**. (**a**, **b**) Axial CBCT images show normal-sized cochlea with a "cork-screw" appearance, with partial ISS (arrowhead) but without modiolus, directly located at the lateral end of the IAC almost in a straight line, with defective cochlear aperture (long arrow), the facial nerve (short arrow) is located above the cochlea. *Abbreviations*: CBCT = cone-beam computed tomography, IAC = internal auditory canal, ISS = interscalar septum

Cochlear hypoplasia (CH) is defined when the cochlea has dimensions smaller than a normal cochlea (see Table 4.1 for reference linear measurements). There are four types of CH:

- *CH type I*: (bud-like cochlea): round/ovoid-shaped cochlea with absent internal architecture; the modiolus and interscalar septa (ISS) cannot be identified, and the bony partition between the cochlea and the IAC may be absent (Fig. 4.27).
- *CH type II*: cochlea with smaller dimensions but almost normal external morphology; the modiolus is completely or partially defective, often creating a wide connection with the IAC, and the ISS may be absent or hypoplas-

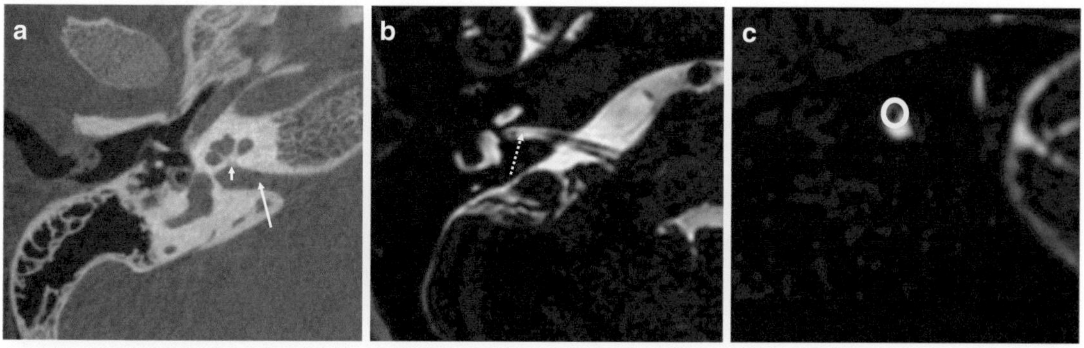

Fig. 4.37 Hypoplasic cochlear aperture. (**a**) Axial CBCT image shows narrow IAC (long arrow) and absence of cochlear aperture (short arrow), where the canal is completely replaced by bone; (**b**) axial and (**c**) sagittal oblique MR images show the absence of the cochlear nerve in the antero-inferior part of the IAC fundus (dashed arrow), and only the facial nerve (circle) is visible. *Abbreviations*: CBCT = cone-beam computed tomography, IAC = internal auditory canal, MR = magnetic resonance

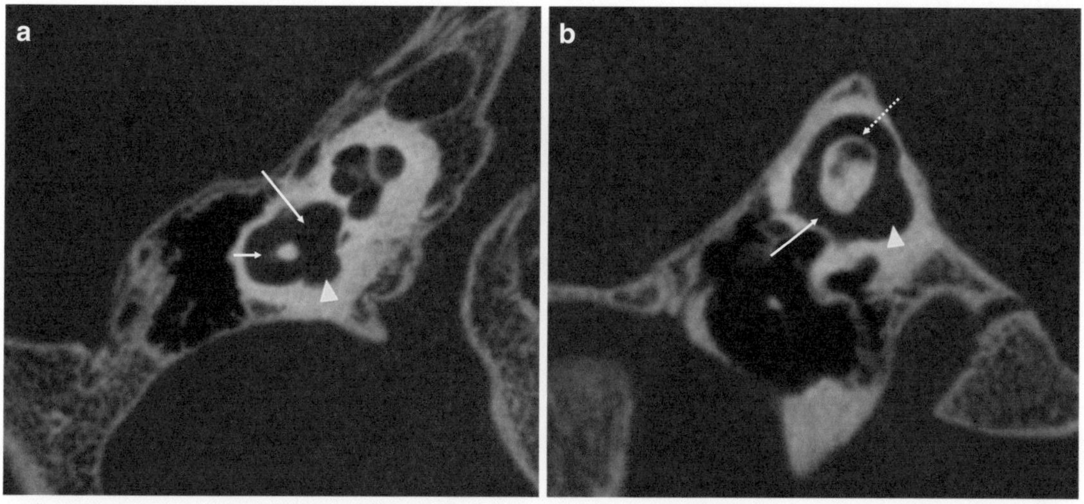

Fig. 4.38 Posterior semicircular canal aplasia. (**a**) Axial and (**b**) coronal plane CBCT images show malformed vestibulum (long arrow), short and dilated with slightly flattened appearance on the coronal plane; a small pouch cavity replaces the posterior SCC (arrowhead). Lateral SSC (short arrow) is short and widened, and the superior SCC (dotted arrow) is regular. *Abbreviations*: CBCT = cone-beam computed tomography, SCC = semicircular canal

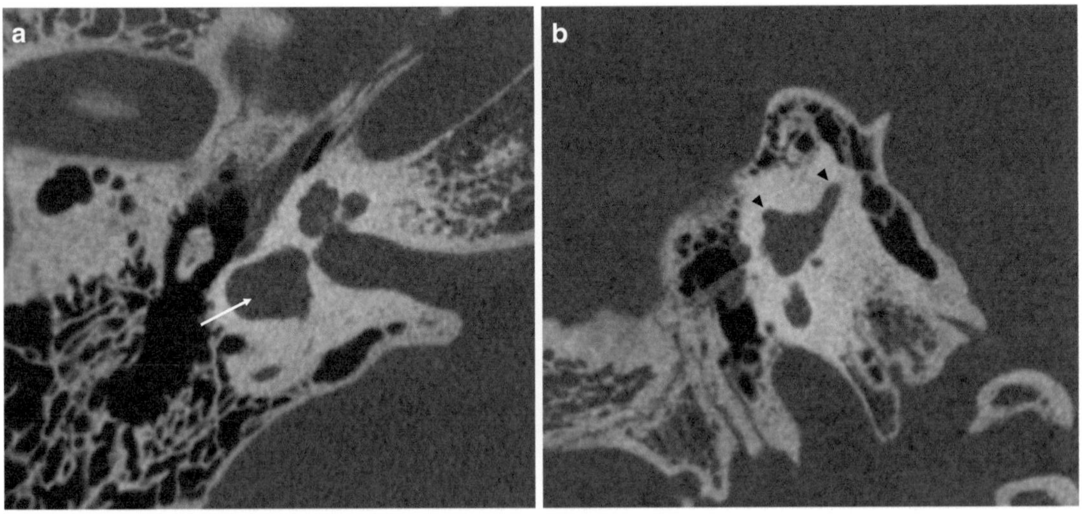

Fig. 4.39 Superior and lateral semicircular canal dysplasia. (**a**) axial CBCT image shows lateral SCC aplasia (arrow) with a broad and cystic space confluent with vestibule, that appears widened; the bony island is absent; (**b**) oblique coronal plane reconstruction CBCT shows partial aplasia of posterior SCC with missing anterior arch (black arrowheads). *Abbreviations*: CBCT = cone-beam computed tomography, SCC = semicircular canal

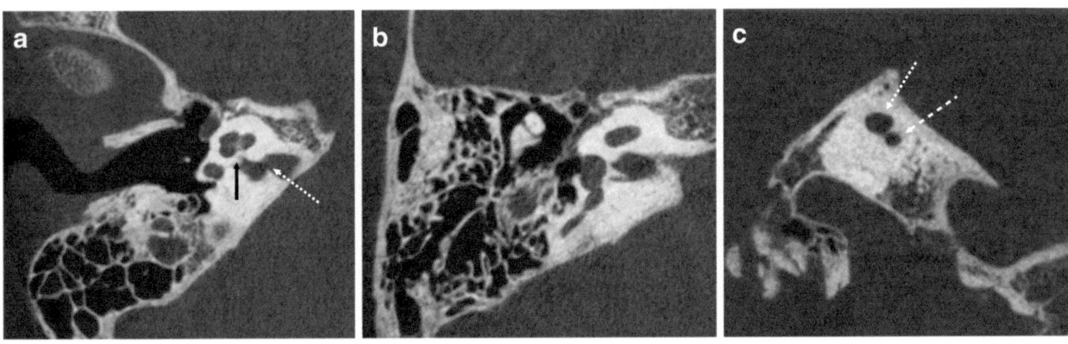

Fig. 4.40 Duplicated IAC and cochlear canal aplasia. (**a**, **b**) Axial and (**c**) oblique coronal CBCT images show duplicated IAC (dotted arrows) and absent cochlear canal (black arrow). *Abbreviations*: CBCT = cone-beam computed, IAC = internal auditory canal

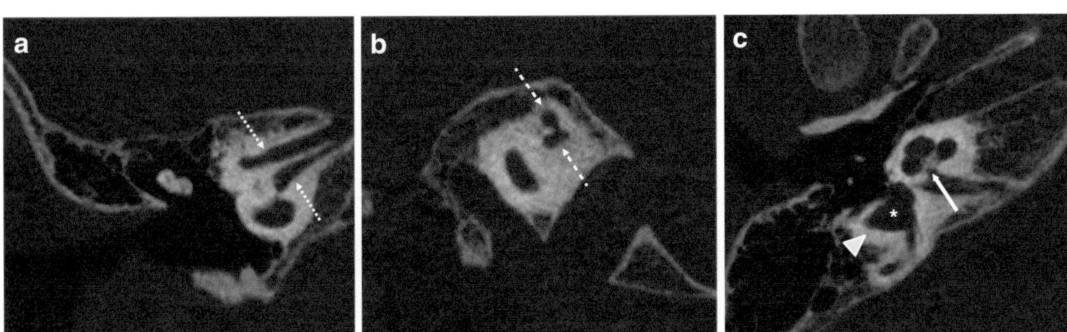

Fig. 4.41 Duplicated IAC and cochlear canal aplasia. (**a**) Coronal, (**b**) sagittal, and (**c**) axial CBCT images show duplicated IAC (dotted arrows) and absent cochlear canal (arrow) and enlarged vestibule (asterisk) with lateral SCC aplasia (arrowhead). *Abbreviations*: CBCT = cone-beam computed tomography, IAC = internal auditory canal, SCC = semicircular canal

tic, giving the cochlea a rounder shape than normal (Fig. 4.28).

- *CH type III*: cochlea with normal architecture but fewer turns (approximately one and a half); the modiolus and ISS are normal, while the most extreme variant consists of only a small basal turn and modiolus without middle and apical turns (Figs. 4.29 and 4.30).
- *CH type IV*: cochlea with a normal basal turn but hypoplastic middle and apical turns, which are located anterosuperiorly (Fig. 4.31).

Incomplete partition (IP) anomalies are characterized by a cochlea with normal external dimensions but abnormal internal architecture:

- *IP type I*: absent modiolus and ISS, cystic appearance of the cochlea, and grossly dilated vestibule (Fig. 4.33)
- *IP type II*: the apical part of the modiolus and the corresponding ISS are defective, with middle and apical turns coalescing to form a cystic apex. The medial border of the cochlea is more rounded than normal. It is part of the Mondini triad, associated with dilatation of the vestibule and enlarged vestibular aqueduct (Figs. 4.34 and 4.35).
- *IP type III*: ISS is partially present while the modiolus is absent; the cochlea is directly located at the lateral end of the IAC, almost in a straight line. The otic capsule around the cochlea is thin, and the facial nerve is located above the cochlea. It is associated with X-linked deafness (Fig. 4.36).

Malformations of the vestibule rarely occur in isolation and are commonly characterized by mild or globose dilatation of the vestibule with partial or complete assimilation of the semicircular canals into the vestibule (see Figs. 4.26–4.28, 4.33, 4.35, 4.38, 4.39, 4.41).

Malformation of SCC encompasses aplasia and dysplasia of the SCC. Dysplastic canals are usually short and wide, though they may be narrow. In extensive malformations, the vestibule is dilated, forming a common lumen with the lateral canal (i.e., lateral semicircular canal-vestibule dysplasia). Measurement of the width of the central bony islands of the superior and lateral semicircular canals on high-resolution CT images has been proposed as a means to identify subtle abnormalities (see Table 4.1 for reference linear measurements, Figs. 4.38 and 4.39).

Enlarged vestibular aqueduct (EVA) is one of the most frequent inner ear malformations and is bilateral in as many as 90% of cases. The vestibular aqueduct is considered enlarged when its diameter, measured midway between the common crus and the external aperture, is greater than 1.5 mm on CT images. A simple way to define it is when the diameter exceeds that of the adjacent ascending portion of the posterior semicircular duct.

IAC abnormalities include stenotic IAC (less than 2 mm in diameter), atretic IAC, or a bony septum that divides it into two or more separate canals (Figs. 4.40 and 4.41).

Cochlear nerve (CN) abnormalities are best seen on sagittal oblique MR images perpendicular to the long axis of the IAC. The CN is defined as normal in size when it is similar to the contralateral normal CN. According to Casselmann et al. [13], the size of the CN is larger than the ipsilateral facial nerve (FN) (Fig. 4.37).

Three types of cochlear nerve anomalies have been described:

- *Type 1*: absent VIII nerve and a stenotic IAC.
- *Type 2*: VIII nerve is recognizable with hypoplasia or aplasia of its cochlear branch:
  - *2A*: associated with other inner ear malformations
  - *2B*: isolated malformation.

Hypoplasia of the bony canal of the CN (Rosenthal canal) is characterized by bony covering at the site of the cochlear aperture [12] (Fig. 4.37 and 4.41).

We also provide a flowchart of an imaging algorithm useful for radiologists in defining malformations (Fig. 4.42).

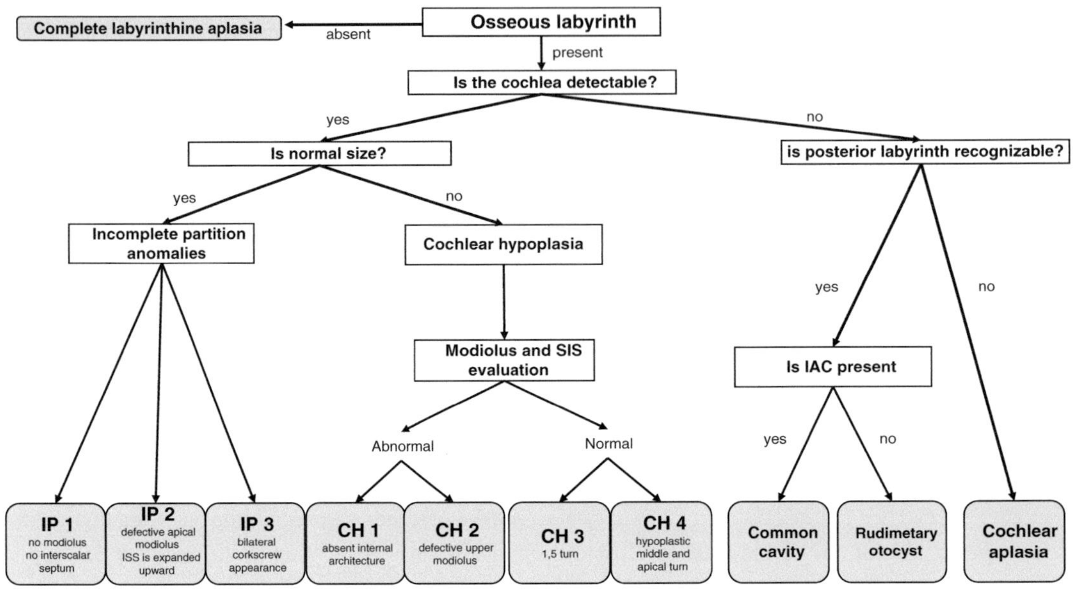

Fig. 4.42 Flowchart of an imaging algorithm to define inner ear malformations

References

1. Bartel-Friedrich S, Wulke C. Classification and diagnosis of ear malformations. GMS Curr Top Otorhinolaryngol Head Neck Surg. 2007;6:Doc05.
2. Gautam R, Kumar J, Pradhan GS, Meher R, Arya S. Congenital aural atresia: what the radiologist needs to know? Curr Probl Diagn Radiol. 2022;51(4):599–616.
3. Yeakley JW, Jahrsdoerfer RA. CT evaluation of congenital aural atresia: what the radiologist and surgeon need to know. J Comput Assist Tomogr. 1996;20(5):724–31.
4. Saylisoy S, Incesulu A, Kaya E, Pinarbasli O, Adapinar B. The round window diameter in congenital aural atresia and comparison with sensorineural hearing loss and control group. J Comput Assist Tomogr. 2014;38(3):461–3. https://doi.org/10.1097/RCT.0000000000000060.
5. Nordstrom CK, Laurell G, Rask-Andersen H. The human vestibular aqueduct: anatomical characteristics and enlargement criteria. Otology & Neurotology. 2016;37:1637–45.
6. Teissier N, Van Den Abbeele T, Sebag G, Elmaleh-Berges M. Computed tomography measurements of the normal and the pathologic cochlea in children. Pediatr Radiol. 2010;40(3):275–83.
7. Saliba I, Sbeity S, El-Zir E, Yammine FG, Noun CT, Haddad A. Down syndrome: an electrophysiological and radiological profile. Laryngoscope. 2014;124(4):E141.
8. Shim HJ, Shin JE, Chung JW, Lee KS. Inner ear anomalies in cochlear implantees: importance of radiologic measurements in the classification. Otol Neurotol. 2006;27(6):831–7.
9. Blaser S, Propst EJ, Martin D, Feigenbaum A, James AL, Shannon P, Papsin BC. Inner ear dysplasia is common in children with down syndrome (trisomy 21). Laryngoscope. 2006;116(12):2113–9.
10. Jahrsdoerfer RA, Yeakley JW, Aguilar EA, Cole RR, Gray LC. Grading system for the selection of patients with congenital aural atresia. Am J Otol. 1992;13(1):6–12.
11. Sennaroglu L. Histopathology of inner ear malformations: do we have enough evidence to explain pathophysiology? Cochlear Implants Int. 2016;17(1):3–20.
12. Joshi VM, Navlekar SK, Kishore GR, Reddy KJ, Kumar EC. CT and MR imaging of the inner ear and brain in children with congenital sensorineural hearing loss. Radiographics. 2012;32(3):683–98.
13. Casselman JW, Offeciers FE, Govaerts PJ, Kuhweide R, Geldof H, Somers T, D'Hont G. Aplasia and hypoplasia of the vestibulocochlear nerve: diagnosis with MR imaging. Radiology. 1997;202(3):773–81.

Traumatic Temporal Bone Imaging

5

Guido Del Vecchio, Elisa Scola, Lorenzo Maria Gaini, Francesco Maria Lo Russo, Fabio Triulzi, Diego Zanetti, and Giorgio Conte

Temporal bone fractures are rare as they require a significant impact, such as in road accidents or assaults. They are associated with a high risk of significant morbidity or mortality due the injury of vital structures. This chapter is structured to cover discussions on normal anatomy and pseudo-fractures, followed by sections on temporal bone fractures and complications arising from temporal bone injury.

5.1 Classification

Temporal bone fractures are traditionally classified as either longitudinal or transverse reflecting their orientation relative to the long axis of the petrous bone [1–3] (Fig. 5.1).

Longitudinal fractures are the most common type (70–90%) and occur due to a lateral blow to the temporoparietal region. The fracture line is parallel to the long axis of the petrous bone. These fractures are often associated with fractures of the squamous portion of the temporal bone.

Transverse fractures are less common and typically result from frontal or occipital trauma. The fracture line is perpendicular to the short axis of the petrous bone defect.

In most cases, however, fracture lines have an oblique or complex course.

The fracture classification can be based on involvement of the otic capsule [1, 4, 5] giving important prognostic information.

Otic capsule-violating fractures are associated with a less favorable prognosis due to involvement of jugular foramen, internal auditory canal (IAC), and foramen lacerum and affect the labyrinth and facial canal with the development of

G. Del Vecchio (✉) · E. Scola · F. M. Lo Russo
Neuroradiology Unit, Fondazione IRCCS Ca' Granda Ospedale Maggiore Policlinico, Milan, Italy
e-mail: guido.delvecchio@policlinico.mi.it; elisa.scola@policlinico.mi.it; francesco.lorusso@policlinico.mi.it

L. M. Gaini
Department of Otolaryngology and Head and Neck Surgery, Fondazione IRCCS Ca' Granda Ospedale Maggiore Policlinico, Milan, Italy
e-mail: lorenzo.gaini@policlinico.mi.it

F. Triulzi · G. Conte
Neuroradiology Unit, Fondazione IRCCS Ca' Granda Ospedale Maggiore Policlinico, Milan, Italy

Department of Pathophysiology and Transplantation, University of Milan, Milan, Italy
e-mail: fabio.triulzi@policlinico.mi.it; giorgio.conte@policlinico.mi.it

D. Zanetti
Audiology Unit, Department of Specialistic Surgical Sciences Fondazione IRCCS Ca' Granda, Ospedale Maggiore Policlinico Milan, Milan, Italy

Department of Clinical Sciences and Community Health University of Milan, Milan, Italy
e-mail: diego.zanetti@policlinico.mi.it

G. Conte et al. (eds.), *Atlas of Normal and Pathological Findings in Otoneuroradiology*, https://doi.org/10.1007/978-3-032-08232-9_5

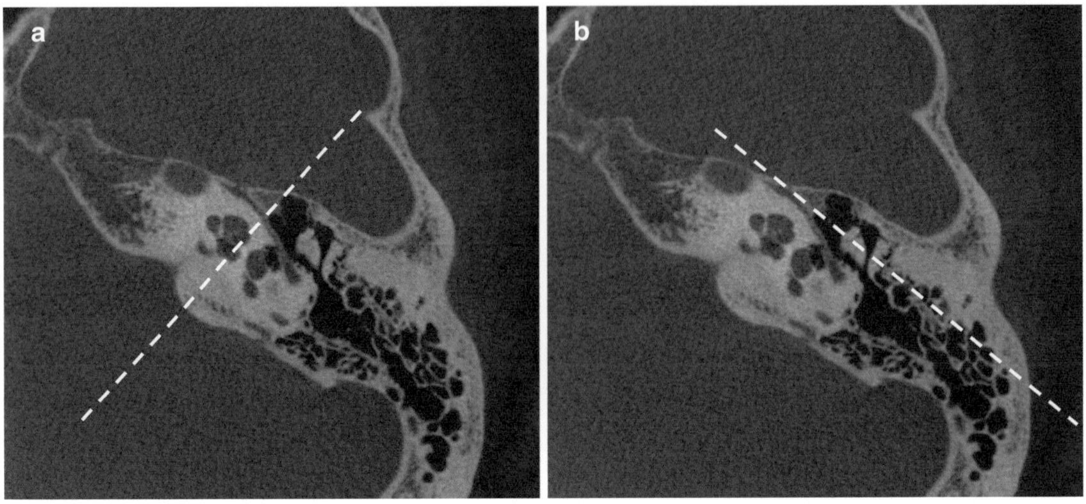

Fig. 5.1 Classification of temporal bone fractures. Temporal bone fractures are traditionally classified as either transverse or longitudinal, reflecting their orientation relative to the long axis of the petrous bone. Transverse fractures (**a**) are less common, typically resulting from frontal or occipital trauma, and are perpendicular to the short axis of the petrous bone. Longitudinal fractures (**b**) -the most common type (70–90%)- are parallel to the long axis of the petrous bone, and are often associated with fractures of the squamous portion of the temporal bone. In most cases, however, fracture lines have an oblique or complex course. CBCT image shows a transverse fractures. Transverse fractures usually involve the otic capsule. CBCT image shows a longitudinal fractures which usually spare the otic capsule. *Abbreviation:* CBCT cone beam computed tomography

facial paralysis, cerebrospinal fluid (CSF) leakage, and hearing loss.

Otic capsule-sparing fractures commonly involve the squamous temporal bone and the posterosuperior wall of the external auditory canal (EAC), passing through the mastoid air cells, middle ear, tegmen mastoideum, and tegmen tympani. These fractures may affect the ossicular chain, leading to conductive hearing loss (CHL) or mixed hearing loss.

EAC fracture may be the result of an extending fracture line from the temporal bone or a direct impaction of the mandibular condyle into the posterior wall of the temporomandibular joint (TMJ). Tympanic plate is a "u"-shaped anterior wall of the auditory canal. Fracture of the tympanic plate may result in EAC stenosis or trismus.

Oblique CT views (Pöschl view) is better to detect EAC fractures [8].

5.2 Imaging Evaluation

CT imaging with multiplanar reconstruction at a section thickness of 0.6 mm or less is the optimal imaging modality for accurate detection of fracture lines and complications [1, 3, 5]. In patients with head trauma, the fluid collection in the middle ear and/or mastoid cells as well as pneumocephalus, air in mastoid process, temporomandibular joint, styloid process, and dural sinus suggest the presence of the temporal bone fracture, even if it is not clearly depicted on CT imaging. It is sometimes recommended to repeat CT scan after some weeks when intratympanic hemorrhage is totally absorbed. Magnetic resonance (MR) imaging should be performed in cases of suspected labyrinthine injury, such as concussion, or associated cranial nerves palsy. CT angiography is recommended when vascular injuries are suspected, for example, in case the fracture line involves the carotid channel, the jugular foramen, and the sigmoid sulcus [1].

5.3 Pitfalls and Pearls

Many normal structures in the temporal bone, such as aqueducts, canaliculi, grooves, sutures, fissures, and other entities, may mimic fracture lines [1, 2]. Knowing these anatomic entities allows excluding the so-called pseudo-fractures; furthermore, comparing the contralateral side can be helpful as these structures are typically symmetrical [2]. The structures that may mimic a fracture are listed hereinafter:

- *The cochlear aqueduct* connects the subarachnoid space and the scala tympani of the cochlea (Fig. 5.2, see also Fig. 2.19).
- *The vestibular aqueduct* contains the endolymphatic duct and sac, originating from the posterosuperior part of the vestibule and reaching the posteroinferolateral aspect of the posterior surface of the petrous portion of the temporal bone (Fig. 5.3, see also Figs. 2.19) and 2.21).
- *The subarcuate canaliculus* is a small canal that contains the subarcuate artery (Fig. 5.4, see also Fig. 2.16).
- *The singular canal* contains the posterior ampullary nerve and connects the bottom of the IAC and the ampulla of the posterior semicircular canal.
- *The canal of the superior vestibular nerve* originates from the vestibule.
- *The canal for the chorda tympany* contains the chorda tympani nerve and posterior tympanic artery (Fig 5.4, see also Figs. 2.13 and 2.14).
- *The groove of the greater superficial petrosal nerve* contains the greater petrosal nerve and the temporal branch of the middle meningeal artery.
- *The mastoid canaliculus* contains the auricular branch of the vagus nerve (Arnold nerve) (Fig 5.5).
- *The inferior tympanic canaliculus* contains the inferior tympanic branch of the glossopharyngeal nerve (Jacobson nerve) (Fig 5.5, see also Fig. 2.15).

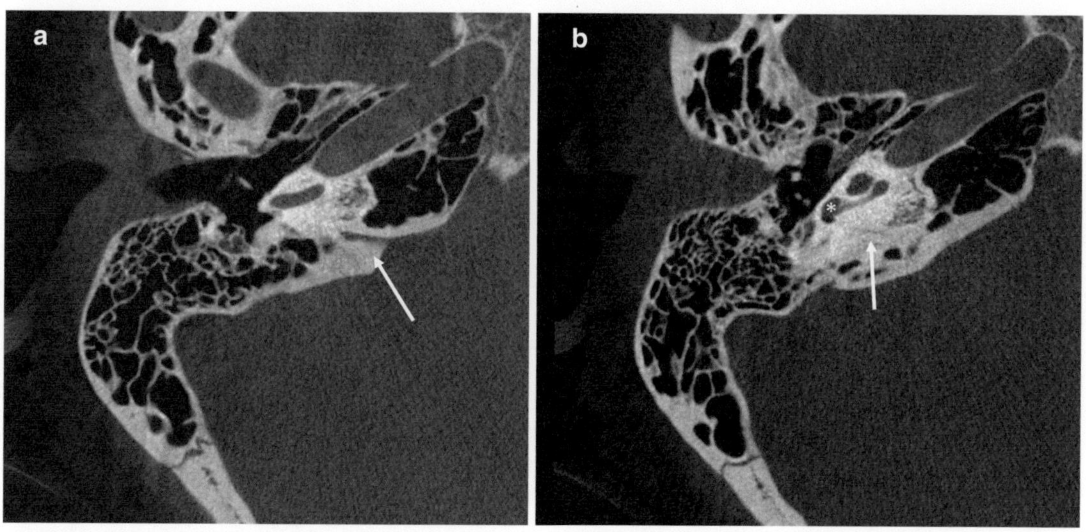

Fig. 5.2 Fracture mimics: cochlear aqueduct. The cochlear aqueduct connects the subarachnoid space and the scala tympani of the basal turn of the cochlea. It is a bony canaliculus that contains the perilymphatic duct wich drains the perilymph into the cerebrospinal fluid. The medial end of cochlear aqueduct opens in the posterior cranial fossa, cranial to the petrosal fossula. (**a**) Axial reformatted CBCT image shows the cochlear aqueduct (arrow) as a thin line parallel to IAC. (**b**) Axial reformatted CBCT image shows the cochlear aqueduct (arrow) through the temporal bone to scala tympani of the basal turn of cochlea (asterisk). *Abbreviations:* CBCT cone beam computed tomography, IAC internal auditory canal

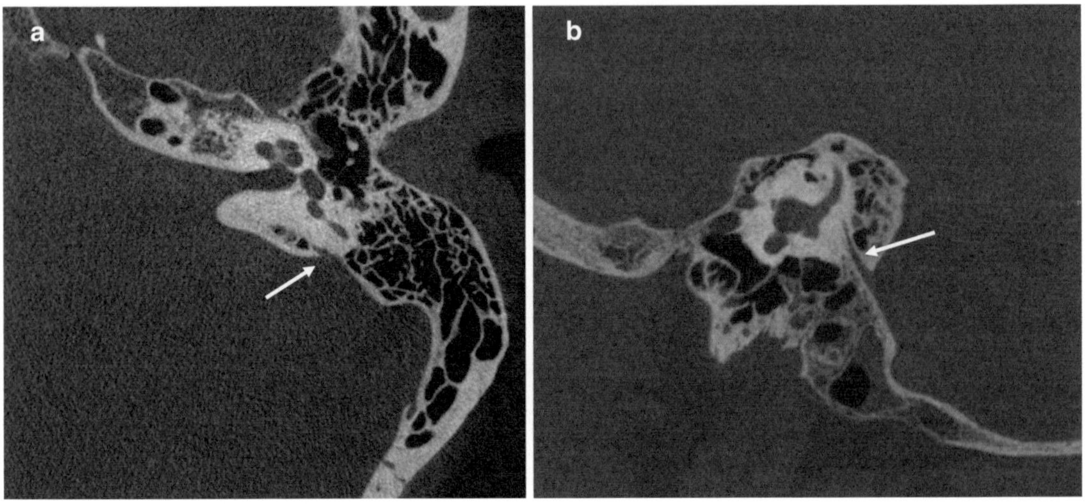

Fig. 5.3 **Fracture mimics: vestibular aqueduct.** The vestibular aqueduct is a bony canal containing the endolymphatic duct and sac. It is part of the labyrinth and originates from the posterosuperior part of the vestibule and reaches the posteroinferolateral aspect of the posterior surface of the petrous portion of the temporal bone. It is usually very thin, and its midpoint part can be hardly detected on CT scan. (**a**) Axial reformatted CBCT image shows the operculum of the vestibular aqueduct (arrow) along the posterior surface of the petrous portion of the temporal bone. (**b**) Oblique reformatted CBCT image oriented parallel to the superior semicircular canal (Pöschl plane) allows the proper visualization of vestibular aqueduct (arrow). *Abbreviation*: CBCT cone beam computed tomography

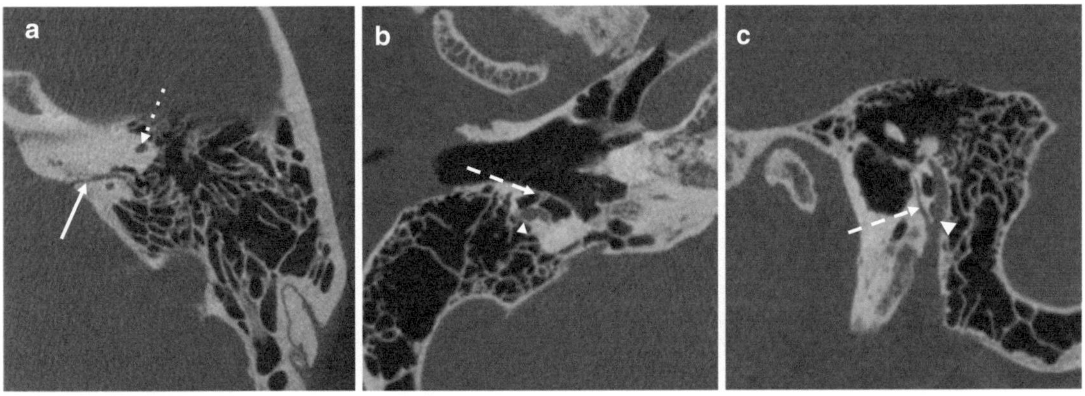

Fig. 5.4 **Fracture mimics: subarcuate canaliculus and canal of the chorda tympani:** (**a**) Axial reformatted CBCT image shows the subarcuate canaliculus as a thin canal (arrow) at the level of the superior semicircular canal (dotted arrow). The arcuate canal contains the subarcuate artery. (**b**) Axial and (**c**) sagittal reformatted CBCT images show the canal of the chorda tympani (dashed arrow) that contains the posterior tympanic artery and chorda tympani nerve which originates from the mastoid part of the facial nerve (arrowhead). *Abbreviation:* CBCT cone beam computed tomography

- *The petrosphenoidal fissure* between the posterior border of the greater wing of the sphenoid bone and the anterior border of the petrous part of the temporal bone, extending posterolaterally from the foramen lacerum (Fig. 5.6).
- *The occipitomastoid suture* runs between the posterior border of the petrous portion of the temporal bone and the occipital bone. It continues to the lambdoid suture (Fig. 5.6).
- *The tympanosquamous fissure* is located between the tympanic and squamous parts of the temporal bone. It connects to the petrosphenoidal fissure medially.
- *Persistent foramen tympanicum* (or Huschke's foramen) is a congenital anatomical variant

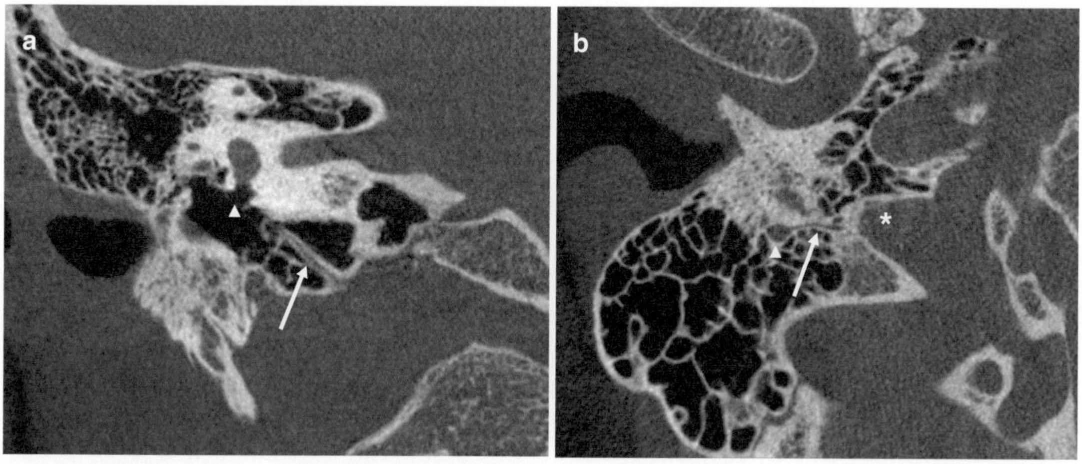

Fig. 5.5 **Fracture mimics: inferior tympanic and mastoid canaliculi.** (**a**) Coronal reformatted CBCT image at the level of the niche of the round window (arrowhead) shows the inferior tympanic canaliculus (arrow) that contains the inferior tympanic branch of the glossopharyngeal nerve (Jacobson nerve) and the inferior tympanic branch of the ascedent pharyngeal artery. (**b**) Axial reformatted CBCT image shows the mastoid canaliculus (arrow) that contains the auricular branch of the vagus nerve (Arnold nerve), connecting the foramen jugulare (asterisk) to the mastoid portion of the facial nerve (arrowhead). *Abbreviation:* CBCT cone beam computed tomography

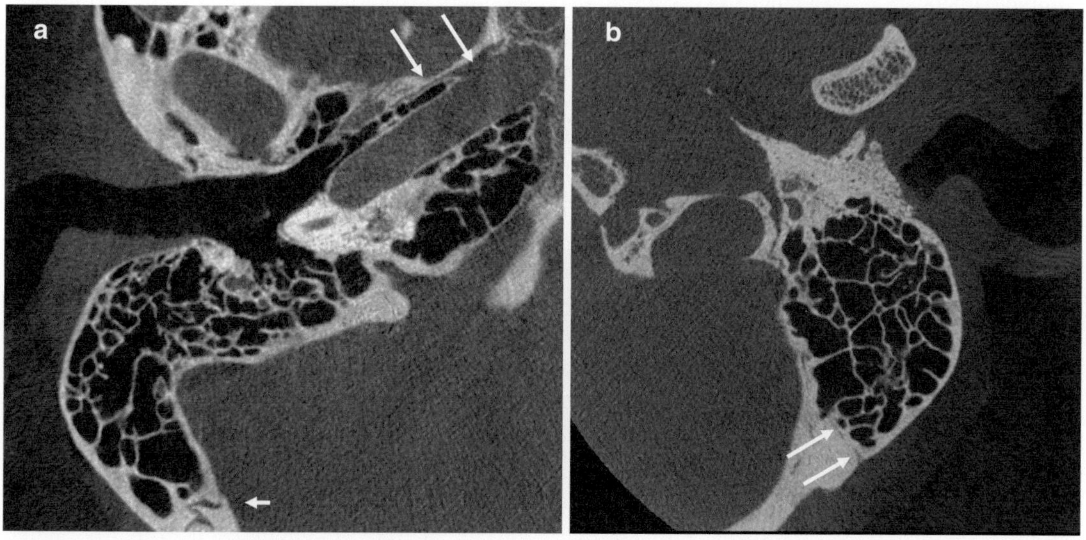

Fig. 5.6 **Fracture mimics: normal sutures.** (**a**) Axial reformatted CBCT image shows the petrosphenoidal fissure (arrows) between the posterior border of the greater wing of the sphenoid bone and the anterior border of the petrous part of the temporal bone, extending posterolaterally from the foramen lacerum. Occipitomastoid suture is also seen (short arrow). (**b**) Axial reformatted CBCT image shows the occipitomastoid suture (arrows) running between the posterior border of the petrous portion of the temporal bone and the occipital bone, and continues superiorly to the lambdoid suture. *Abbreviation:* CBCT cone beam computed tomography

characterized by the persistence of an opening in the floor of the EAC, which normally closes during embryonic development.

- *The petro-occipital fissure* is located between the petrous part of the temporal bone and the basilar part of the occipital bone.
- *The cochlear cleft* is located in the anterior portion of the oval window. It is detected on CT images at 41% of pediatric examinations. The incidence of this cleft decreases with age.

5.4 Complications of Temporal Bone Fractures

Ossicular injury includes ossicular fracture and ossicular dislocation. The latter are more common than ossicular fractures, and they frequently occur with longitudinal fractures. The most common sites are (in order of frequency) incudostapedial joint, incudomalleolar junction, and complete dislocation of the incus [1]. These injuries lead to conductive hearing loss. If a conductive hearing loss persists beyond 6–8 weeks after resolution of edema and hemotympanum, ossicular chain damage should be suspected. The incus is most frequently dislocated, whereas the stapes tends to fracture (Figs 5.7, 5.8, 5.9, 5.10, and 5.11).

In the setting of *facial nerve lesion*, presenting with paralysis, the radiologist should carefully look for a bony fragment or spicules in the facial canal which requires early surgical decompression. In presence of a facial paralysis with negative CT scan, MR imaging can be obtained to rule out swelling of the nerve and/or hematoma, wich usually improves spontaneously and can often be treated conservatively with steroids and observation [1, 2, 4] (Figs. 5.12, 5.13, and 5.14).

Perilymphatic fistula is an abnormal communication between the labyrinth and the tympanic cavity. The most common cause is rupture of the oval window or round window with post-traumatic fistula. CT scan often can be not conclusive, and pneumolabyrinth or unexplained fluid collection may suggest an abnormal connection between the middle ear and the membranous labyrinth [1]. A 4-hour delayed post-contrast MR imaging with 3D fluid-attenuated inversion recovery (FLAIR) images can depict the perilymph leakage through the round or oval window [6] (Figs. 5.13 and 5.15).

Traumatic CSF leakage due to temporal bone fracture occurs four times more commonly with otic capsule-violating fractures and is more common with longitudinal fractures than with transverse fractures [1]. At imaging, any fluid collection in the tympanic cavity and/or mastoid air cells should be carefully scrutinized. Approximately 10% or fewer patients with CSF leakage develop meningitis in the subacute phase [1]. MR imaging can be useful to detect cephalocele.

Vascular injury is a common complication in the presence of temporal bone fracture. If the fracture line extends beyond the carotid canal, an internal carotid artery (ICA) lesion can occur as intimal flap, irregular narrowing, stenosis, thrombosis or pseudoaneurysm. Fractures involving the jugular foramen or sigmoid sinus and jugular bulb can lead to venous injury [1, 2, 5] (Fig. 5.16).

Fracture of the otic capsule is associated with sudden sensorineural hearing loss (SNHL), vertigo, and tinnitus. When the fracture line extends through the fundus of IAC, a transection of the cochlear nerve can occur [1]. Pneumolabyrinth strongly suggests fracture of the otic capsule, even when a fracture line is not apparent [1]. In addition to temporal bone fracture, MR imaging can be useful to detect intralabyrinthine bleeding for concussion [2]. Chronically, intralabyrinthine hemorrhage may result in labyrinthitis ossificans, which is a cause of permanent SNHL [1].

EAC stenosis: Post-traumatic EAC stenosis ranges from mild to complete occlusion, causing varying degrees of conductive hearing loss. It can result from comminution and displacement of the tympanic plate, callus formation, or fibrous inflammation [7].

Cholesteatoma: Post-traumatic cholesteatomas occur rarely as a complication of EAC displaced fracture or tympanic perforation. They result from keratinous epithelium implant, can occur in the EAC, tympanic cavity, and mastoid, and may involve the ossicular chain, facial nerve,

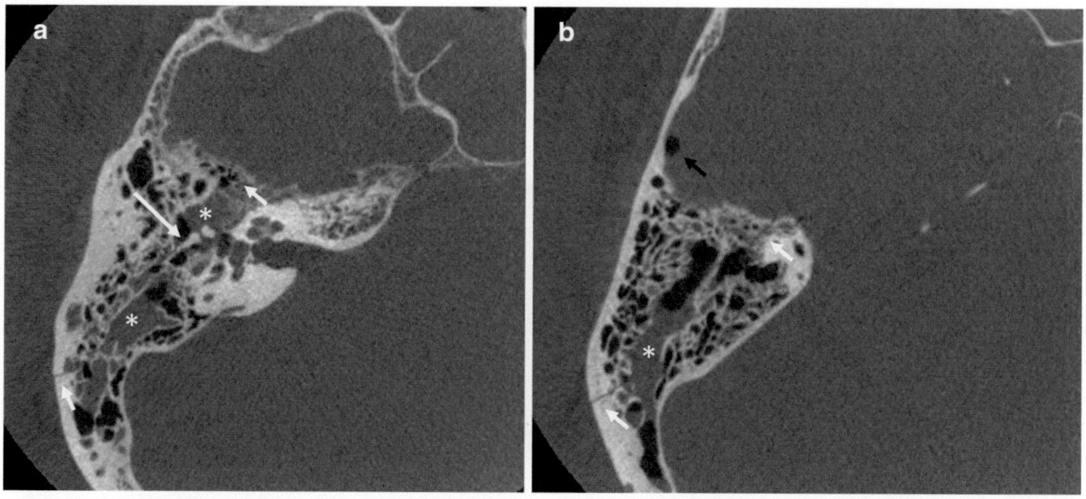

Fig. 5.7 Longitudinal fractures. (**a**) Axial reformatted CBCT image shows fracture line (short arrows) passing through the long axis of the temporal bone. There is also fluid collection (asterisk) in mastoid cells and middle ear due the trauma. There is also incudomalleolar disarticulation (arrow). (b) Axial reformatted CBCT scan passing through the epitympanum shows the fracture line (short arrows), fluid collection (asterisk) in antrum, and pneumocephalus (black arrow). *Abbreviation:* CBCT cone beam computed tomography

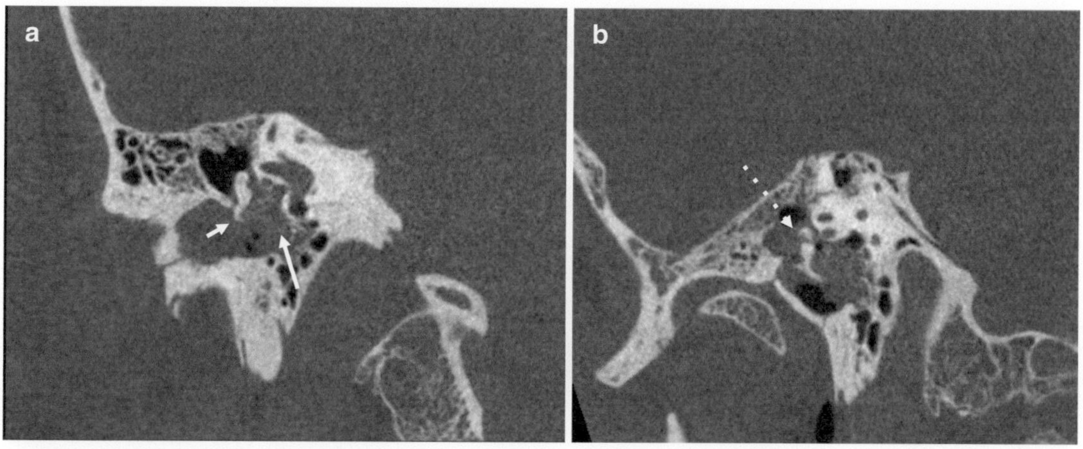

Fig. 5.8 Complications of longitudinal fractures: ossicular injuries. One of the complications of longitudinal fractures is the ossicular injuries. These injuries lead to conductive hearing loss. (**a**) Coronal CBCT reformatted image passing through the incus shows the dislocation of the incus, with fracture of its long process (short arrow) and disarticulation of the incudostapedial joint as suggested by the widening of the space between the incus and the stapes (arrow). (**b**) Coronal oblique CBCT image shows the dislocation of the malleus and the fracture of its head (dotted arrow). *Abbreviation:* CBCT cone beam computed tomography

and labyrinth. Long-term follow-up is crucial, as cholesteatomas can develop years later [5]

Two-panel CBCT images labeled 'a' and 'b' showing inner ear structure. Arrows in panel 'a' and 'b' point to the same structure in two sequential axial scans. Asterisk in panel 'b' indicates a different structure.

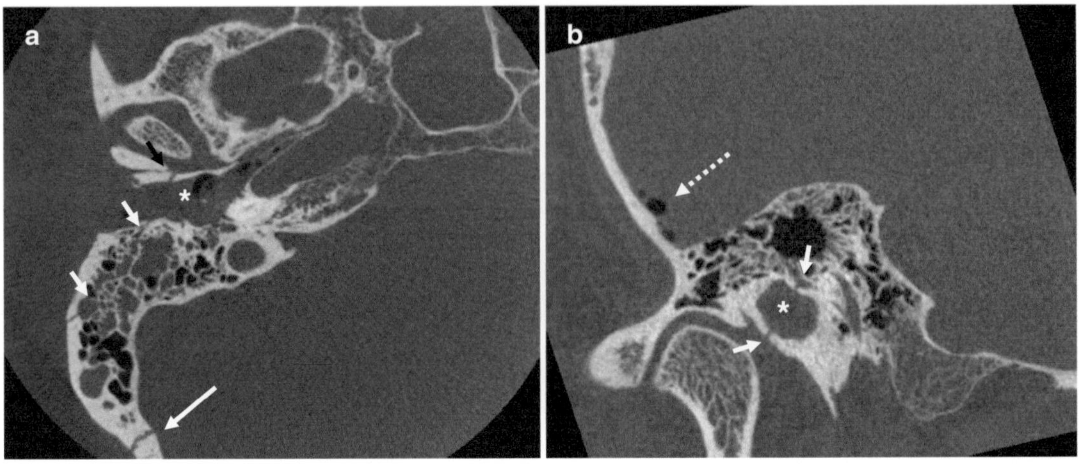

Fig. 5.9 Longitudinal fracture with EAC involvement. (**a**) Axial CBCT image shows a longitudinal fracture (short arrows) with involvement of the tympanic plate (black short arrow) with fluid filled EAC (asterisk). Do not confuse the occipitomastoid suture (arrow) for a fracture line. (**b**) Oblique sagittal CBCT image shows a fracture line (short arrows) through the anterior and posterior walls of the EAC, with fluid within the EAC (asterisk). This CBCT image shows also pneumocephalus (dotted arrow). *Abbreviations:* CBCT cone beam computed tomography, EAC external auditory canal

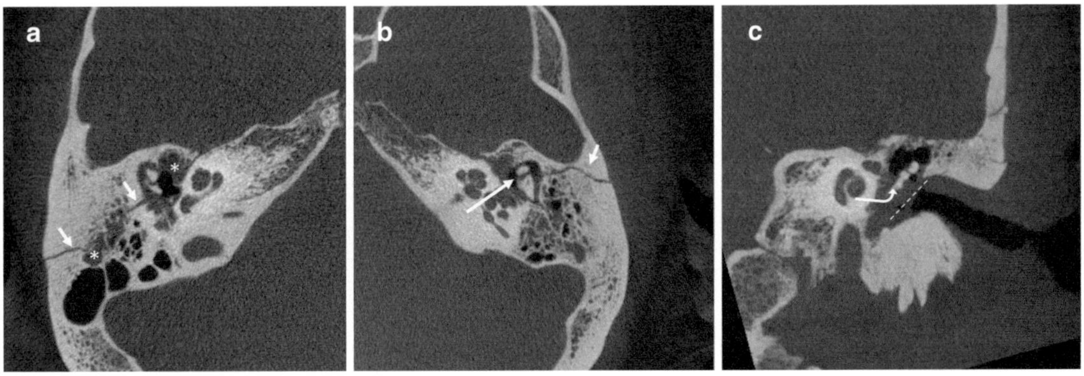

Fig. 5.10 Longitudinal fracture with ossicular injury. (**a**) Axial reformatted CBCT shows a longitudinal fracture, (short arrows) there is also fluid collection (asterisk) in mastoid cells and middle ear, the otic capsule is not involved. (**b**) Axial CBCT image shows a longitudinal fracture (short arrow) sparing the otic capsule, with incudomalleolar joint subluxation (arrow). (**c**) Coronal CBCT image shows the medial dislocation of the malleus (curved arrow) which is no longer articulated with the tympanic membrane (dashed line). *Abbreviation:* CBCT cone beam computed tomography

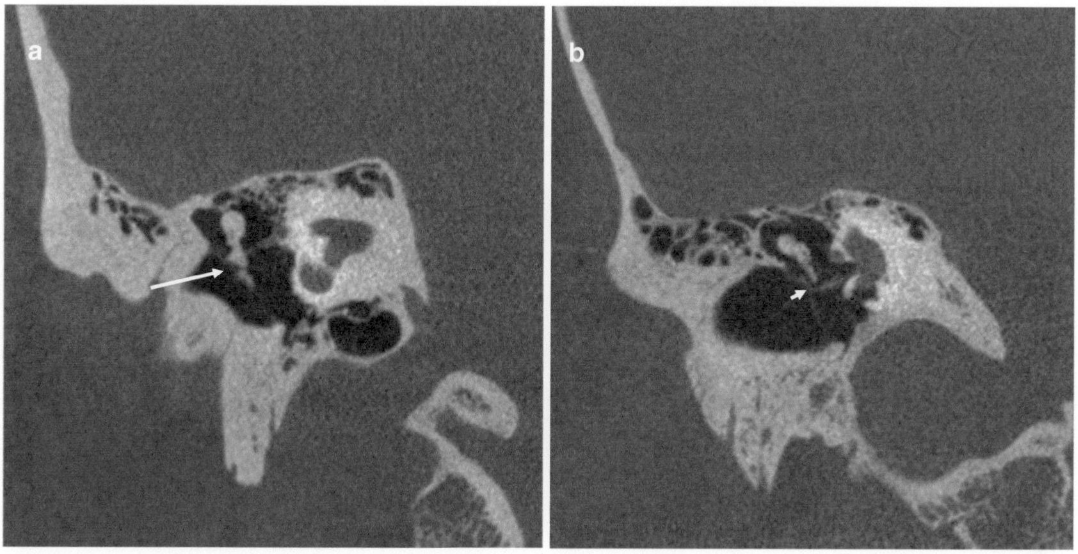

Fig. 5.11 Longitudinal fracture with ossicular injury. (**a, b**) Coronal oblique CBCT images show facture of the malleolar handle (long arrow) and of the long process of the incus with incudostapedial disjunction (short arrow). *Abbreviation:* CBCT cone beam computed tomography

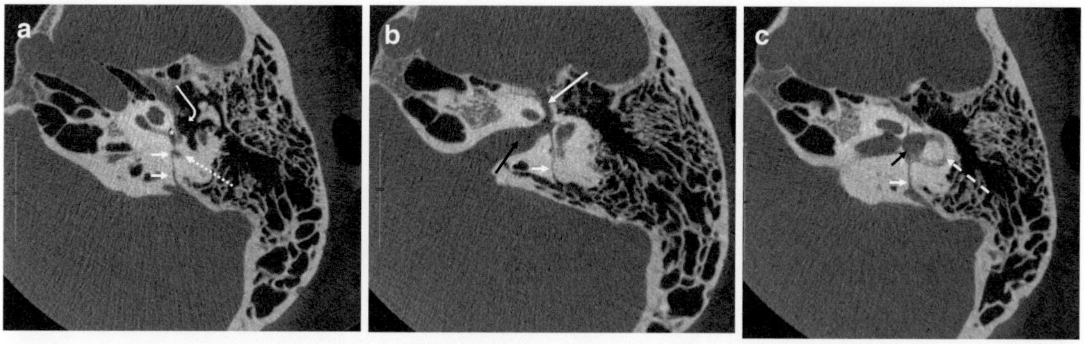

Fig. 5.12 Transverse fractures. (**a,b,c**) Axial CBCT images show a transvere fracture (white short arrows) of the temporal bone involving the basal turn of the cochlea (asterisk), the posterior semicircular canal (dotted line), the oval window (curved arrow), the IAC (long black arrow), the labyrinthine segment of the facial canal (long white arrow), the vestibule (short black arrow) with hyperdensity in the lateral semicircular canal suggesting intralabyrinthine hemorrhage (dashed arrow). *Abbreviations:* CBCT cone beam computed tomography, IAC internal auditory canal

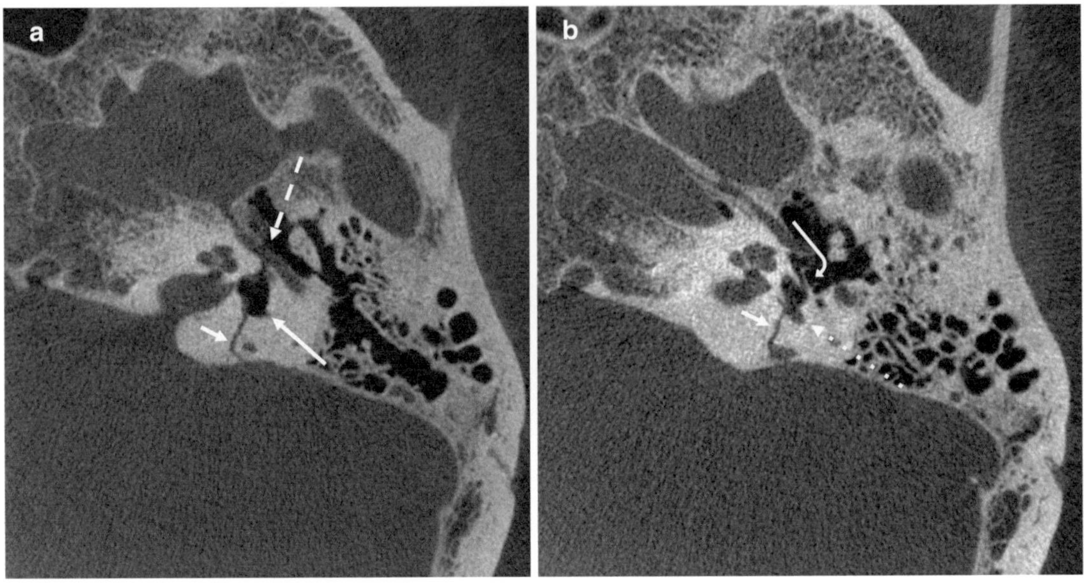

Fig. 5.13 **Transverse fracture with perilymphatic fistula.** (**a, b**) Axial reformatted CBCT images show the fracture line (short arrow) involving the vestibule (arrow) which is air filled suggesting pneumolabyrinth, the tympanic segment of the facial nerve (dashed arrow), the superior semicircular canal (dotted line) and the oval window (curved arrow) suggesting communication between the labyrinth and the tympanic space (i.e. perilymphatic fistula). *Abbreviation:* CBCT cone beam computed tomography

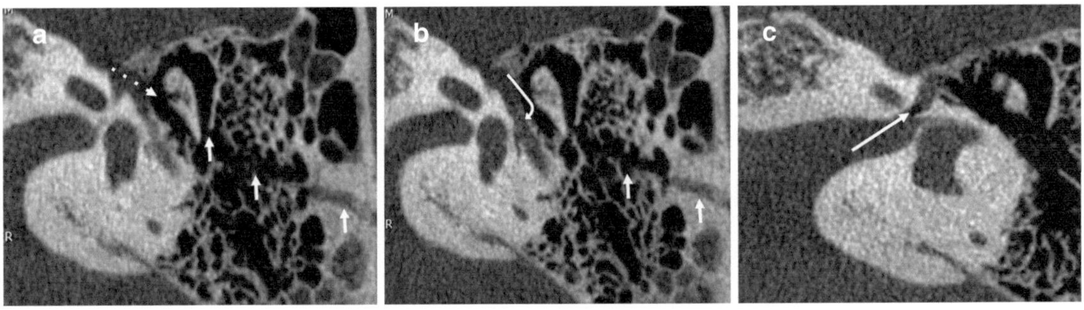

Fig. 5.14 **Longitudinal fracture with facial nerve involvement**. (**a, b**) Axial reformatted CBCT images show the fracture (short arrows) causing incus body fracture (dotted line) and involving the tympanic part of the facial nerve (curved line). (**c**) Axial reformatted CBCT passing through the IAC shows a small air bubble (arrow) in the labyrinthine segment of the facial nerve suggesting the traumatic involvement of facial nerve canal. *Abbreviation:* CBCT cone beam computed tomography

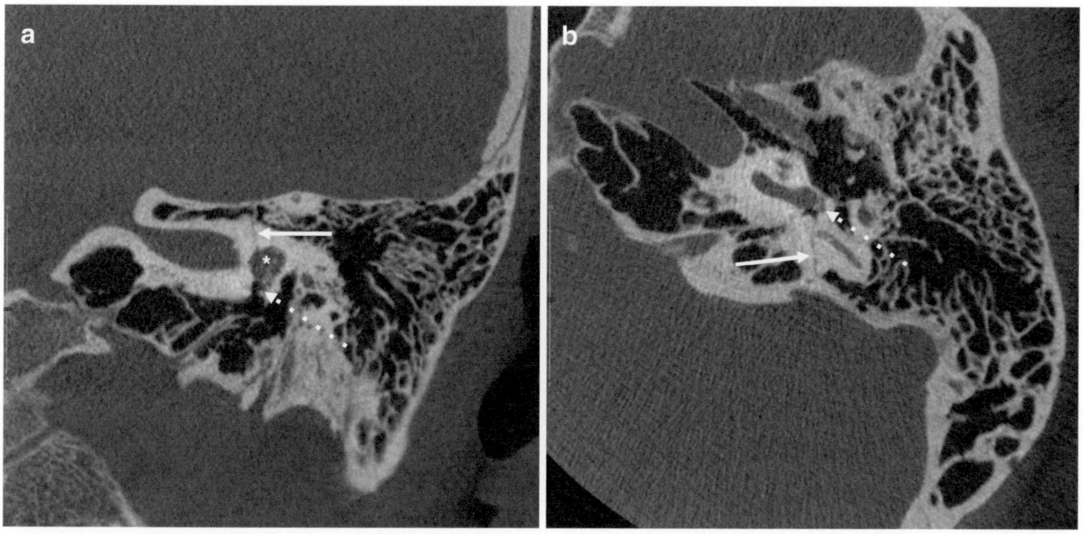

Fig. 5.15 **Transverse fracture with perilymphatic fistula.** (**a**) Axial and (**b**) coronal reformatted CBCT images show fracture line (arrow) involving the vestibule (asterisk) and the round window (dotted arrow) causing a communication between the cochlea and the tympanic space (i.e. perilymphatic fistula). *Abbreviations:* CBCT cone beam computed tomography, IAC internal auditory canal

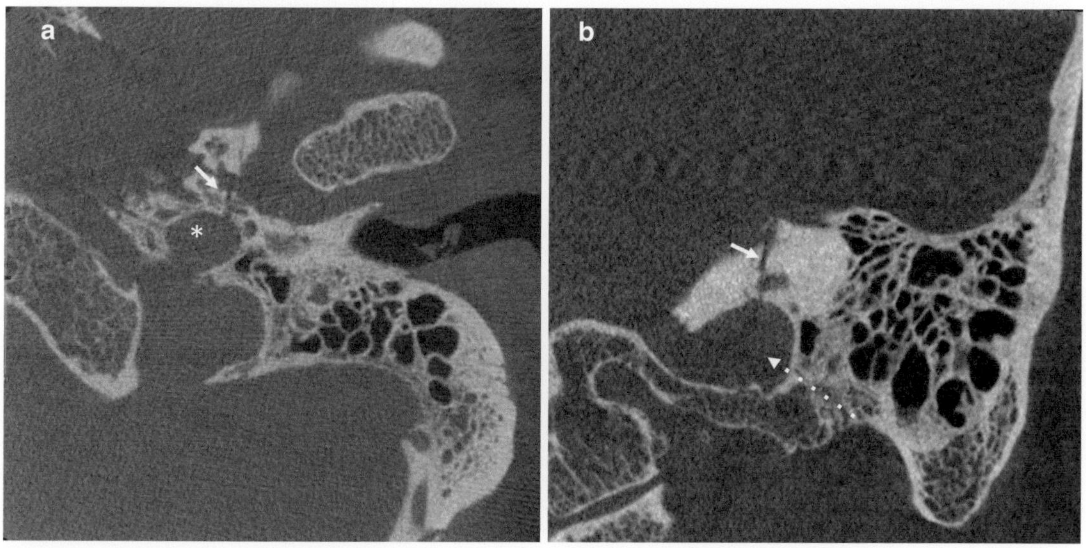

Fig. 5.16 **Transverse fracture with involvement of the vascular structures.** (**a**) Axial reformatted CBCT shows fracture line (short arrow) perpendicular to the temporal bone involving the petrous portion of carotid canal (asterisk). (**b**) Coronal oblique reformatted CBCT shows the fracture line (short arrow) that involves the jugular bulb (dotted line). *Abbreviation:* CBCT cone beam computed tomography

Report checklists are reported in tables:

Emergency setting

Anatomical structures	**What to check?**
Define temporal bone fracture	Orientation: longitudinal/ transverse
	Otic capsule involvement: Yes (pneumolabyrinth?)/ no
Rule out vascular injury	Carotid canal involvement
	Jugular foramen involvement
Rule out facial canal involvement	Bone fragment in facial nerve canal
Rule out associated intracranial injuries	Intracranial bleeding/ hematoma

Sub-acute setting

Clinical findings	**What to check?**
If conductive hear loss	Ossicular chain injury
	Perilymphatic fistula
If sensoneural hear loss	Intralabyrinthine hemorrhage
	Labyrinthitis ossificans sign
	Perilymphatic fistula
If facial nerve paralysis	Facial nerve swelling
If othorrea/ rinoliquorrea	CSF leak
	Meningeal enhancement
	Rule out meningo–/ cephalocele
If vertigo	Perilymphatic fistula/ hydrops
	CUI and cranial nerves

References

1. Kurihara YY, Fujikawa A, Tachizawa N, Takaya M, Ikeda H, Starkey J. Temporal bone trauma: typical CT and MRI appearances and important points for evaluation. Radiographics. 2020;40(4):1148–62. https://doi.org/10.1148/rg.2020190023.
2. Swartz JD, Kang MD. Trauma to the temporal bone. In: Swartz MJD, Loevner MA, editors. Imaging of the temporal bone. 4th ed. Thieme; 2009.
3. Patel A, Groppo E. Management of temporal bone trauma. Craniomaxillofacial trauma and reconstruction. 2010;3(2):105–13. https://doi.org/10.1055/s-0030-1254383.
4. Patel A, Lofgren DH, Varacallo M. Temporal fracture continuing education activity. NCBI Bookshelf; n.d. Retrieved from https://www.ncbi.nlm.nih.gov/books/NBK535391/
5. Dreizin D, et al. CT of skull base fractures: classification systems, complications, and management. Radiographics. 2021;41(3):762–82. https://doi.org/10.1148/rg.2021200189.
6. Dubrulle F, Chaton V, Risoud M, et al. The round window sign: a sensitive sign to detect perilymphatic fistulae on delayed postcontrast 3D-FLAIR sequence. European Radiology. 2020;30(11):6303–10. https://doi.org/10.1007/s00330-020-06924-4.
7. Wood CP, Hunt CH, Bergen DC, Carlson ML, Diehn FE, Schwartz KM, McKenzie GA, Morreale RF, Lane JI. Tympanic plate fractures in temporal bone trauma: prevalence and associated injuries. American Journal of Neuroradiology. 2014;35(1):186–90. https://doi.org/10.3174/ajnr.A3609.
8. Tsuno NSG, Tsuno MY, Coelho Neto CAF, Noujaim SE, Decnop M, Pacheco FT, Souza SA, Fonseca APA, Garcia MRT. Imaging the external ear: practical approach to normal and pathologic conditions. RadioGraphics. 2022;42(2):522–40.

6 Acquired Pathology of the External Ear

Silvia Casale, Eleonora Piccin, Antonia Valentina Genovese, Elena Caloro, Elisa Massullo, Elisa Scola, Giorgio Conte, Lorenzo Maria Gaini, Diego Zanetti, and Fabio Triulzi

6.1 Introduction

The external auditory canal (EAC) consists of an outer cartilaginous part and an inner osseous segment, formed by the tympanic portion of the temporal bone. The tympanosquamous and the tympanomastoid fissures lie, respectively, anteriorly and posteriorly to the EAC running parallel to it. They separate the tympanic part from the squamous and the mastoid portion of the temporal bone. The EAC is divided into the lateral one-third fibrocartilaginous portion and the medial two-third bony portion, which terminates with the tympanic annulus, a bone ridge anchoring the tympanic membrane. The isthmus, representing the narrowest part of the EAC, separates these two segments. The skin lining the bony EAC is continuous with the outer layer of the tympanic membrane.

A variety of acquired conditions may affect the external ear (EE) and EAC including traumatic injuries, inflammatory and infectious conditions, benign or malignant neoplasms, and vascular anomalies. The diagnosis is often clinical. Nevertheless, the same clinical features may derive from different pathologic conditions. Thus, imaging may be required for the differential diagnosis and for the detection of potential complications. Preoperative imaging is crucial to delineate lesion extent, guide surgi-

S. Casale (✉) · E. Piccin · A. V. Genovese
E. Massullo · E. Scola
Neuroradiology Unit, Fondazione IRCCS Ca' Granda Ospedale Maggiore Policlinico, Milan, Italy
e-mail: silvia.casale@policlinico.mi.it; eleonora.piccin@policlinico.mi.it; valentina.genovese@policlinico.mi.it; elisa.massullo@policlinico.mi.it; elisa.scola@policlinico.mi.it

E. Caloro
Postgraduation School in Radiodiagnostics, Università Degli Studi di Milano, Milan, Italy

G. Conte · F. Triulzi
Neuroradiology Unit, Fondazione IRCCS Ca' Granda Ospedale Maggiore Policlinico, Milan, Italy

Department of Pathophysiology and Transplantation, University of Milan, Milan, Italy
e-mail: giorgio.conte@policlinico.mi.it; fabio.triulzi@policlinico.mi.it

L. M. Gaini
Department of Otolaryngology and Head and Neck Surgery, Fondazione IRCCS Ca' Granda Ospedale Maggiore Policlinico Milan, Milan, Italy

Department of Clinical Sciences and Community Health, Università Degli Studi di Milano, Milan, Italy
e-mail: lorenzo.gaini@policlinico.mi.ti

D. Zanetti
Department of Clinical Sciences and Community Health, Università Degli Studi di Milano, Milan, Italy

Audiology Unit, Fondazione IRCCS Ca' Granda Ospedale Maggiore Policlinico Milan, Milan, Italy
e-mail: diego.zanetti@policlinico.mi.it

G. Conte et al. (eds.), *Atlas of Normal and Pathological Findings in Otoneuroradiology*,
https://doi.org/10.1007/978-3-032-08232-9_6

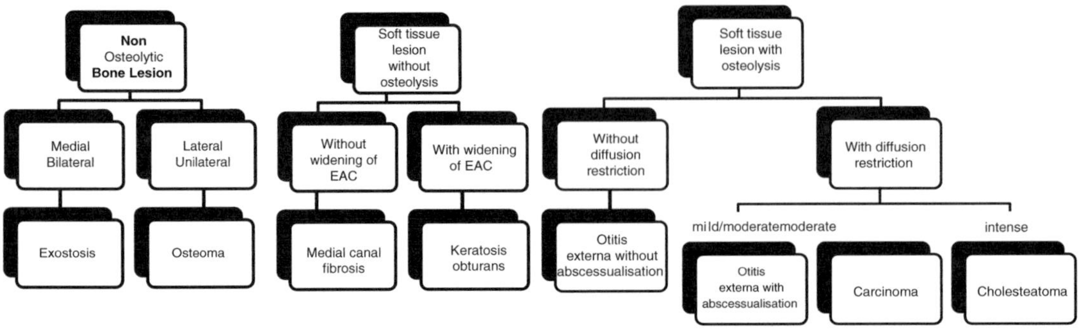

Fig. 6.1 Flow chart for the differential diagnosis of EAC lesions. *Abbreviation*: EAC external auditory canal

Table 6.1 The most common pathologies involving the EE

Inflammatory and infectious diseases	Otitis externa Necrotizing otitis externa Polypoid granulomatosis of TM EAC cholesteatoma Keratosis obturans
Osseous lesions	Exostosis and osteoma Osteopetrosis Fibrous dysplasia
Benign neoplasms	Aural polyps Benign cutaneous neoplasms
Malignant neoplasms	Metastasis Squamous cell carcinoma Melanoma Adenoid cystic carcinoma Mucoepidermoid carcinoma Lymphoma
Miscellaneous conditions	Fractures Foreign body Cephalocele

cal planning, and assess the feasibility of resection. For the differential diagnosis, the flowchart shown in Fig. 6.1 can be helpful. In the evaluation of EAC pathology, the first step is to define whether the lesion primarily involves bony or soft tissue structures. Then the presence of osteolysis, as assessed by computed tomography (CT), is a main feature that can narrow the differential diagnosis. Magnetic resonance imaging (MRI) is particularly effective in differential diagnosis between malignant and benign conditions. Malignancies usually present low to moderate signal intensity on T2-weighted images and pronounced enhancement on post-contrast T1-weghted images, whereas cholesteatomas typically appear with higher signal on T2-weighted images, with intense restriction on diffusion-weighted imaging (DWI), without post-contrast enhancement [3].

The most common pathologies involving EE are listed in Table 6.1, we also provide a flowchart for the differential diagnosis in Fig. 6.1.

6.2 Inflammatory and Infectious Diseases

6.2.1 Otitis Externa

Otitis externa refers to inflammation of the EAC, with possible involvement of the auricle and the tympanic membrane. It is a common disease, especially in swimmers, usually with an infective etiology, mostly caused by *Pseudomonas aeruginosa*, *Staphylococcus epidermidis*, and *Staphylococcus aureus* [1]. Radiological exams are usually not required, except for immunocompromised patients, lack of treatment response, and in suspicion of adjacent tissue involvement, as seen in complications such as necrotizing otitis externa.

When imaging is performed, CT scans may reveal thickening of cutaneous lining of EAC and tympanic membrane. Calcifications are rare findings in otomycosis, as a probable reaction against topical antifungal drugs [2] (Fig. 6.2).

The presence of intraluminal soft tissue within the bony portion of the EAC may suggest a diagnosis of medial canal fibrosis induced by ongoing inflammation [3].

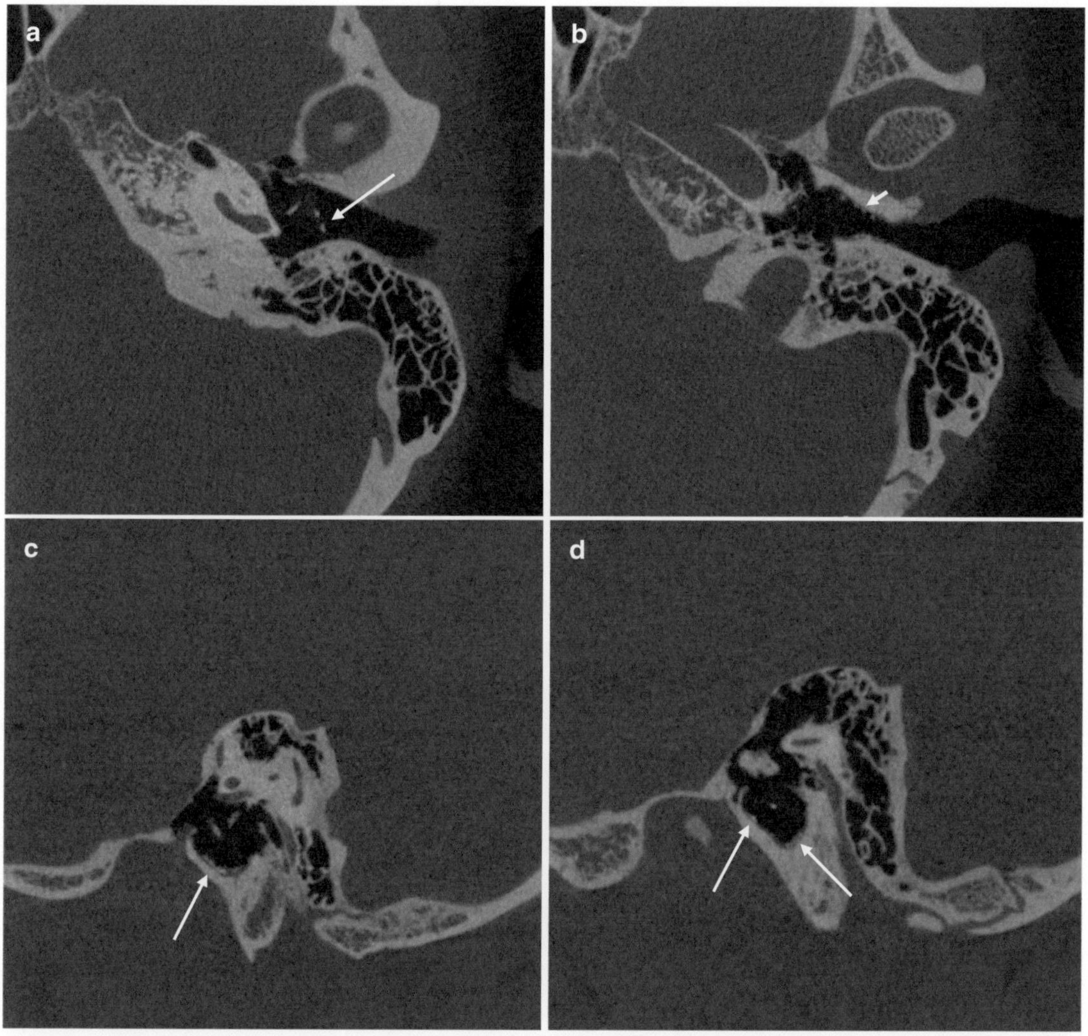

Fig. 6.2 **Fungal external otitis.** External otitis is most often infectious in origin, typically diagnosed through clinical and otoscopic evaluation. Imaging, such as CBCT, is reserved for immunocompromised patients, those unresponsive to therapy, or when extension beyond the EAC is suspected. In cases of otomycosis, calcifications are an uncommon finding, hypothesized to result from reactive changes secondary to antifungal treatment. (**a, b**) Axial CBCT images show microcalcifications within a mildly thickened tympanic membrane (arrow) and the skin (short arrow) in the medial EAC. (**c, d**) Sagittal CBCT reconstructions confirm skin thickening and the presence of microcalcifications along the EAC (arrows). *Abbreviations:* CBCT cone beam computed tomography, EAC external auditory canal

The erosion of the osseous segment of the EAC can be associated with chronic erosive otitis [4] or necrotizing otitis externa (NOE), depending on the presence of infection spreading to the surrounding tissues.

6.2.2 Necrotizing Otitis Externa

NOE also known as malignant otitis externa is a serious complication that can arise from external ear infection, mostly in elderly individuals with diabetes or weakened immune systems. If untreated, NOE is associated with a high mortality, and this is due to its tendency to spread to the temporal bone and the nearby structures. In this clinical subset, MRI can be useful, in addition to CT examination, to exclude possible routes of intracranial propagation of the infection [5] (Figs. 6.3, 6.4, and 6.5).

6.2.3 Otitis Caused by Mycobacterial Infection

Tuberculous otitis externa has been characterized by a punched-out ulcerative lesion on the tragus, accompanied by edema and inflammation of the EAC or by a purulent, non-mucoid otorrhea that may be associated with facial nerve palsy. Tuberculous involvement of the mastoid, petrous apex, and middle ear also occurs. Radiologically, tuberculosis manifests as an aggressive, osteolytic lesion with bone destruction (Fig. 6.6).

6.2.4 Polypoid Granulomatosis of Tympanic Membrane

Polypoid granulomatous tissue results from chronic inflammation that typically arises from the middle ear, extending into the EAC through a defect in the tympanic membrane. Clinical otoscopy is usually enough to make a diagnosis, and imaging can be used in such cases to study the precise extension. CT reveals soft tissue thickening or a polypoid mass within the external auditory canal. Bony involvement is not usually present, unless chronic inflammation has led to erosion. CT scans demonstrate the presence of a

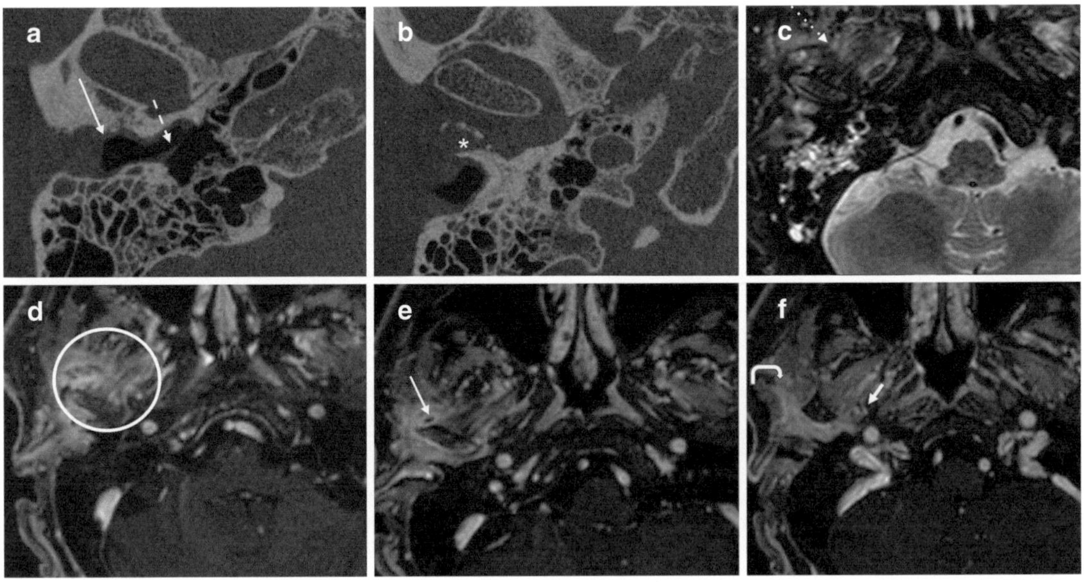

Fig. 6.3 Right-sided necrotizing otitis externa. NOE is a life-threatening complication of EE infection; it predominantly affects elderly patients with diabetes or immunosuppression. If untreated, it can progress to skull base osteomyelitis and adjacent deep neck space involvement, with significant morbidity and mortality. (**a, b**) CBCT images reveal inflammatory thickening of the EAC skin (arrow) and tympanic membrane (dashed arrow), with associated bony erosion of the anterior EAC wall (asterisk in fig. **b**). (**c**) Axial TSE T2W with fat suppression demonstrates abnormal signal intensity of the soft tissues surrounding the EAC, extending into the masticator space (dotted arrow); fluid is present within the mastoid air cells. (**d, e**) Axial contrast enhanced 3D FFE T1w with fat suppression images show involvement of the temporomandibular joint and lateral pterygoid muscle, along with a small adjacent abscess near the mandibular condyle (arrow). (**f**) Axial contrast enhanced 3D FFE T1w with fat suppression image depicts extension into the parapharyngeal space (short arrow) and parotid space (curved arrow). *Abbreviations:* CBCT cone-beam computed tomography, EAC external auditory canal, FFE fast field echo, NOE necrotizing otitis externa, TSE turbo spin echo

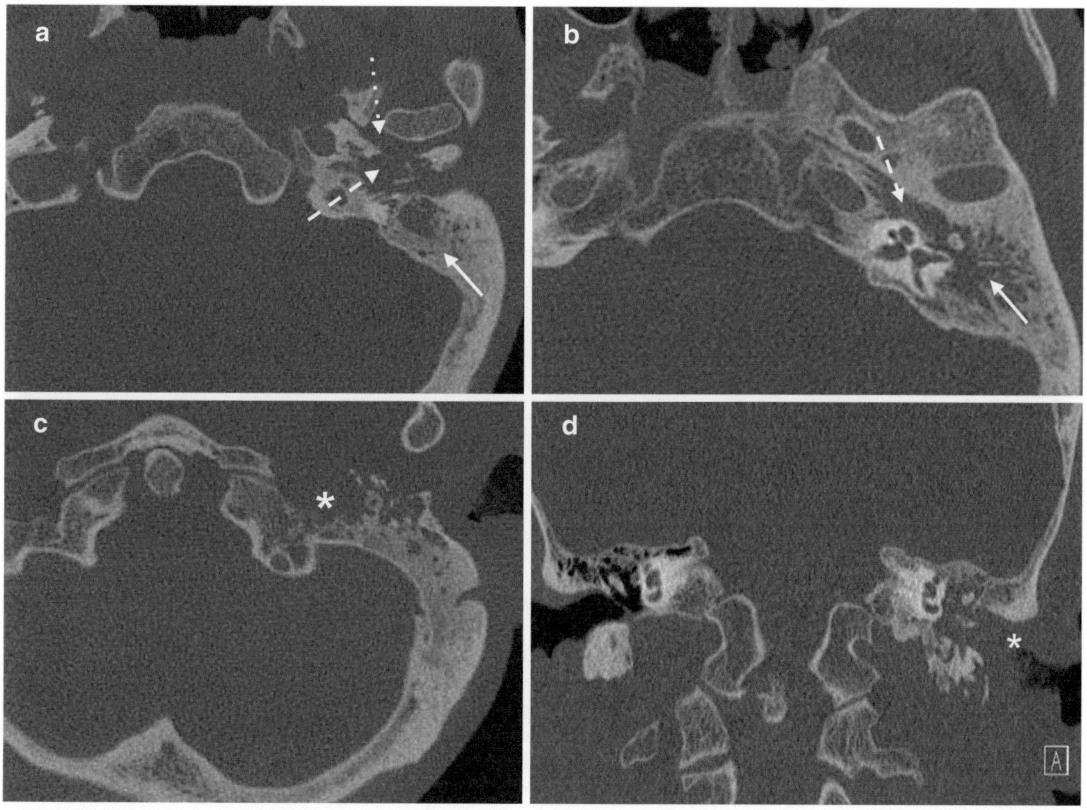

Fig. 6.4 **Left-sided necrotizing otitis externa with sull-base involvement.** (**a, b**) Axial MDCT images show complete opacification of the left mastoid air cells (arrows) and middle ear cavity (dashed arrows), with osseous erosion of the petrous portion of the temporal bone. The erosion involves the anterior margin and extends into the glenoid cavity of the temporomandibular joint (dotted arrow). (**c**) Axial MDCT image reveals bone erosion at the infero-anterior margin of the petrous temporal bone, adjacent to the jugular bulb (asterisk). (**d**) Coronal MDCT image demonstrates opacification of the EAC (asterisk) and erosion partially involving the ossicular chain. *Abbreviations*: EAC external auditory canal, MDCT multi-detector computed tomography

tissue density lesion with well-defined margins adherent to the tympanic membrane [6] (Fig. 6.7). On MRI, the lesion shows low-intermediate signal on T1w images, high signal on T2w, moderate to marked enhancement on post-contrast T1w images, and absence of diffusion restriction. Additionally the tympanic membrane can be affected by myringosclerosis which is characterized by calcification and fibrosis of the tympanic membrane (Fig. 6.8).

6.2.5 Keratosis Obturans

Keratosis obturans is an accumulation of keratin debris within the EAC due to hyperstimulation of ceruminous glands. There is not any enclosing sac of stratified squamous epithelium, and it is a separate entity than cholesteatoma. It is usually bilateral and occurs in younger patients than EAC cholesteatoma. It causes otalgia and conductive hearing loss due to inflammation, EAC expansion, and remodeling but no bony erosion. On MRI keratosis obturans shows overlapping features with cholesteatoma with DWI restriction [7].

6.2.6 EAC Cholesteatoma

A cholesteatoma is characterized by a sac of keratinizing stratified squamous epithelium filled

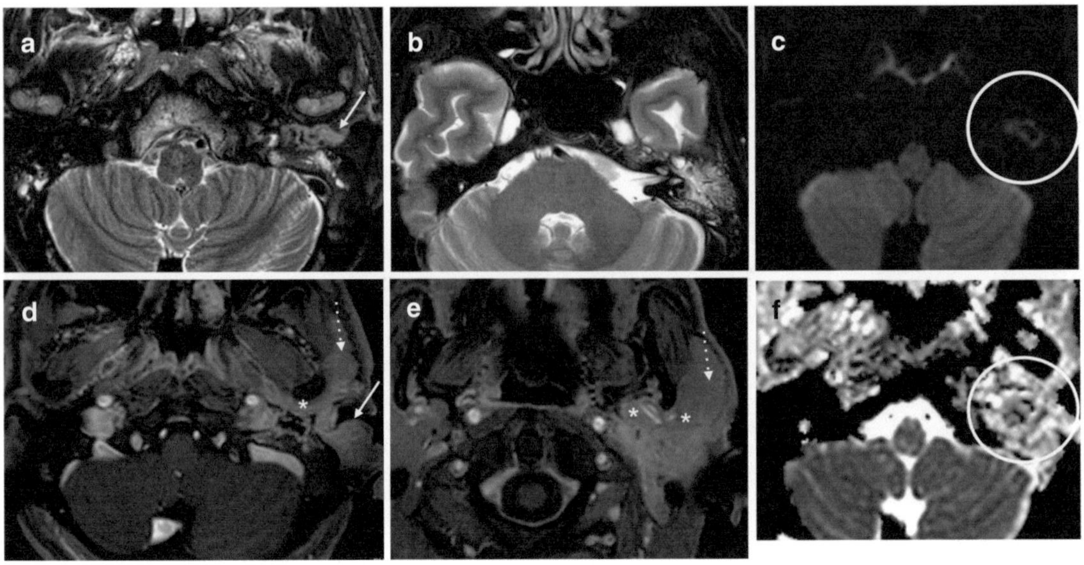

Fig. 6.5 Left-sided necrotizing otitis externa with skull-base involvement (continued from Fig. 6.4). (**a, b**) Axial TSE T2W with fat suppression images show complete obliteration of the mastoid air cells, consistent with ongoing otomastoiditis (arrow in fig. **a**). (**c**) Axial DWI and (**f**) ADC map reveal mild diffusion restriction within the middle ear cavity (white circles), suggesting inflammatory or early abscess-related changes. (**d, e**) Axial contrast enhanced 3D FFE T1w with fat suppression images demonstrate extensive involvement of the left otomastoid region, with altered signal intensity and enhancement of the obliterated EAC (arrow), extending into the adjacent periauricular soft tissues, parotid space (dotted arrow), and masticator space (asterisks), notably surrounding the ascending ramus of the left mandible. *Abbreviations:* ADC apprent diffusion coefficient, DWI diffusion-weighted imaging, EAC external auditory canal, FFE fast field echo, TSE turbo spin echo

with defoliating keratin debris. Cholesteatomas are usually acquired and rarely congenital. In rare cases cholesteatomas occur in the EAC and are more often idiopathic. Secondary EAC cholesteatomas can be due to radiation therapy, surgery, trauma to the canal, or EAC stenosis or obstruction. It often causes periostitis and erosion of the bony portion of the EAC leading to otorrhea and chronic pain. EAC cholesteatomas are usually unilateral and occur in older patients than keratosis obturans. On MRI cholesteatoma shows overlapping features with keratosis obturans with DWI restriction (Fig. 6.9). Similarly to EAC of the middle ear, it is important to report the extension into the middle ear, mastoid, facial nerve canal, or tegmen tympani [8, 9].

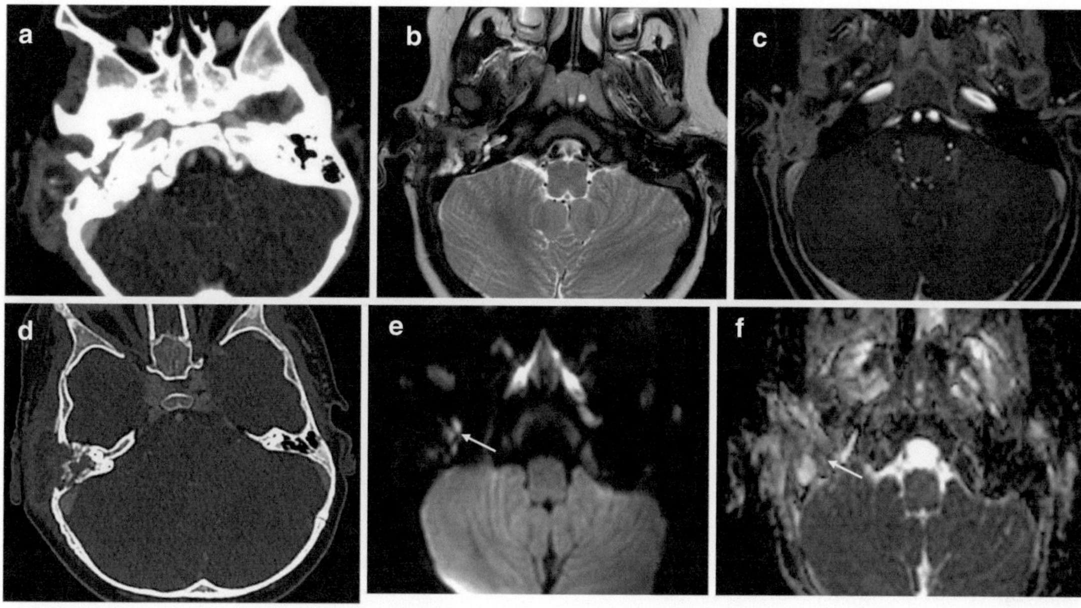

Fig. 6.6 Right-sided otomastoiditis associated with *Mycobacterium avium* infection. (**a**, **d**) Axial post-contrast MDCT images demonstrate extensive necrotic collection within the right perauricular soft tissues, with associated erosion of the mastoid, involvement of the EAC, and extension into the tympanic cavity. (**b**) Axial TSE T2w and (**c**) contrast-enhanced 3D FFE T1w with fat suppression MR images obtained following antibiotic therapy reveal significant reduction in inflammatory changes and enhancement within the otomastoid region, indicating treatment response. (**e**, **f**) Axial DWI and ADC map show persistent mild diffusion restriction in the right mastoid, suggestive of residual inflammatory activity (arrows). *Abbreviations:* ADC apparent diffusion coefficient, DWI diffusion weighted imaging, EAC external auditory canal, FFE fast field echo, MDCT multi-detector computed tomography, TSE turbo spin echo

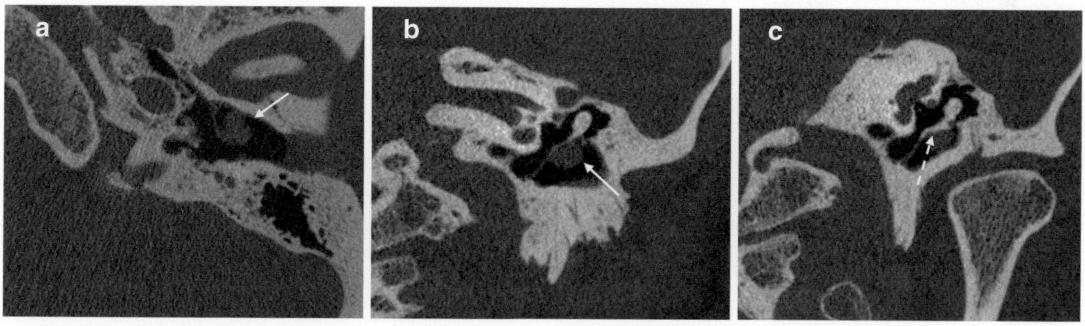

Fig. 6.7 Polypoid granulomatous lesion of the tympanic membrane. These lesions result from chronic inflammatory processes and usually do not cause bone erosion; biopsy is essential to exclude neoplastic conditions such as squamous or basal cell carcinoma. (**a**, **b**) Axial and coronal CBCT images show a well-circumscribed, soft tissue–density, polypoid lesion (arrows) adherent to the tympanic membrane. (**c**) Malleus-oriented coronal CBCT demonstrates fine erosion of the handle of the malleus adjacent to the lesion (dashed arrow), with no evidence of ossicular erosion. *Abbreviation:* CBCT cone-beam computed tomography

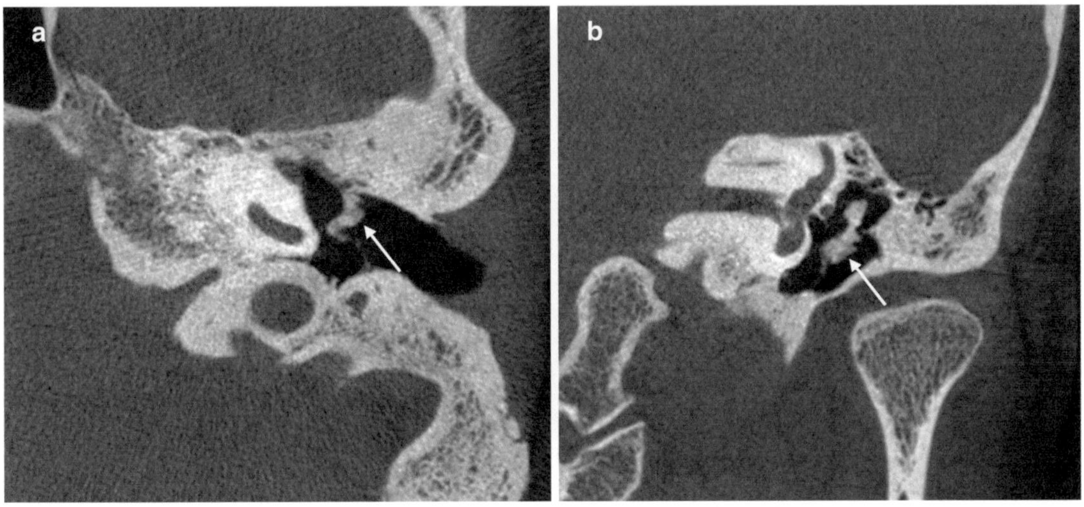

Fig. 6.8 **Myringosclerosis.** Myringosclerosis is characterized by calcification and fibrosis of the tympanic membrane. It is distinct from tympanosclerosis, in which calcium deposits involve not only the tympanic membrane but also the middle ear structures. This condition can impair the function of the eardrum, potentially leading to conductive hearing loss. (**a**, **b**) Axial and coronal CBCT images demonstrate areas of increased bone density along the tympanic membrane, with calcifications adherent to the malleus (arrows). *Abbreviation:* CBCT cone-beam computed tomography

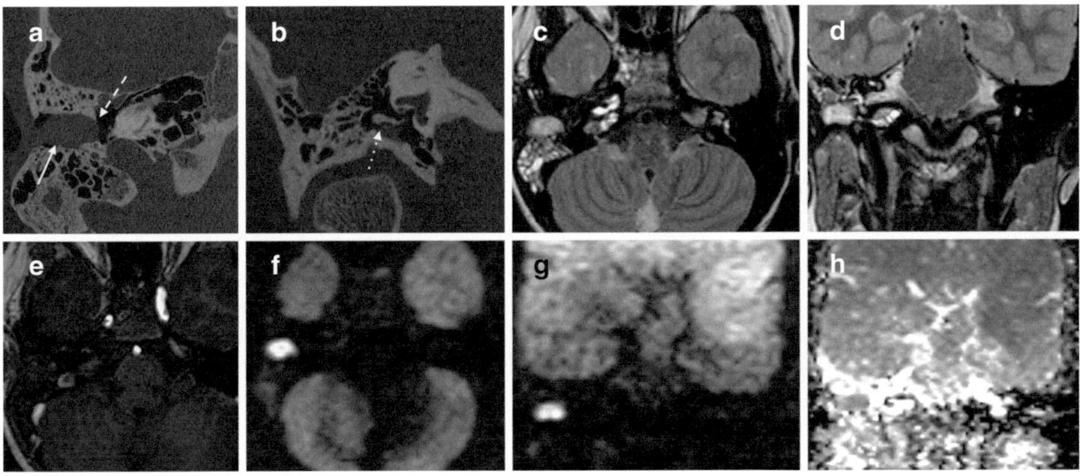

Fig. 6.9 **Cholesteatoma of the right external auditory canal.** Cholesteatoma most commonly arises in the middle ear but can rarely involve the EAC, a presentation more frequently observed in elderly individuals. Due to its low incidence and indolent progression, diagnosis is often delayed, potentially resulting in bone erosion and compression of adjacent structures. (**a**, **b**) Axial and incus-oriented coronal CBCT images demonstrate a cholesteatoma of the EAC (arrow) associated with partial atresia of the canal. The lesion causes complete canal occlusion and scalloping of the bony floor. It also exerts pressure on the tympanic membrane (dashed arrow) and protrudes into the tympanic cavity, indenting the incus (dotted arrow). (**c**, **d**) On axial and coronal TSE T2w MR images, the lesion shows high signal. (**e**) On axial 3D FFE T1w image the lesion shows low signal. (**f**, **g**) non-echo-planar DWI and (**h**) ADC map show the characteristic diffusion restriction due to the presence of desquamated keratinizing squamous epithelium. *Abbreviations:* ADC apparent diffusion coefficient, CBCT cone-beam computed tomography, DWI diffusion weighted imaging, FFE fast field echo, TSE turbo spin echo

6.3 Osseous Lesions

6.3.1 Exostosis and Osteoma

Exostoses of the EAC are reactive bone thickening of the walls of EAC, thought to result from prolonged and repeated exposure to cold water and wind—hence the term “surfer’s ear” (Figs. 6.10 and 6.11). Unlike exostoses, osteomas are true benign slow-growing neoplasms, solitary, typically unilateral, and pedunculated, commonly arising from the tympanosquamous or tympanomastoid suture lines, laterally to the isthmus [10] (Fig. 6.12).

6.3.2 Osteopetrosis

Osteopetrosis, also known as Albers-Schönberg disease or marble bone disease, is a rare hereditary bone disorder characterized by defective osteoclast-mediated bone resorption, leading to abnormally dense and brittle bones that can affect also the EAC.

High-resolution CT is the preferred imaging modality and typically shows diffuse bony sclerosis and narrowing of the EAC, which may result in stenosis or complete obliteration of the canal [11] (Figs. 6.13 and 6.14).

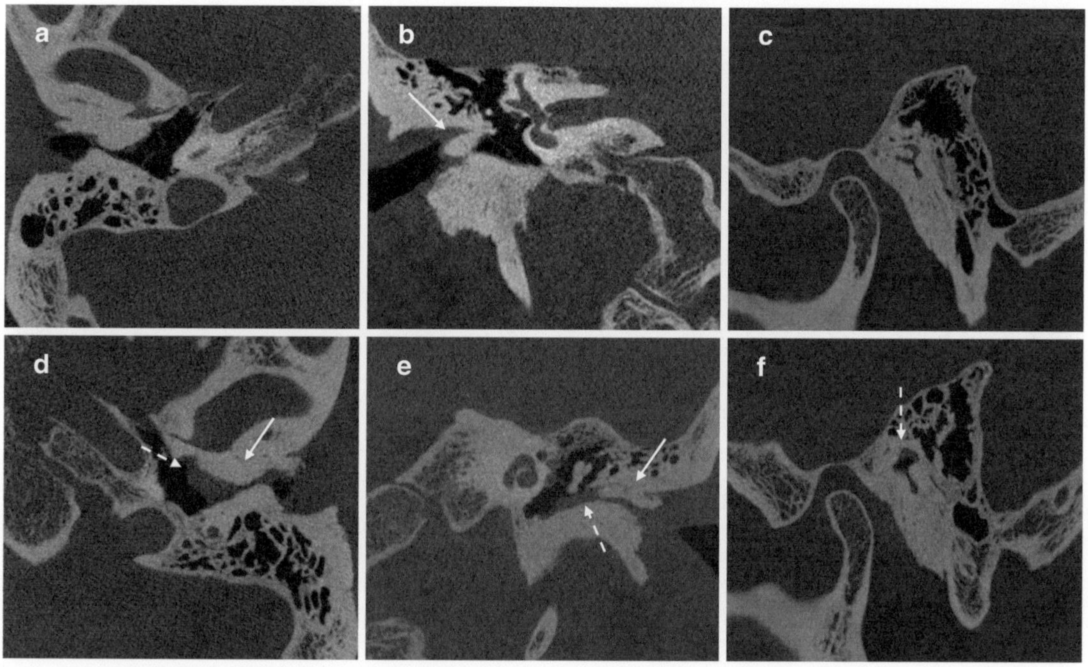

Fig. 6.10 Exostoses of the external auditory canal. EAC exostoses are typically bilateral, multiple, reactive bony overgrowths. They are distinct from osteomas, which are true benign neoplasms that tend to be unilateral, solitary, and pedunculated. (**a–c**) Axial, coronal, and sagittal CBCT images of the right ear demonstrate pseudonodular thickening of the bony walls of the EAC (arrow), with mild overlying skin thickening at the same level. (**d–f**) Axial, coronal, and sagittal CBCT images of the left ear show similar pseudonodular bony thickening (arrows), with soft tissue–density material partially obliterating the EAC (dashed arrow). *Abbreviations:* CBCT cone-beam computed tomography, EAC external auditory canal

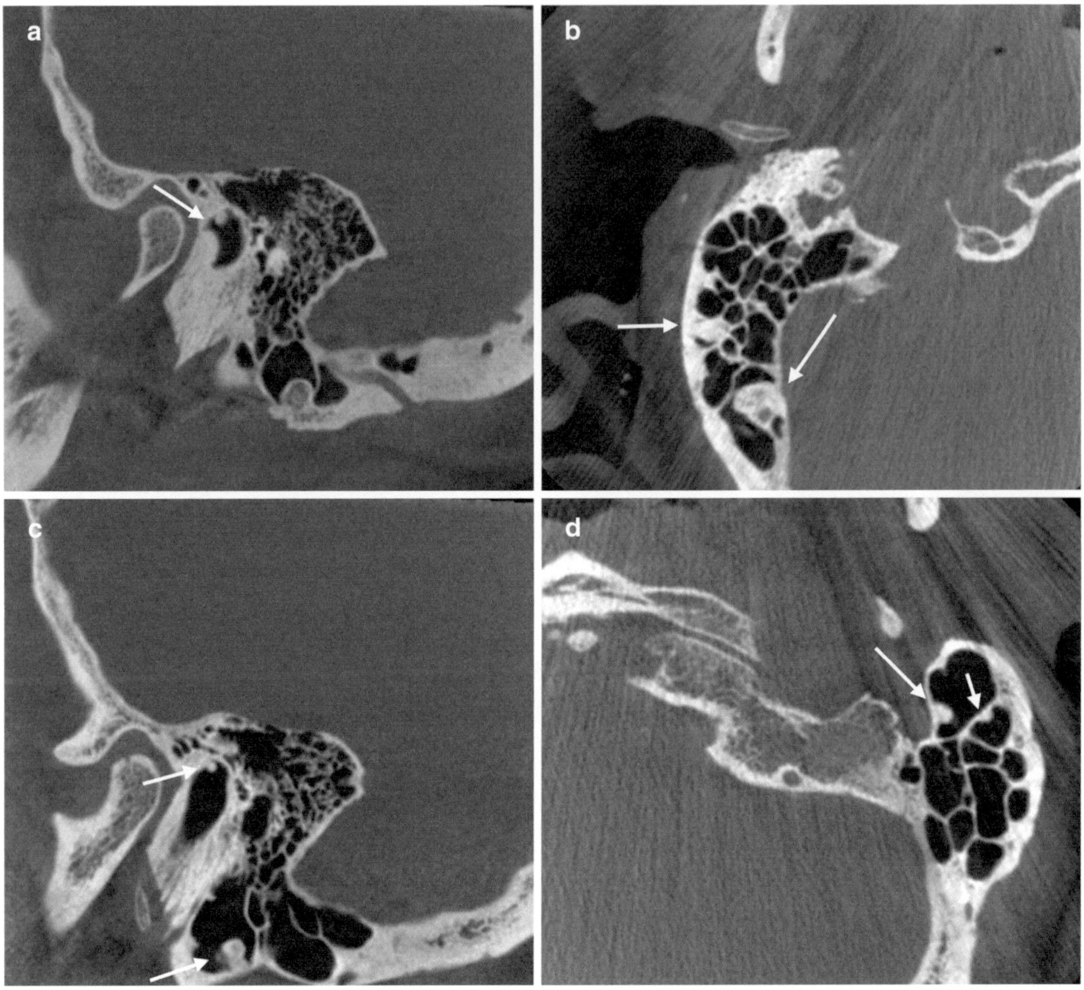

Fig. 6.11 **Exostoses of the external auditory canal** (continued from Fig. 6.10). (**a**, **b**) Sagittal and axial CBCT images of the right ear demonstrate pseudonodular thickening of the bony walls of the EAC and within the mastoid air cells (arrows). (**c**, **d**) Sagittal and axial CBCT images of the left ear similarly show pseudonodular bony thickening of the EAC and mastoid air cells (arrows). *Abbreviation:* CBCT cone-beam computed tomography, EAC external auditory canal

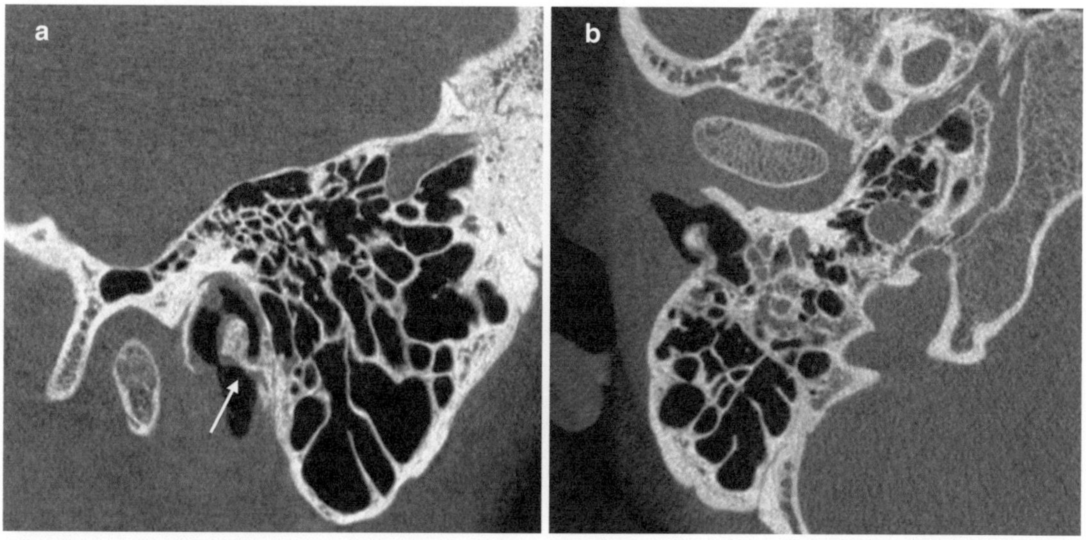

Fig. 6.12 **Osteoma of the external auditory canal.** Osteomas of the EAC are rare, typically solitary and unilateral, pedunculated bony lesions. They commonly originate at the bony-cartilaginous junction, particularly from the tympanosquamous or tympanomastoid suture lines. These lesions are distinct from exostoses, which present as bilateral, multiple, reactive bony overgrowths. (**a**) Sagittal CBCT image demonstrates a pedunculated bony lesion arising from the tympanomastoid suture (arrow). (**b**) Axial CBCT image confirms narrowing of the EAC. *Abbreviations:* CBCT cone-beam computed tomography, EAC external auditory canal

6.3.3 Fibrous Dysplasia

Fibrous dysplasia is a benign skeletal disorder where normal bone is replaced by fibro-osseous tissue, leading to structural weakness and deformity. Involvement of the temporal bone occurs in less than 10% of patients. When the disease involves the temporal bone, the EAC is the area most commonly affected, causing canal narrowing or stenosis. Non-contrast high-resolution MDCT is the study of choice, showing three possible patterns: pagetoid, sclerotic, and cystic. The most common, the pagetoid type, presents a "ground-glass" appearance, reflecting the mixture of fibrous and osseous components [12] (Figs. 6.15 and 6.16). Genetic disorders such as McCune Albright syndrome (MAS) are associated with polyostotic fibrous dysplasia.

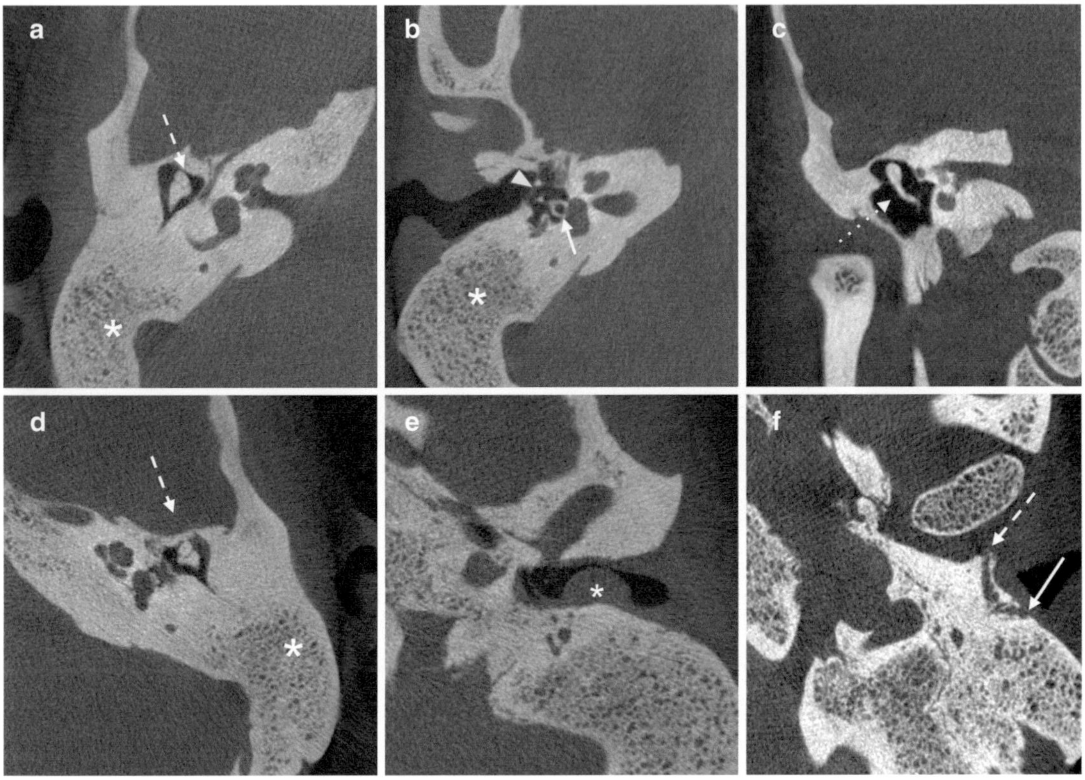

Fig. 6.13 Osteopetrosis with ring-like appearance of the stapes and fibroepithelial polyp of the external auditory canal. Osteopetrosis is a group of genetically determined skeletal disorders characterized by excessive deposition of immature bone due to osteoclast dysfunction. Involvement of the temporal bone can result in conductive and sensorineural hearing loss, ossicular chain fixation, chronic otitis media, facial nerve palsy, and vertigo. (**a**, **b**) Axial CBCT images of the right ear show absence of mastoid pneumatization (asterisk) and a hypoplastic tympanic cavity consistent with osteopetrosis. The stapes appears with a characteristic ring-like morphology (arrow), and the head of the malleus is in contact with the anterior wall of the epitympanic recess (dashed arrows). Mild thickening of the tympanic membrane is also noted (arrowhead). (**c**) Coronal CBCT image oriented to the malleus demonstrates absence of the lateral process, with preservation of the remaining ossicular structures (dotted arrow). (**d**) Axial CBCT of the left ear shows similar absence of mastoid pneumatization (asterisk) and hypoplastic tympanic cavity, with the head of the malleus abutting the anterior wall of the epitympanic recess (dashed arrows). (**e**, **f**) Axial CBCT images of the left ear demonstrate obstruction of the EAC in its middle third, with circumferential wall thickening caused by a fibroepithelial polyp (asterisk). The lesion induces erosion of the posterior-inferior bony canal wall (arrow), with an apparent communication with the adjacent glenoid cavity (dashed arrow). *Abbreviations:* CBCT cone-beam computed tomography, EAC external auditory canal

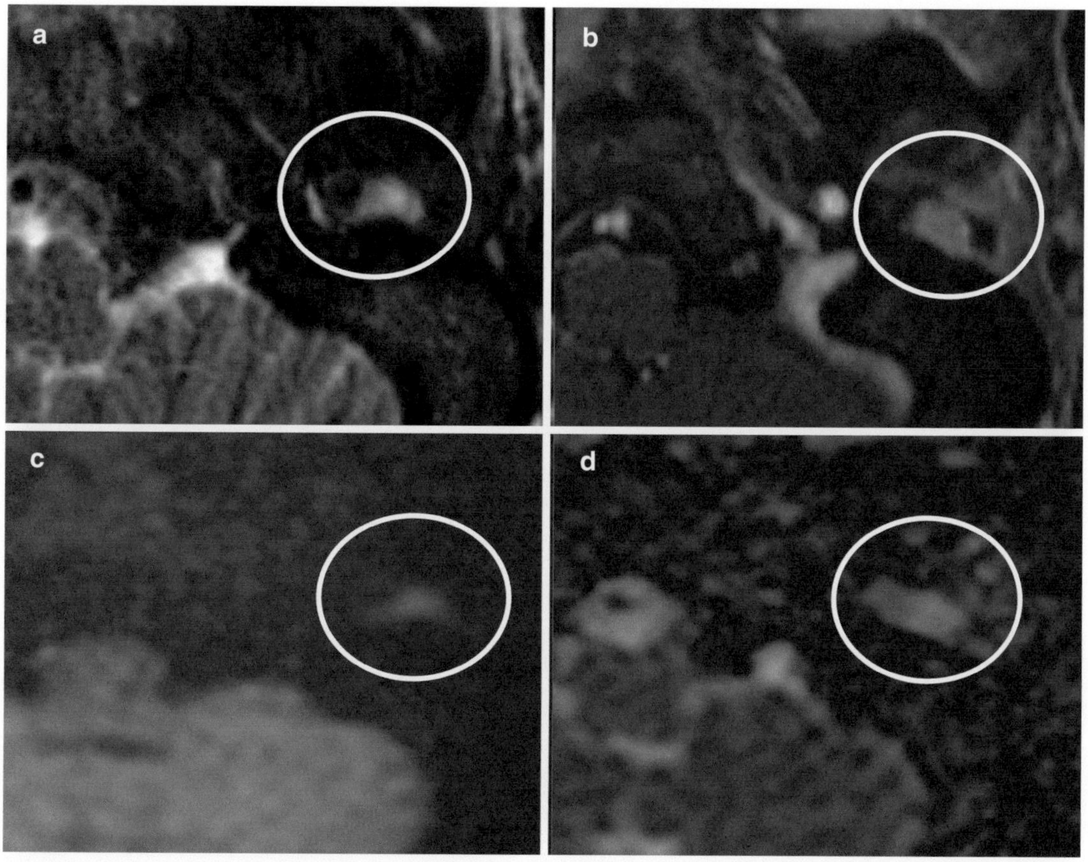

Fig. 6.14 Osteopetrosis with ring-like appearance of the stapes and fibroepithelial polyp of the external auditory canal (continued from Fig. 6.13). (**a**) On axial TSE T2w the lesion show high signal. (**b**) On contrast-enhanced 3D FFE T1w with fat suppression MR image the lesion shows homogeneous contrast-enhancement. (**c**) Axial DWI and (**d**) ADC map show minimal diffusion restriction of the lesion. *Abbreviations:* ADC apparent diffusion coefficien, DWI diffusion weighted imaging, FFE fast field echo, TSE turbo spin echo, FFE fast field echo

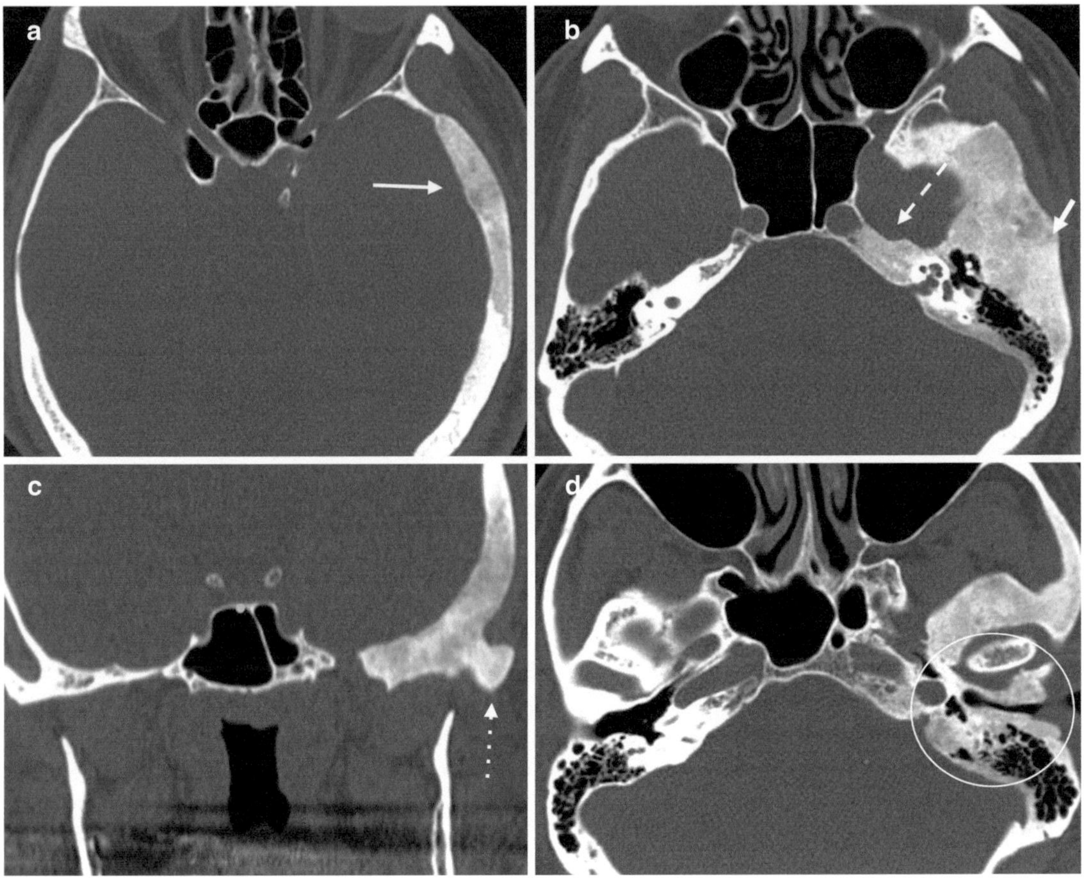

Fig. 6.15 Fibrous dysplasia. MDCT is the imaging modality of choice for evaluating fibrous dysplasia, which is characterized by a variety of osseous changes including ground-glass opacities, homogeneous sclerosis, and cystic components. Typically, affected bone is expanded with well-defined margins and an intact cortical outline. (**a**, **b**) Axial MDCT images of the brain demonstrate thickening and a ground-glass appearance involving the squama (arrow), petrous (dashed arrow), and mastoid (short arrow) portions of the left temporal bone. (**c**) Coronal MDCT image shows thickening and ground-glass opacity of the zygomatic process of the left temporal bone (dotted arrow). (**d**) Axial MDCT image reveals stenosis of the bony portion of the left EAC (white circle). *Abbreviations:* EAC external auditory canal, MDCT multi-detector computed tomography

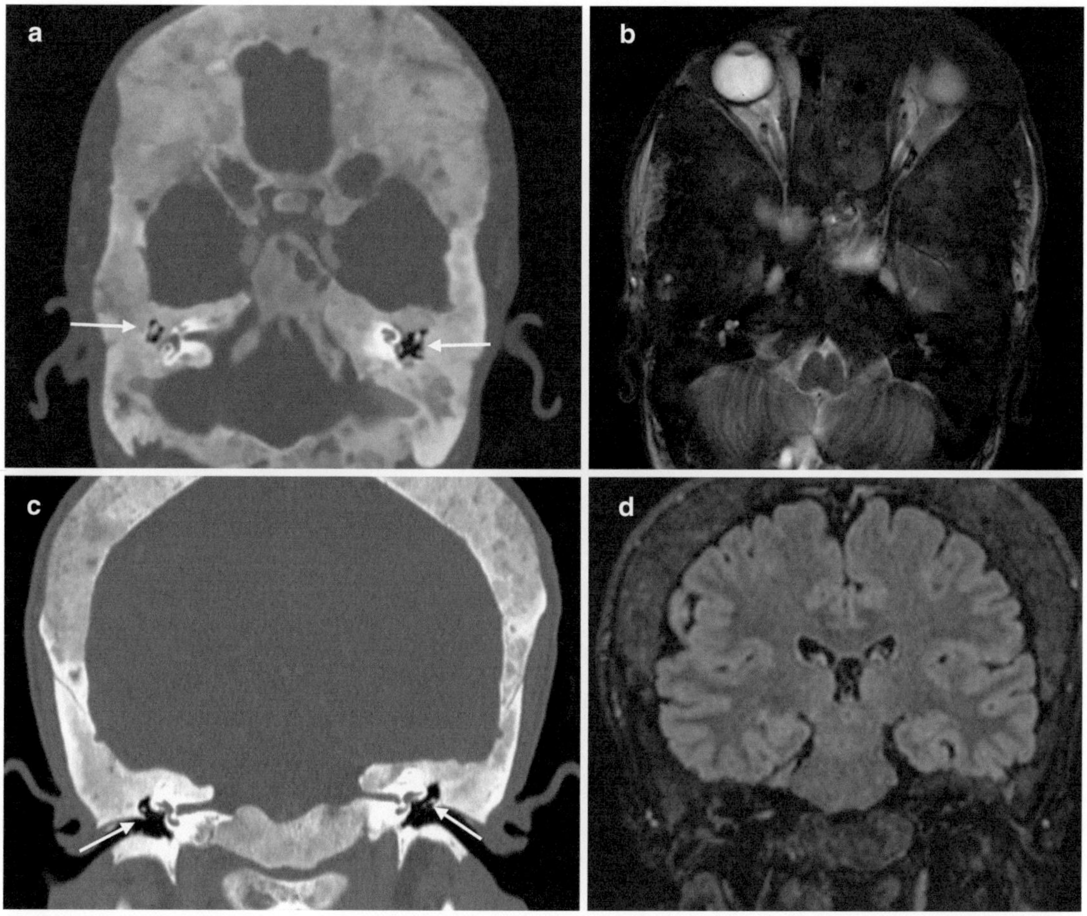

Fig. 6.16 **Fibrous dysplasia in McCune-Albright syndrome**. MAS is a rare neurocutaneous disorder characterized by polyostotic fibrous dysplasia. (**a**, **b**) Axial and coronal MDCT images demonstrate thickening and ground-glass appearance of the skull bones, with marked narrowing of the tympanic cavity (arrow), more prominent on the right side. (**c**, **d**) Axial TSE T2w and coronal 3D FLAIR MR images reveal low and heterogeneous signal intensity within the affected bones. *Abbreviations:* FLAIR fluid attenuated inversion recovery, MAS McCune-Albright syndromoe, MDCT multi-detector computed tomography, TSE turbo spin echo

6.4 Benign Neoplasms

6.4.1 Benign Cutaneous Neoplasms

The World Health Organization has recognized a distinct subset of benign neoplasms that arise specifically in the EAC, from the ceruminous glands of the cartilaginous segment. This group includes rare entities such as ceruminous adenoma, ceruminous pleomorphic adenoma, and syringocystadenoma papilliferum.

The EAC can also be affected by common benign skin neoplasms including nevi and actinic keratoses, as other parts of the body [13]. Neurofibroma can rarely present as a primary lesion of the external auditory canal (Fig. 6.17).

6.4.2 Malignant Neoplasms

Malignant neoplasms can be primary, when originating directly from EE itself, or secondary, resulting from metastasis from elsewhere (often adjacent sites, such as parotid gland). Secondary involvement is more common than primary malignancies of the EE.

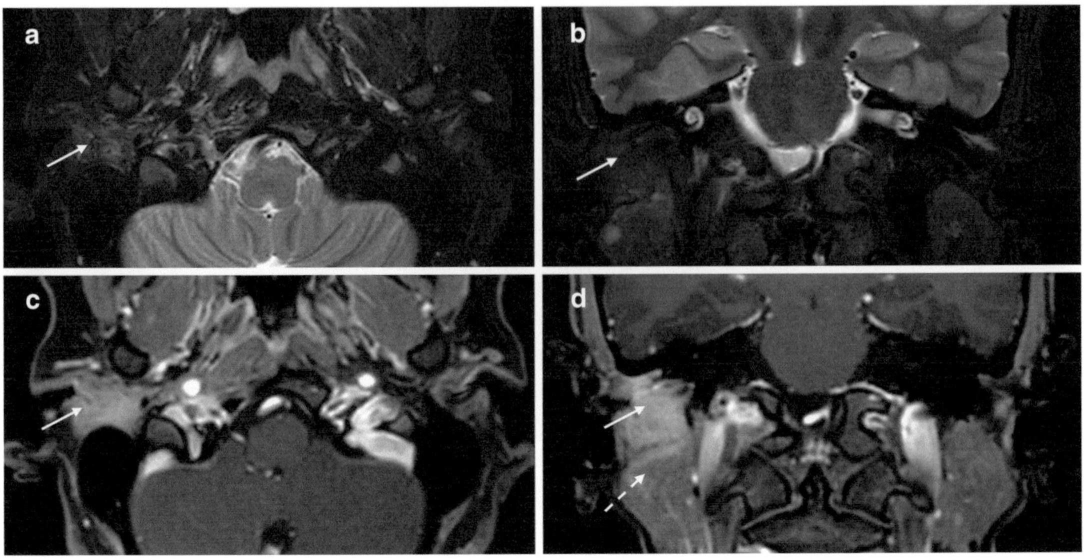

Fig. 6.17 Neurofibroma of the right external auditory canal. Neurofibroma is a benign tumor arising from the connective tissue of peripheral nerves. These tumors most commonly occur in the distal extremities and head and neck region and are frequently associated with neurofibromatosis type 1. However, solitary neurofibromas confined exclusively to the EAC are exceedingly rare. (**a**, **b**) Axial and coronal TSE T2w with fat suppression MR images demonstrate a soft tissue mass (arrow) with intermediate signal intensity occupying the right EAC. (**c**, **d**) Axial and coronal contrast-enhanced 3D FFE T1w with fat suppression images show homogeneous enhancement of the lesion (arrow), which extends into the pre- and post-auricular soft tissues and contacts the parotid gland (dashed arrow). *Abbreviations:* EAC external auditory canal, FFE fast field echo, TSE turbo spin echo

The most common malignant skin neoplasms are basal cell and squamous cell carcinomas (Figs. 6.18 and 6.19), followed by melanoma. lymphoma, Kaposi sarcoma, and adnexal carcinoma (including ceruminous adenocarcinoma and adenoid cystic carcinoma) are other less common primary malignancies of the EAC [14].

While erosion of the bony EAC is often an early indicator of tumor spread, caution is needed when interpreting bony changes in the anteroinferior canal wall. This region may display a pseudo-defect due to natural anatomical variations found in healthy individuals, such as focal thinning (35%) or the presence of the foramen of Huschke (10%).

MRI provides a better evaluation in identification of extra-ear spreading signs, like the replacement of normal T1 bright fatty adjacent tissue with T1 intermediate signal of tumor tissue, contrast enhancement, and restricted diffusion. Intracranial involvement and perineural spread along cranial nerves VII and VIII are clearly depicted on T1-weighted fat-suppressed images after contrast administration.

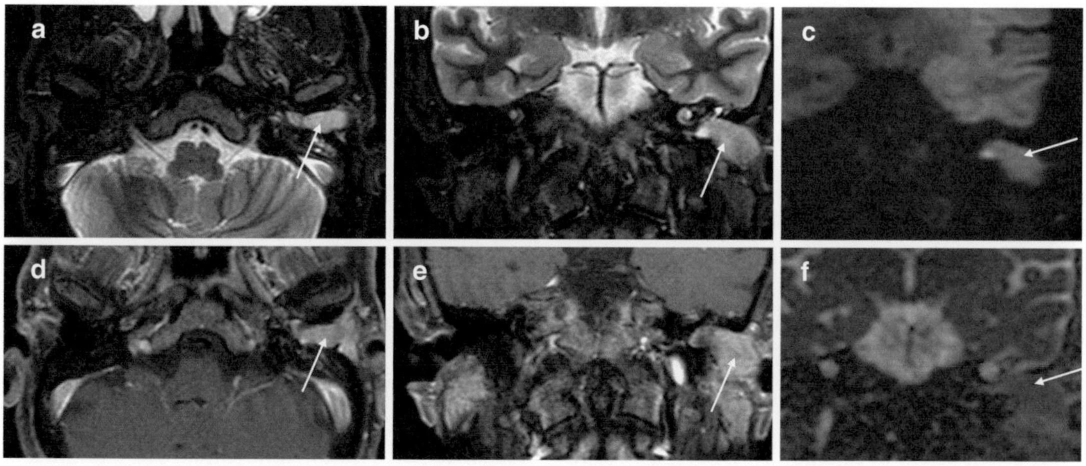

Fig. 6.18 Squamous cell carcinoma of the external auditory canal. SCC of the EAC is rare but represents one of the most common primary malignancies affecting the temporal bone. The tumor often arises in the setting of chronic inflammation. (**a**, **b**) Axial and coronal TSE T2w with fat suppression MR images reveal a soft tissue mass (arrow) with intermediate to high signal intensity occupying the left EAC. (**d**, **e**) Axial and coronal contrast-enhanced 3D FFE T1w with fat suppression images demonstrate homogeneous enhancement of the lesion (arrow). (**c**) Coronal DWI and (**f**)ADC map show moderate diffusion restriction of the lesion (arrow). *Abbreviations:* ADC apparent diffusion coefficient, DWI diffusion weighted imaging, EAC external auditory canal, FFE fast filed echo, TSE turbo spin echo

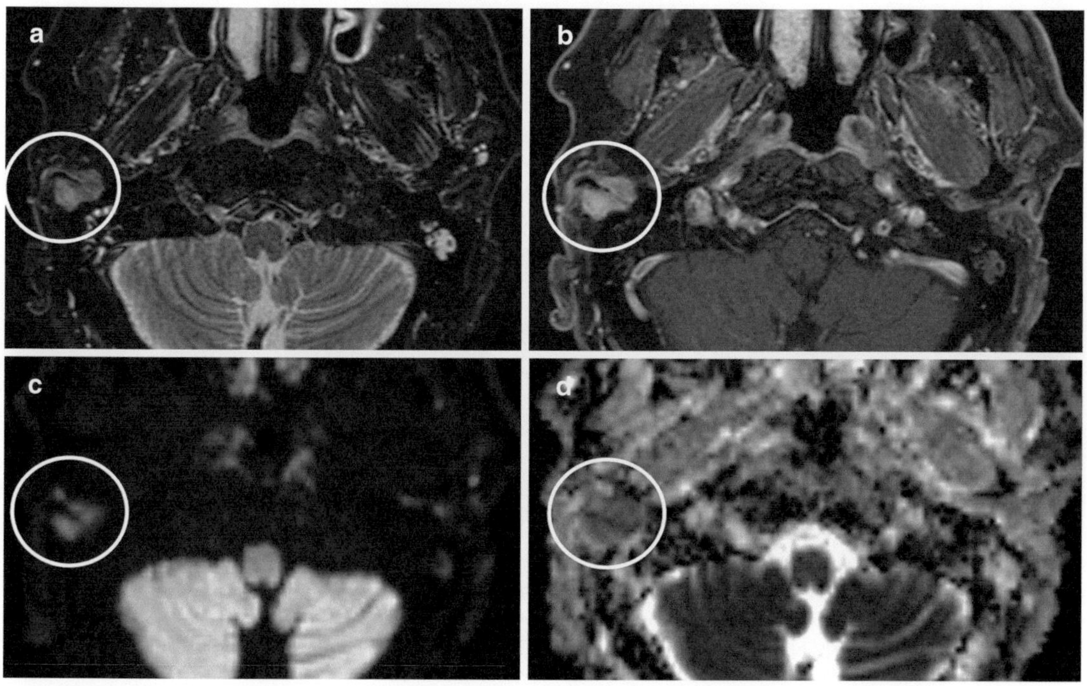

Fig. 6.19 Squamous cell carcinoma of the external auditory canal. (**a**, **b**) Axial TSE T2w with fat suppression and contrast-enhanced 3D FFE T1w with fat suppression MR images reveal a soft tissue mass with intermediate signal intensity arising from the right EAC and extending into adjacent tissues (white circle). (**c**, **d**) Axial DWI and ADC map demonstrate moderate diffusion restriction of the lesion (white circle). *Abbreviations:* ADC apparent diffusion coefficient, DWI diffusion weighted imaging, EAC external auditory canal, FFE fast field echo, TSE turbo spine echo

6.5 Other Conditions

6.5.1 Fractures

Fractures of the EAC often occur as extension of a fracture line of another region of temporal bone or as a consequence of the traumatic impact of the mandibular condyle to the posterior wall of the temporomandibular joint.

Fracture of EAC can be transverse, longitudinal, or both, and when the tympanic plate is involved, narrowing of EAC and trismus can be observed.

It is important to distinguish a persistent foramen tympanicum or tympanosquamous and tympanomastoid fissures from true fractures [3].

6.5.2 Foreign Body

Foreign bodies in the ear are frequent reasons for emergency department access by children.

Clinical examination is usually enough; anyway radiological imaging can help to detect retained foreign bodies and complications such as granuloma formation, tissue lacerations, and tympanic membrane perforations.

The choice of imaging modality depends on the nature of the suspected foreign material, but CT is regarded as the gold standard for foreign body detection because it provides precise anatomical localization of both radiopaque and radiolucent materials. Foreign body-induced otomastoiditis without early management can lead to important intracranial complications (Figs. 6.20 and 6.21).

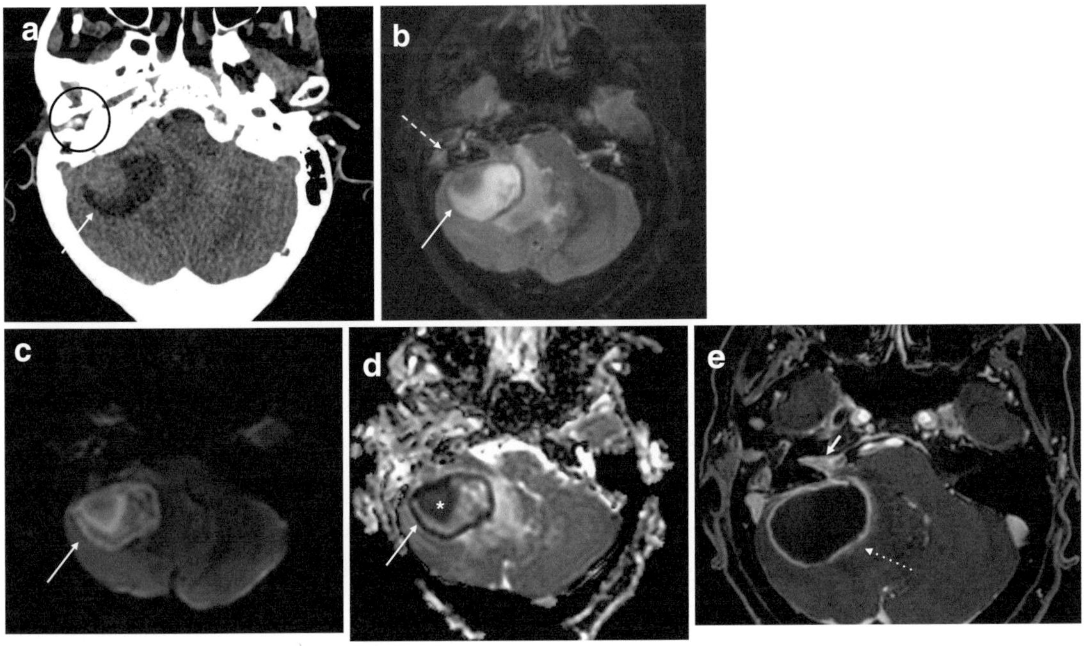

Fig. 6.20 Right-sided foreign body-induced otomastoiditis complicated by cerebellar abscess. Foreign body-induced otomastoiditis, if not promptly and effectively managed, can lead to serious intracranial complications. In cases of chronic ear discharge, it is crucial to consider and exclude the presence of a foreign body, which must be completely removed if identified. Early detection and treatment are essential to minimize the risk of infectious complications. (**a**) Axial CT image shows hyperdense soft tissue in the right EAC representing granulation tissue surrounding a foreign body (cotton) (circle). The image also demonstrates a right cerebellar abscess (arrow). (**b**) Axial TSE T2w with fat suppression MR image reveals right otomastoiditis (dashed arrow) and a right cerebellar abscess with surrounding edema (arrow). (**c**) Axial DWI and (**d**) ADC maps show intense diffusion restriction of the cerebellar abscess (arrow), particularly in the central nodule (asterisk). (**e**) Axial contrast-enhanced 3D FFE T1w with fat suppression image demonstrates ring-enhancing contrast of the right cerebellar abscess (dotted arrow) and enhancement of the internal auditory canal (short arrow), consistent with meningeal involvement. *Abbreviations:* ADC apparent diffusion coefficient, DWI diffusion weighted imaing, FFE fast filed echo, MDCT multi-detector computed tomography, TSE turbo spin echo

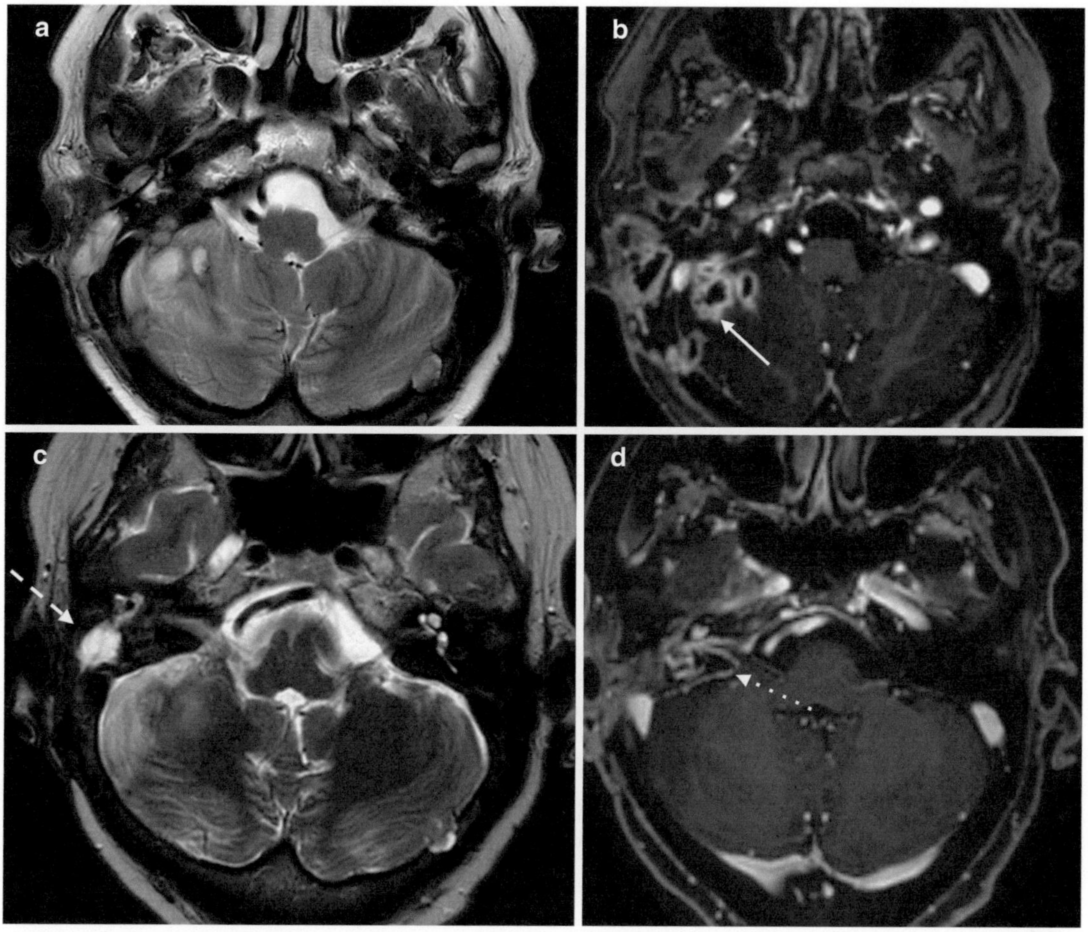

Fig. 6.21 **Right-sided foreign body-induced otomastoiditis complicated by cerebellar abscess** (continued from Fig. 6.20). (**a**) Axial TSE T2w and (**b**) contrast-enhanced 3D FFE T1w with fat suppression MR images at 1-month follow-up show reduced cerebellar edema and multiple smaller cerebellar abscesses following surgical drainage. (**c**) Axial TSE T2w and (**d**) contrast-enhanced 3D FFE T1w with fat suppression MR images at 3-month follow-up demonstrate resolution of otomastoiditis with a residual fluid collection within the mastoid antrum (dashed arrow). Improvement of intracranial complications is evident with resolution of the cerebellar abscess; however, residual dural enhancement is observed along the internal auditory canal and the dura of the pontine-cerebellar angle cistern (dotted arrow). *Abbreviations:* FFE fast field echo, TSE turbo spin echo

6.5.3 Cephalocele

Temporal bone cephalocele refers to the protrusion of intracranial structures—such as the meninges and sometimes brain tissue—into spaces like the middle ear, mastoid air cells, petrous apex, or, less commonly, the external auditory canal, sometimes associated with cerebrospinal fluid (CSF) leaks. This condition can arise spontaneously (idiopathic), as a result of surgical intervention (iatrogenic), or following trauma. CT scanning is ideal for detecting the bony defects responsible for the herniation, while MRI provides superior visualization of the soft tissue contents.

References

1. Roland PS, Stroman DW. Microbiology of acute otitis externa. Laryngoscope. 2002;112(7):1166–77. https://doi.org/10.1097/00005537-200207000-00005.

2. Hoshino T, Matsumoto M. Otomycosis: subdermal growth in calcified mass. Eur Arch Otorrinolaringol. 2006;263(9):875–8. Available from: https://pubmed.ncbi.nlm.nih.gov/16799802/.
3. Tsuno NSG, Tsuno MY, Neto CAFC, Noujaim SE, Decnop M, Pacheco FT, et al. Imaging the external ear: practical approach to Normal and pathologic conditions. Radiographics. 2022;42(2):522–40. https://doi.org/10.1148/rg.210148.
4. Nguyen LT, Harris JP, Nguyen QT. Erosive external otitis: a novel distinct clinical entity of the external Auditory Canal in nonimmunosuppressed individuals. Otol Neurotol. 2010;31(9):1409. Available from: https://pmc.ncbi.nlm.nih.gov/articles/PMC3364102/.
5. Mehrotra P, Elbadawey MR, Zammit-Maempel I. Spectrum of radiological appearances of necrotising external otitis: a pictorial review. J Laryngol Otol. 2011;125(11):1109–15. Available from: https://pubmed.ncbi.nlm.nih.gov/21846417/.
6. Prasad KC, Varsha GI, Mohammadi K, Gupta A, Jose DA. A clinicopathological study of aural polyps: a retrospective analysis in a tertiary care hospital. Int Arch Otorhinolaryngol. 2024;28(3):e368–73. https://doi.org/10.1055/s-0043-1777418.
7. Shinnabe A, Hara M, Hasegawa M, Matsuzawa S, Kanazawa H, Yoshida N, et al. A comparison of patterns of disease extension in keratosis obturans and external auditory canal cholesteatoma. Otol Neurotol. 2013;34(1):91–4. Available from: https://pubmed.ncbi.nlm.nih.gov/23235551/.
8. Heilbrun ME, Salzman KL, Glastonbury CM, Harnsberger HR, Kennedy RJ, Shelton C. External auditory canal cholesteatoma: clinical and imaging spectrum. AJNR Am J Neuroradiol. 2003;24(4):751. Available from: https://pmc.ncbi.nlm.nih.gov/articles/PMC8148678/.
9. Baráth K, Huber AM, Stämpfli P, Varga Z, Kollias S. Neuroradiology of cholesteatomas. Am J Neuroradiol. 2011;32(2):221–9. Available from: https://pubmed.ncbi.nlm.nih.gov/20360335/.
10. Carbone PN, Nelson BL. External auditory Osteoma. Head Neck Pathol. 2011;6(2):244. Available from: https://pmc.ncbi.nlm.nih.gov/articles/PMC3370017/
11. Kumar S, Singh P, Verma R, et al. Imaging spectrum of osteopetrosis: a pictorial review. Indian J Radiol Imaging. 2024;34(1):1–10. https://doi.org/10.4103/ijri.IJRI_24_23.
12. Jethanamest D, Roehm P. Fibrous dysplasia of the temporal bone with complete canal stenosis and Cholesteatoma. Otol Neurotol. 2011;32(7):e52. Available from: https://pmc.ncbi.nlm.nih.gov/articles/PMC4513648/.
13. Sand M, Sand D, Brors D, Altmeyer P, Mann B, Bechara FG. Cutaneous lesions of the external ear. Head Face Med. 2008;4(1). Available from: https://pubmed.ncbi.nlm.nih.gov/18261212/.
14. Samara P, Athanasopoulos M, Goulioumis A, Athanasopoulos I. Malignant tumors of the external auditory canal: diagnosis, treatment, genetic landscape, biomarkers, and clinical outcome. Explor Target Antitumor Ther. 2023;4(5):801. Available from: https://pmc.ncbi.nlm.nih.gov/articles/PMC10645464/.

Otitis Media and Cholesteatoma

7

Elisa Scola, Luca Gambardella,
Margherita Bevilacqua, Fabio Triulzi,
Lorenzo Maria Gaini, Diego Zanetti, Silvia Casale,
and Giorgio Conte

7.1 Acute and Chronic Otomastoiditis

Acute otomastoiditis (AOM) refers to the purulent infection of the tympanic cavity due to bacteria; it is often associated with the obstruction of the eustachian tube (ET) or of the antrum. Purulent effusion in the tympanic cavity often spreads to the mastoid through the aditus ad antrum or other cellular traits, with subsequent acute mastoiditis, considered by some authors as a complication of AOM. AOM is more common in children due to the short length and horizontal orientation of the ET and to the prominent adenoidal tissue that act as predisposing factors to middle ear effusion and are a reservoir of bacteria. Intratemporal complications of AOM are middle ear effusion, cochleo-labyrinthitis, facial nerve palsy, subperiosteal abscess, and petrous apicitis; intracranial complications include meningitis, intracranial abscesses, and dural sinus venous thrombosis. The inflammatory material may drain through the perforation of tympanic membrane, or on the contrary the infection may persist in the antrum, making the placement of a transtympanic drainage necessary [1, 2].

E. Scola (✉) · S. Casale
Neuroradiology Unit, Fondazione IRCCS Ca' Granda Ospedale Maggiore Policlinico, Milan, Italy
e-mail: elisa.scola@policlinico.mi.it; silvia.casale@policlinico.mi.it

L. Gambardella
School in Radiodiagnostics, Università degli Studi del Molise, Campobasso, Italy
e-mail: l.gambardella@studenti.unimol.it

M. Bevilacqua
Postgraduate School in Radiodiagnostics, Università degli Studi di Milano, Milan, Italy
e-mail: marghe.bevilacqua@gmail.com

F. Triulzi · G. Conte
Neuroradiology Unit, Fondazione IRCCS Ca' Granda Ospedale Maggiore Policlinico, Milan, Italy

Department of Pathophysiology and Transplantation, University of Milan, Milan, Italy
e-mail: fabio.triulzi@policlinico.mi.it; giorgio.conte@policlinico.mi.it

L. M. Gaini
Department of Otolaryngology and Head and Neck Surgery, Fondazione IRCCS Ca' Granda Ospedale Maggiore Policlinico, Milan, Italy
e-mail: lorenzo.gaini@policlinico.mi.it

D. Zanetti
Audiology Unit, Department of Specialistic Surgical Sciences, Fondazione IRCCS Ca' Granda Ospedale Maggiore Policlinico, Milan, Italy

Department of Clinical Sciences and Community Health, Università degli Studi di Milano, Milan, Italy
e-mail: diego.zanetti@policlinico.mi.it

G. Conte et al. (eds.), *Atlas of Normal and Pathological Findings in Otoneuroradiology*,
https://doi.org/10.1007/978-3-032-08232-9_7

Chronic otomastoiditis (COM) is the inflammation of the middle ear associated with long-standing eustachian tube dysfunction and characterized by persistence or recurrence: it usually lasts for 12 weeks. COM usually causes irreversible damage to the ossicular chain and tympanic membrane, with perforation. Complications of COM partially overlap with AOM complications but also include tympanic membrane retractions, ossicular fixation and erosion, granulation tissue, cholesterol granuloma, and acquired cholesteatoma. Additionally, poor mastoid pneumatization can be a consequence of COM in infancy, and it is found to be correlated with deficit of middle ear aeration [1].

Usually imaging is not needed in AOM. Computer tomography (CT) scan may display fluid levels in the middle ear and mastoid with the integrity of the ossicular chain, mastoid septa and the internal and external mastoid cortex. Middle ear effusion (MEE) often leads to a collection of fluid in the mastoid. It should be noted that the presence of fluid in mastoid air cells is quite commonly seen in magnetic resonance imaging (MRI) both in children and in adults despite the absence of a history of infection. Therefore, it is preferable to use the term "nonspecific mastoid fluid or debris" rather than "mastoiditis." Imaging is needed in case of coalescent mastoiditis where the inflammation and infection involve the bone with osteoclastic disruption of the bone septa and the development of an intramastoid empyema. When the external or internal mastoid cortex is eroded, an exteriorized mastoiditis can ensue, and a subperiosteal abscess or an intracranial abscess and meningitis may develop. If the bone erosion occurs in the mastoid tip, the subperiosteal abscess may spread lateral (pseudo-Bezold's abscess) or medial and deep to the insertion of the digastric and sternocleidomastoid muscles or even medial and deep to the insertion of the digastric muscle (Mouret's abscess); the two latter may be not clinically palpable. Mastoid abscess are dangerous as they may extend to the laterocervical spaces and mediastinum [3].

COM often appears on CT with opacification of the tympanic cavity and mastoid. While erosions of the ossicular chain are relatively infrequent in case of chronic non-cholesteatomatous otitis, ossicular interruption by septic necrosis or ossicular fixation ("tympanosclerosis") is a common post-inflammatory consequence which may be due to deposition of fibrous tissue, hyalinized collagen, or new bone formation (Figs. 7.1, 7.2, and 7.3) [1, 4].

The tympanic membrane and middle ear can be involved by infectious processes also in case of necrotizing otitis externa (NOE). NOE is a serious complication that can arise from external ear infection, mostly in elderly individuals with diabetes or weakened immune systems. NOE has tendency to spread to the middle ear and to the nearby structures. In NOE, MRI can be useful, in addition to a previously performed CT examination, to exclude possible routes of propagation of the infection to intracranial compartment and in particular to the intracranial venous sinuses which can lead to the development of thrombophlebitic phenomena (Figs. 7.4 and 7.5) [3].

7.2 Cholesteatoma

Cholesteatomas can be defined as enlarging cysts consisting of an inner wall of stratified squamous epithelium ("matrix") and an outer layer of loose areolar tissue rich of osteoclasts and Langerhans cells releasing osteolytic enzymes ("perimatrix"), which surround a collection of keratin debris. Cholesteatomas are more common in males and can be congenital (see later in the paragraph). More often, middle ear cholesteatomas are acquired (up to 98% of cases). Acquired cholesteatomas are primary or secondary. Primary acquired cholesteatoma derives from chronic middle ear dysventilation causing the retraction pocket of the tympanic membrane. Secondary acquired cholesteatoma is the consequence of the migration of the epithelium through a marginal perforation of tympanic membrane or of epithelial squamous metaplasia in the tympanic cavity caused by chronic infection (Figs. 7.6 and 7.7). Cholesteatoma may arise from either the pars tensa or flaccida of the tympanic membrane [5].

In a patient who presents extensive opacification of the middle ear, the presence of a cholesteatoma hidden among effusive material can be extremely difficult to detect as they have almost identical density on CT scan. The suspicion of cholesteatoma usually arise from the clinical examination. However, there are some CT signs that may suggest the presence of a cholesteatoma such as the presence of erosions affecting the tympanic tegmen and ossicular chain, scutum blunting or the retraction of the tympanic membrane. Therefore, cholesteatoma may be suspected in the presence of erosions of the ossicular chain and/or the walls of the tympanic cavity in an untreated patient with compatible clinical symptoms. On the contrary, diagnosing cholesteatoma recurrence in a patient who has undergone surgery and presents with a poorly aerated middle ear due to extensive soft-tissue opacities poses significant diagnostic challenges: in case of postoperative follow-up, CT scans do not allow to distinguish between different soft-tissue density materials. Soft-tissue density materials can be attributed to inflammation, fibrous or granulation tissue or the recurrence of cholesteatoma. The diagnostic dilemma may be resolved by performing an MRI with the use of non-echo planar diffusion weighted imaging (non-EPI DWI) sequences, which are helpful in identifying even small diffusion restrictions caused by cholesteatoma of a few millimeters in size [5–7].

Cholesteatomas are usually hypointense/isointense on T1-weighted images and hyperintense on T2-weighted images compared with brain tissue and do not enhance with gadolinium injection, but these characteristics are not specific. On the other hand, they show a typical high signal on DWI, which presumably can be partly attributed to restriction of the diffusion of water molecules between the keratinous debris of the cholesteatoma contents and to a T2 shine-through effect. The DWI images interpretation should be integrated with the apparent diffusion coefficient (ADC) map evaluation: ADC maps are free from T2 shine-through effect, and a true diffusivity restriction is seen with low signal on ADC maps. Inflammation, granulation tissue, fluid and in general non-cholesteatomatous soft tissue have high signal on the ADC map. Non-EPI DWI is preferable to EPI-DWI in detecting cholesteatoma because it is less sensitive to air-bone susceptibility artifact and distortion at petrous bones (Figs. 7.8, 7.9, and 7.10) [6, 7].

Complications of cholesteatoma are due to bone erosion and include ossicular chain, facial nerve canal erosion, tympanic erosion, labyrinthine fistula, extension to petrous apex and automastoidectomy when the outer walls of mastoid are involved [6, 8].

Ossicular erosion is much more common in cholesteatoma than in chronic otitis media. Usually the ossicular chain is spared in less than one third of middle ear cholesteatoma cases; this proportion is even lower in cases of pars tensa cholesteatoma. In cholesteatoma arising from the pars tensa, the long process of the incus and the stapes are eroded together with malleus handle. In cholesteatoma arising from the pars flaccida, the long process and body of the incus and the malleus head are typically eroded. In reporting it is very important to highlight if the cholesteatoma is located medially or laterally to the ossicular chain. This information is crucial for the surgeon in the planning of surgical approach and technique for the preservation of the ossicular chain. Childhood cholesteatoma is more aggressive and causes more frequent ossicular erosion, in particular of stapes superstructure, compared to adults. If the platina of the stapes is eroded, there is a higher risk of perilymphatic leakage in the middle ear [11]. Facial nerve dehiscence may occur after cholesteatoma bone erosion of bone wall canal, and it is a predisposing factor to damage of the nerve during surgery, usually occurring at the level of the mid-tympanic segment. Patients with cholesteatoma complaining of episodic vertigo should be suspected for labyrinthine fistula. Labyrinthine fistula usually occurs in the lateral semicircular canal, in case of atticoantral cholesteatoma, and less often in the other semicircular canals and in cochlea. Cochlea fistula is usually associated with pars tensa cholesteatoma (posterior tympanic) and is usually located in the promontory between the oval and the round window. A typical clinical sign of labyrinthine fistula is the Tullio phenomenon consisting in nystagmus (conjugate eye movements) induced by sound or pressure and is the consequence of the erosion of semicircular canals or labyrinthine fistula. Fistula staging is based on the severity of otic capsule destruction. The first stage is characterized only by bone erosion of otic capsule but the endosteal membrane is intact; in the second stage the cholesteatoma enters in contact with the perilymphatic space but the membranous labyrinth is spared; in the third stage the membranous labyrinth is directly involved [8]. MRI may be useful in the presurgical evaluation of the semicircular canal, when involved by cholesteatoma: if fibrosis of the semicircular canal is already present before surgery, a more aggressive surgical approach can be considered. Fibrosis is demonstrated as a disappearance of physiological high T2 signal intensity in semicircular canals.

Erosion of the tegmen tympani should always be considered, as the bony defect places the cholesteatoma into direct contact with the meninges of the middle cranial fossa MRI is mandatory when an erosion of the tegmen tympani is detected in order to exclude the presence of meningocele or encephalocele, to describe their location and to alert the surgeon about a possible cerebrospinal fluid (CSF) leak (Figs. 7.11, 7.12, and 7.13) [8]. Colesteastoma has a high risk of recurrence after surgery. In postoperative follow-up non-EPI DWI may reduce the need of second-look surgery in detecting recurrent disease. This changed dramatically the management of follow-up of cholesteatoma. Nevertheless, non-EPI DWI technique has limitations in sensitivity and specificity: false negatives include small cholesteatoma pearls less than 3 mm that can be missed, and false positives include the presence of postoperative materials such as silastic sheet; false positives have been also reported in cases of cholesterol granuloma or proteinaceous fluid (Figs. 7.14, 7.15, 7.16, 7.17, 7.18, and 7.19) [6, 7]

Acquired cholesteatomas quite rarely extend to the petrous apex; therefore, alternative diagnoses should be taken into account. Contrast-enhanced MRI may help in the differential diagnosis as aggressive tumors typically enhance while cholesteatoma does not [9, 10].

Congenital cholesteatoma can be associated to external auditory canal (EAC) atresia or congenital aural atresia is a complete or incomplete narrowing of bony EAC. It is more often monolateral but can be bilateral. It is often isolated but can be depicted in syndromic cases (Crouzon, Goldenhar, Pierre Robin, and Treacher Collins syndromes) in which the malformation is more severe than in isolated cases. In case of incomplete bony atresia, the EAC may be further narrowed by soft tissue (membranous EAC atresia). EAC atresia is often associated with a dysplastic auricle and malformation of middle ear cavity and ossicles due to common embryologic origin of the external and middle ear. On the contrary the internal ear and the internal auditory canal are usually normal because of their earlier embryological formation. EAC atresia can be complicated by the formation of a congenital cholesteatoma behind the atresia plate (Figs. 7.20 and 7.21).

7.3 Cholesterol Granuloma

In the differential diagnosis of petrous bone lesions, the temporal bone cholesterol granuloma (CG) should be considered. CG is a collection of cholesterol crystals lined by fibrous connective tissue that can be located in the petrous apex, in the middle ear or in the mastoid. CG is a cell granulomatous chronic reaction to cholesterol crystals that derive from red blood cell breakdown. CG pathogenesis is probably linked to eustachian tube dysfunction leading to mucosal edema, vessel damage and stagnation of hemorrhagic contents. Contrary to cholesteatoma, the CG is lined by fibrous connective tissue and not by keratinizing stratified squamous epithelium. CG of the middle ear rarely causes erosion of the bone structure, while CG of the petrous apex is erosive and, due to its location, can be dangerous for carotid canal and cavernous sinus invasion. On CT images the differential diagnosis between cholesteatoma, typical inflammatory granulomatous tissue and CG is not possible. MRI may help in the diagnosis as CG is typically hyperintense in T1 images, while typical granulomatous tissue and cholesteatoma are not. The differential diagnosis between inflammatory granulomatous tissue and cholesteatoma is based on T1-weighted images with gadolinium injection and DWI: the inflammatory granulomatous tissue enhances, while cholesteatoma does not enhances but has restriction on diffusion images. Usually CG does not show diffusion restriction even if some exceptions are reported (Figs. 7.22 and 7.23) [9, 10].

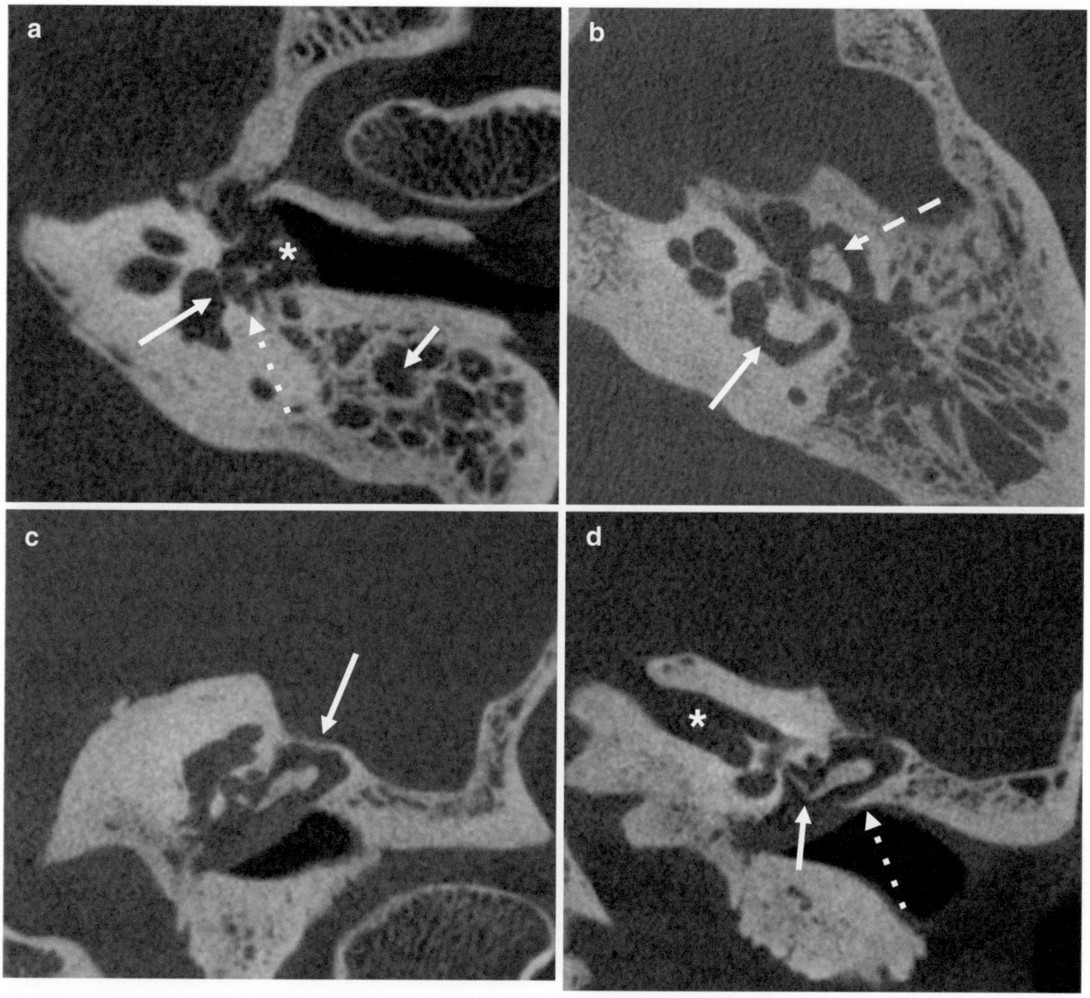

Fig. 7.1 Non-cholesteatomatous chronic otomastoiditis. Chronic otomastoiditis often appears on imaging with opacification of the tympanic cavity and mastoid without evidence of erosion of the ossicular chain and bone walls, which are more typical of cholesteatomatous otitis. CBCT images show a case of non-cholesteatomatous chronic left-sided otomastoiditis. (**a**) Axial reformatted CBCT image passing through the stapes shows the presence of soft-tissue density material that completely obliterates the mesotympanic cavity (asterisk) and mastoid cells (short arrow). It gets in contact with the oval window (arrow) and occupies the sinus tympani (dotted arrow). (**b**) Axial reformatted CBCT image shows the epitympanum. The incudomalleal joint is normally represented (dashed arrow). Regular morphology of the lateral semicircular canal (arrow) is also shown. (**c**) A coronal reformatted CBCT image passing through the incudomalleolar joint shows no clear sign of erosions of the tegmen tympani (arrow). The bony walls of the middle ear, including the scutum, do not appear to be involved by the inflammatory process and do not show sign of erosion. The tegmen tympani may be very thin making the assessment of erosion challenging. (**d**) A coronal reformatted CBCT image passing through the incus with regular visualization of the incudostapedial joint (short arrow). In this case the scutum (dotted arrow) is well represented, whereas it is frequently eroded in case of cholesteatomatous otitis. The normal internal acoustic meatus (asterisk) is included in the scan plane. *CBCT* cone beam computed tomography

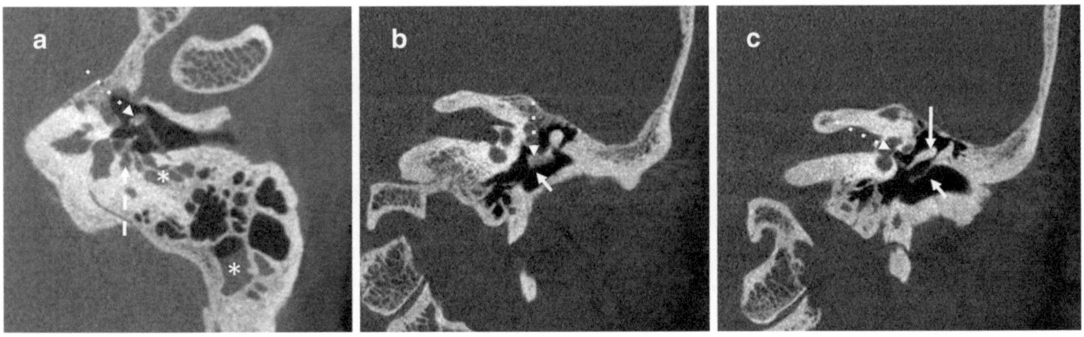

Fig. 7.2 Post-inflammatory changes after non-cholesteatomatous chronic otitis media. While erosions of the ossicular chain are relatively infrequent in case of chronic non-cholesteatomatous otitis, ossicular fixation is a more common post-inflammatory consequence which may be due to deposition of fibrous tissue, hyalinized collagen, or new bone formation. Additionally, ossicular ligaments may calcify. The lateral malleolar ligament fixation can undergo surgery without the sacrifice of the ossicular chain. On the contrary, the antero-superior malleolar ligament fixation can be operated only by removing the ossicular chain. (**a**) Axial reformatted CBCT image passing through the stapes, without sign of erosion. Instead, an important finding consists of the gross calcification clearly visible attached to the manubrium of the malleus (dotted arrow) and constitutes the final result of a probably long-term chronic process. Overall the tympanic cavity and the EAC are normally ventilated, except for a small amount of soft-tissue density material located in the sinus tympani (dashed arrow). This can be attributed either to fibrotic tissue or to inflammatory effusions, but CBCT does not allow a clear differentiation. Small amounts of inflammatory effusions are recognized in some mastoid cells (asterisk). (**b**) A coronal reformatted CBCT image passing through the malleus demonstrates deposition of hyperdense calcified material along the manubrium (dotted arrow) with consequent retraction of the tympanic membrane (short arrow). A similar finding involves the long process and the short process of the incus (not shown), configuring overall a typical example of tympanosclerosis with consequent post-inflammatory ossicular chain fixation. (**c**) A coronal reformatted CBCT image passing through the incus well shows a thickened tympanic membrane (short arrow) due to hyalinization of the intermediate collagen layer. The incus (arrow) and the oval window (dotted arrow) appear regularly represented. *CBCT* cone beam computed tomography, *EAC* external auditory canal

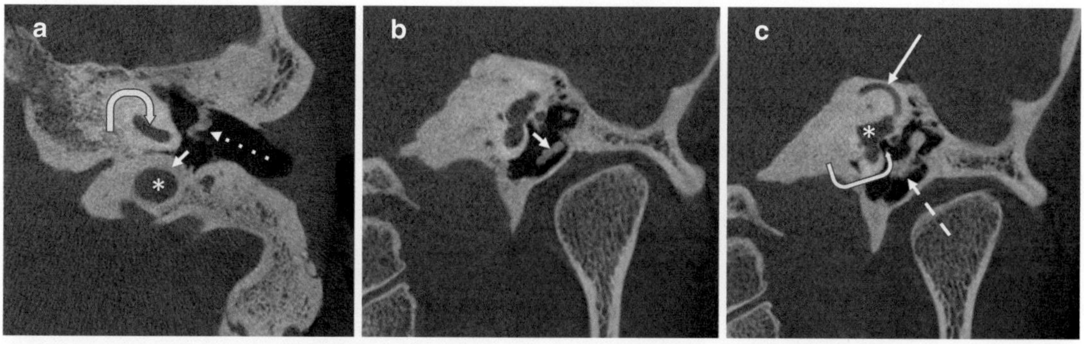

Fig. 7.3 Post-inflammatory changes of the tympanic membrane. (**a**) Axial reformatted CBCT image shows the presence of a gross calcification (dotted arrow) in the anterior portion of the tympanic membrane which also appears retracted. The EAC and the tympanic cavity are normally ventilated. The jugular bulb (asterisk) has an anatomical variant, whereby it is located in a higher position (high riding bulb). There is no unanimous definition of the transverse level above which a jugular bulb is considered high riding, but some authors use the floor of the internal acoustic meatus, the basal turn of the cochlea (curved arrow), or the oval window as a reference point. It may be useful to keep in mind that the procidence of a high riding jugular bulb in the tympanic cavity can be variably associated with pathology, such as pulsatile tinnitus or conductive hearing loss, especially if the bony plate that separates the two structures (known as the sigmoid plate) is very thin or completely absent, as in case of dehiscent jugular bulb. In this case the sigmoid plate (short arrow) is thick and clearly visible. (**b**) This coronal reformatted CBCT image better demonstrates that the calcification of the tympanic membrane extends mainly along its upper portion (short arrow). (**c**) A more posterior coronal reformatted CBCT image shows that the calcifications also include part of the manubrium of the malleus (dashed arrow) which appears thickened. If the calcifications affected only the tympanic membrane, the condition could be defined as "myringosclerosis" instead of the more generic "tympanosclerosis." The oval window is regularly represented (curved arrow). The vestibule (asterisk) and part of the superior semicircular canal (arrow) are also shown. *CBCT* cone beam computed tomography, *EAC* external auditory canal

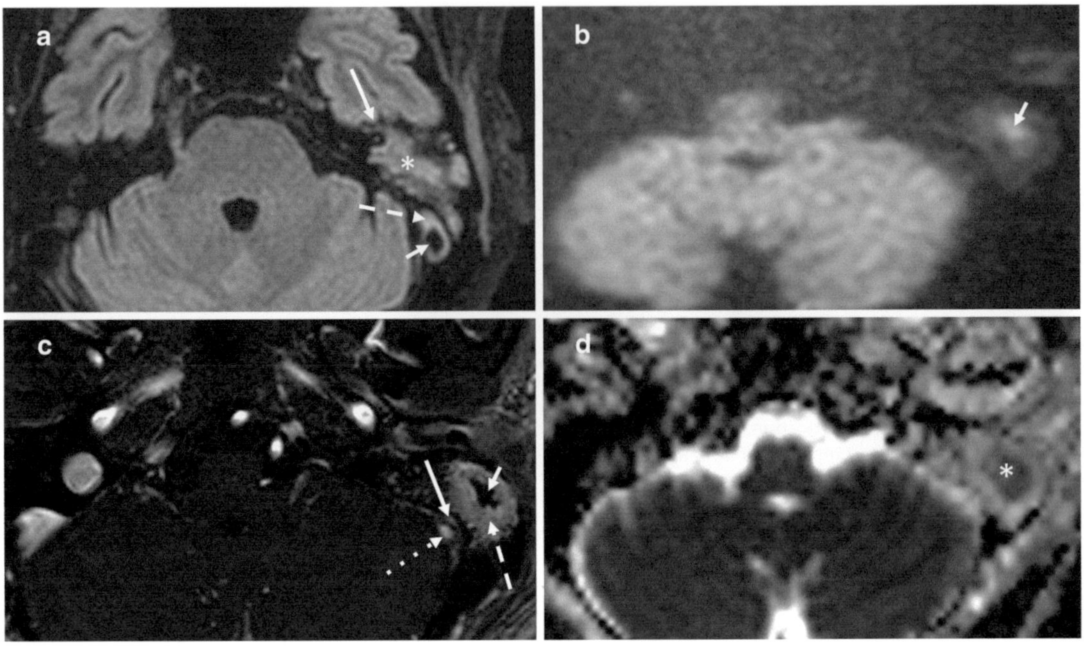

Fig. 7.4 Serratia-related necrotizing otitis externa. NOE is a serious complication that can arise from external ear infection, mostly in elderly individuals with diabetes or weakened immune systems. If untreated, NOE is associated with a high mortality, and this is due to its tendency to spread to the temporal bone and the nearby structures. In this clinical subset, MRI can be useful, in addition to a previously performed CT examination, to exclude possible routes of intracranial propagation of the infection and in the follow-up. (**a**) Axial FLAIR sequence documents the presence of isointense tissue obliterating the mastoid antrum and mastoid cells (asterisk). The tissue is close to the temporal cerebral cortex (arrow), yet without directly invading it as there are no appreciable parenchymal signal alterations. Axial post-gadolinium T1-weighted image (**c**) shows enhancement of the inflammatory tissue in the mastoid (dashed arrow), surrounding a central non-vascularized area (short arrow) compatible with the presence of a small bony sequestrum (see Fig. 7.5). In cases of severe NOE such as the one exposed here, the proximity of the intracranial venous sinuses to the otomastoid must always be taken into consideration because of the possible spread of the infection, which can lead to the development of thrombophlebitic phenomena. Along the internal and posterior surface of the petrous part of temporal bone, the sigmoid sinus can be observed presenting both thickening and weak enhancement of its walls (arrow). In this case, an important finding is that the venous sinuses are still patent, as outlined by the high endoluminal signal intensity due to the presence of gadolinium (dotted arrow). On FLAIR (**a**) the pathological signal hyperintensity of the sigmoid sinus wall can be better appreciated (dashed arrow), while vascular patency is expressed through the typical signal hypointensity inside the vessel due to flow void (short arrow). On b 1000 DWI image (**b**) and on corresponding ADC map (**d**), a respectively hyperintense (short arrow) and hypointense (asterisk) signal alteration is revealed centrally in the mastoid. This finding is compatible with the presence of highly cellular inflammatory infiltrates within the small bone sequestration already described (see Fig. 7.5). *NOE* necrotizing otitis externa, *MRI* magnetic resonance imaging, *CT* computed tomography, *FLAIR* fluid attenuated inversion recovery, *DWI* diffusion-weighted images, *ADC* apparent diffusion coefficient

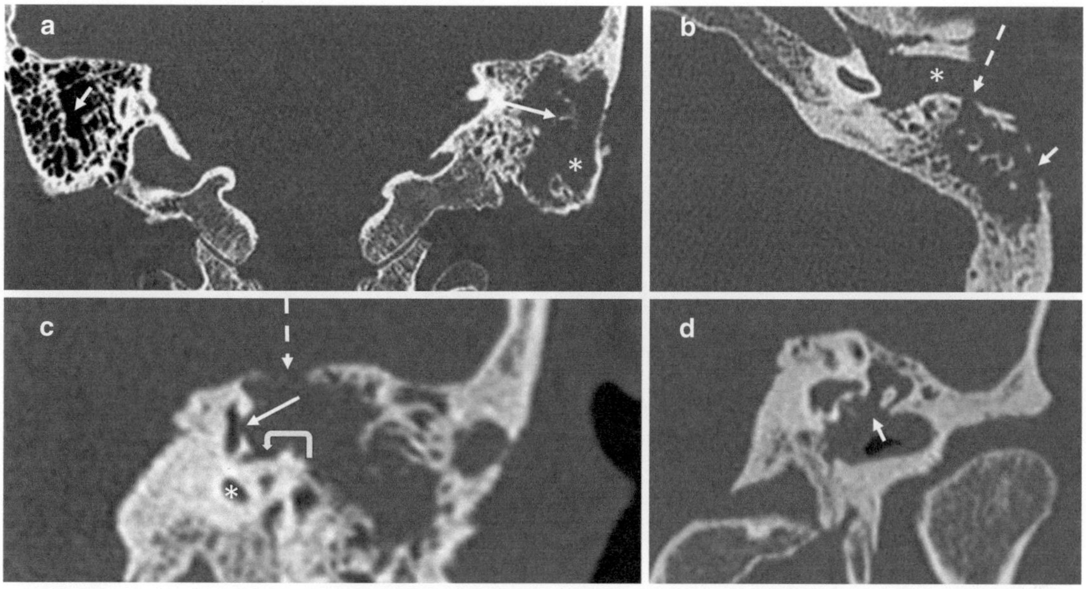

Fig. 7.5 Serratia-related necrotizing otitis externa (continued from Fig. 7.4). (**a**) Coronal reformatted MDCT image shows the cranial base at the level of the mastoid processes. Compared to the normally represented mastoid cells of the right side (short arrow), on the left side the infection markedly subverts the normal bone architecture of the mastoid up to its tip, with bone trabeculae appearing diffusely eroded (asterisk). The whole process seems to develop around a small central bony sequestrum (arrow). (**b**) Axial reformatted MDCT image passing through the EAC demonstrates how it is completely obliterated by soft-tissue density material (asterisk) which directly communicates with the infectious process located in the mastoid through an interruption in the profile of the posterior bone wall of the EAC (dashed arrow). Bone erosions also extensively involve the cranial lateral wall of the mastoid (short arrow). (**c**) Coronal reformatted MDCT image shows the involvement of some structures of the bony labyrinth. In relation to the aggressiveness of the infection in its acute phase, erosive phenomena are expressed through the presence of multiple labyrinthine fistulas, one of which affecting the common crus of superior and posterior semicircular canals (arrow), while a further one affects the horizontal semicircular canal (curved arrow). A normal section of the posterior semicircular canal is also depicted (asterisk). Also note in this image how the tegmen mastoideum (i.e., the bony roof of the mastoid) is largely interrupted (dashed arrow), guaranteeing the infection a dangerous communication route with the middle cranial fossa. (**d**) A coronal reformatted MDCT image passing through the incus and the stapes demonstrates the obliteration of the tympanic cavity which is completely filled with soft-tissue density material, causing severe erosive changes of the incudostapedial joint (short arrow): the long crus of incus and its lenticular process are no longer visible. *MDCT* multidetector computed tomography, *EAC* external auditory canal

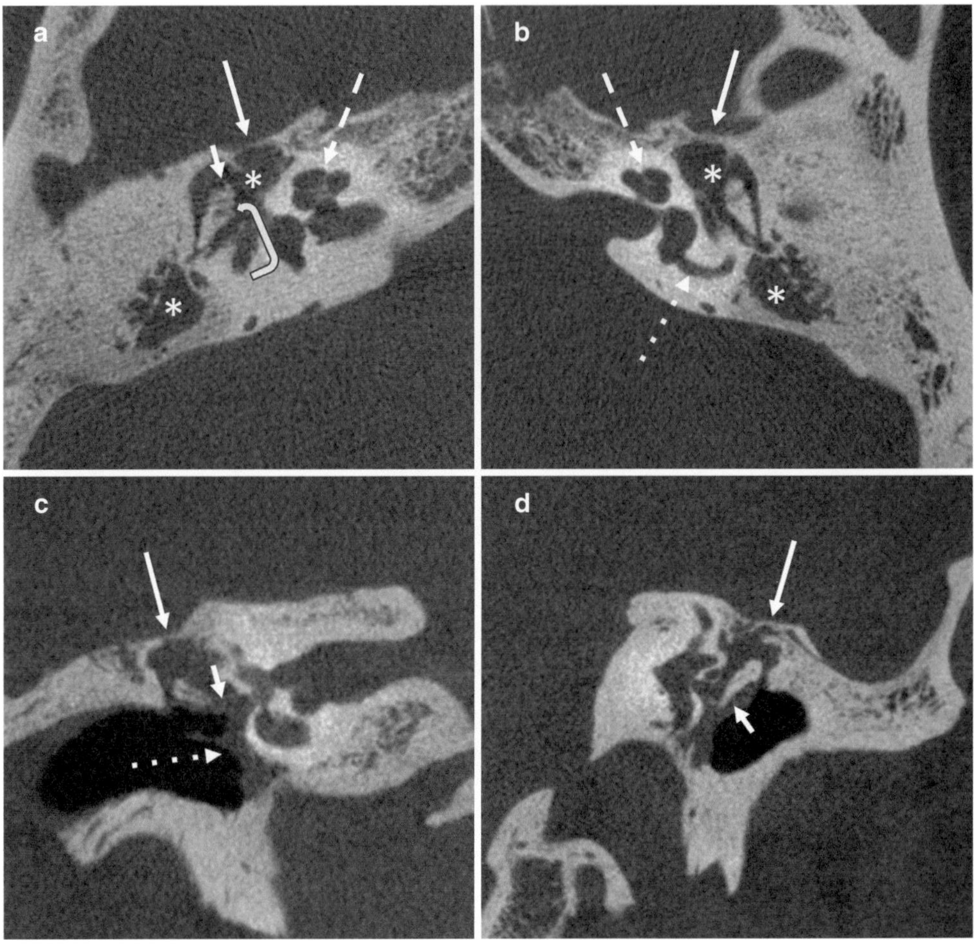

Fig. 7.6 Cholesteatomatous chronic right-sided otomastoiditis and non-cholesteatomatous chronic left-sided otomastoiditis. In a patient who presents extensive opacification of the middle ear, the presence of a cholesteatoma hidden within effusive material can be extremely difficult to detect, as cholesteatoma and inflammatory tissue have almost identical density on CT scan. Therefore, the suspicion of cholesteatoma should necessarily be based on clinical examination. However, there are some CT signs which may suggest the presence of a cholesteatoma even in an otomastoid that is not well ventilated: the presence of erosions affecting the tympanic tegmen and ossicles, the scutum blunting or the retraction of the tympanic membrane. (**a**) Axial CBCT image of the right temporal bone passing through the epitympanum shows the middle ear and the mastoid obliterated by material (asterisks in **a** and **b**) with a density similar to the soft tissues. This finding is associated with bone erosions affecting the head of the malleus (short arrow) and the body of the incus (curved arrow). Furthermore, a slight remodeling of the anterior bony wall of the epitympanum is depicted (arrow), appearing thinner than the respective one on the left side (arrow on image **b**). Overall, these signs may raise suspicions about the presence of an underlying cholesteatoma and should lead to consider further investigation with MRI. (**b**) Axial CBCT image of the left temporal bone passing through the epitympanum depicts the opacification of the tympanic cavity and the mastoid (asterisks) as the only significant finding, without bone erosion, showing a condition compatible with non-cholesteatomatous chronic otomastoiditis. The bony labyrinth is normally represented on both sides: the cochlea is depicted on images **a** and **b** (dashed arrow), and part of the lateral semicircular canal is shown on image **b** (dotted arrow). (**c**) Coronal CBCT image of the right temporal bone shows focal erosive thinning of the tegmen tympani (arrow) and better demonstrates the involvement of the ossicular chain (short arrow) with complete erosion of the long crus of the incus and even the stapes, which has been replaced by soft-tissue density material entirely obliterating the oval window. Finally, the tympanic membrane appears slightly retracted (dotted arrow). (**d**) Coronal reformatted CBCT image of the left temporal bone passing through the incus, which is well represented and free of erosions (short arrow). The tegmen tympani also appears thicker (arrow) when compared to the contralateral side (arrow on image **c**). *CBCT* cone beam computed tomography

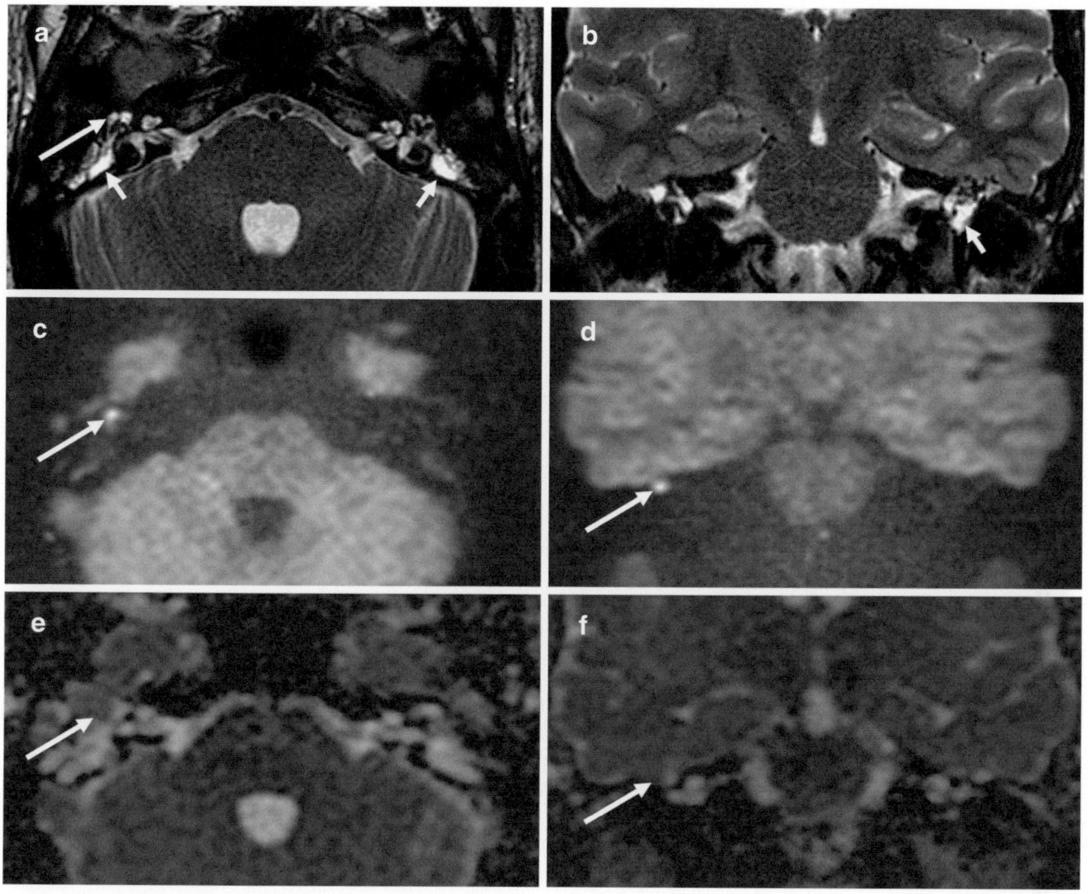

Fig. 7.7 Cholesteatomatous chronic right-sided otomastoiditis and non-cholesteatomatous chronic left-sided otomastoiditis (continued from Fig. 7.6). Due to its better ability to discriminate different soft-tissue components compared to CT scan, MRI is often used as a complementary imaging to CT in the diagnostic evaluation of any clinically suspected cholesteatomas. Cholesteatomas can be defined as enlarging cysts consisting of a wall of stratified squamous epithelium surrounding a collection of keratin debris. They are usually hypointense/isointense on T1-weighted image and hyperintense on T2-weighted image compared with brain tissue, but these characteristics are not specific. On the other hand they show a typical high signal on DWI, which presumably can be partly attributed to restriction of the diffusion of water molecules between the keratinous debris of the cholesteatoma contents. Axial (**a**) and coronal (**b**) TSE T2W images confirm the presence of hyperintense inflammatory tissue (short arrows) affecting the mastoids bilaterally, but since a cholesteatoma (arrow in **a**), which is also typically hyperintense on T2-weighted image, could be hidden inside it, the DWI must also be evaluated. Axial (**c**) and coronal (**d**) b 1000 DWI images passing through the same level demonstrate the presence of a focal signal hyperintensity (arrows) at the transition between the mastoid antrum and the epitympanum on the right side, suggesting the coexistence of a cholesteatoma. Contralaterally, no obvious diffusion alterations are recognized. On axial (**e**) and coronal (**f**) corresponding ADC map images, the small cholesteatoma appears with typical signal hypointensity given by restricted water diffusion (arrows). *CT* computed tomography, *MRI* magnetic resonance imaging, *TSE* turbo spin echo, *DWI* diffusion-weighted imaging, *ADC* apparent diffusion coefficient

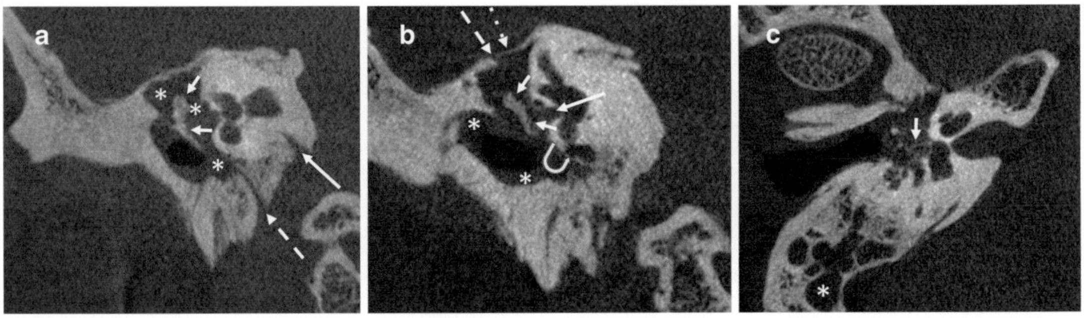

Fig. 7.8 Middle ear atticoantral cholesteatomatous chronic otomastoiditis. (**a**) Coronal CBCT image of the right temporal bone passing through the malleus showing the tympanic cavity entirely obliterated by soft-tissue material of inflammatory significance (asterisks) associated with signs of demineralization and superficial erosion of the malleus (short arrows) affecting its head, neck and manubrium. The tympanic membrane is not recognizable. For educational purposes, the opening of the cochlear aqueduct (arrow) and the inferior tympanic canaliculus (dashed arrow), also referred to as "Jacobson's canal," are illustrated. (**b**) Coronal CBCT image of the right temporal bone passing through the incus demonstrates that this ossicle also shows signs of demineralization and surface erosion (short arrows) affecting its body and the long and the lenticular processes. The tegmen tympani appears thinned (dotted arrow) with small focal interruptions (dashed arrow). The obliteration of the oval window (arrow) and round window niches (curved arrow) are also depicted. Finally, although the EAC appears patent, it is nevertheless affected by a circumferential thickening of its lining epithelium (asterisks). (**c**) Axial CBCT image of the right temporal bone passing through the stapes, which appears to be demineralized in all its portions (short arrow). The obliteration of the mastoid cells is also shown (asterisk). *CBCT* cone beam computed tomography, *EAC* external auditory canal

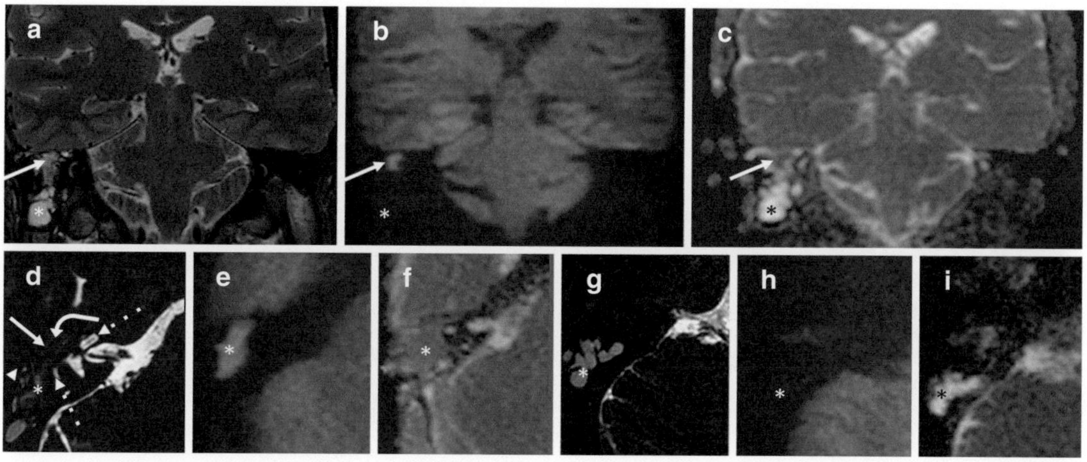

Fig. 7.9 Atticoantral cholesteatoma confirmed on MRI (continued from Fig. 7.8). This represents another example in which diffusion imaging is able to dispel any doubts or suspicions about the presence of a cholesteatoma and to determine how much of the soft-tissue attenuating material actually belongs to a cholesteatoma and how much to tissue of another nature. (**a**–**c**) Coronal MRI images passing through the pontine tegmentum depict the different imaging presentation between the cholesteatomatous tissue and the non-cholesteatomatous inflammatory tissue in the right temporal bone. Caudally the mastoid cells are obliterated by chronic inflammatory effusions showing high hyperintensity on TSE T2W (asterisk in **a**) and free diffusion of water molecules, demonstrated by a hypointense signal on b = 1000 DWI non-EPI (TSE) (asterisk in **b**) and a hyperintense signal on the ADC map (black asterisk in **c**). More cranially, at the level of the posterior portion of the mastoid antrum where the T2 signal appears less hyperintense (arrow in **a**), the cholesteatomatous component is highlighted by a certain restriction of diffusivity supported by marked hyperintensity on DWI (arrow in **b**) and isointensity compared to the brain parenchyma on ADC map (arrow in **c**). (**d**–**f**) Axial MRI images passing through the epitympanum. The cholesteatomatous tissue is indicated by an asterisk on DWI (**e**) and on ADC map (**f**), and, taking advantage of the better anatomical detail of 3D TSE T2W image (**d**), it entirely occupies the mastoid antrum (asterisk in **d**), the aditus ad antrum (arrowhead in **d**), and the epitympanum, including Prussak's space (**d**, arrow) and surrounding the ossicles (**d**, curved arrow) at this level. The structures of the inner ear (dotted arrows in **d**) show regular morphology, without signs of labyrinthine fistulas. (**g**–**i**) Axial MRI images passing through the hypotympanum. At this level the mastoid cells are obliterated by chronic non-cholesteatomatous inflammatory tissue that is highly hyperintense on 3D TSE T2W-sequence (asterisk in **g**) and devoid of diffusion restriction, being hypointense on b = 1000 non-EPI DWI (asterisk in **h**) and hyperintense on ADC map (black asterisk in **i**). Overall, the imaging illustrated the presence of an atticoantral cholesteatoma and describe the typical presentation pattern of cholesteatomas originating from the pars flaccida. When the cholesteatoma occupies Prussak's space and reaches the tegmen tympani, it is important to exclude a possible intracranial extension of the pathology. In this regard, no focal alterations in diffusivity in the adjacent intracranial compartment are recognizable. *MRI* magnetic resonance imaging, *TSE* turbo spin echo, *EPI* echo planar imaging, *DWI* diffusion-weighted imaging, *ADC* apparent diffusion coefficient

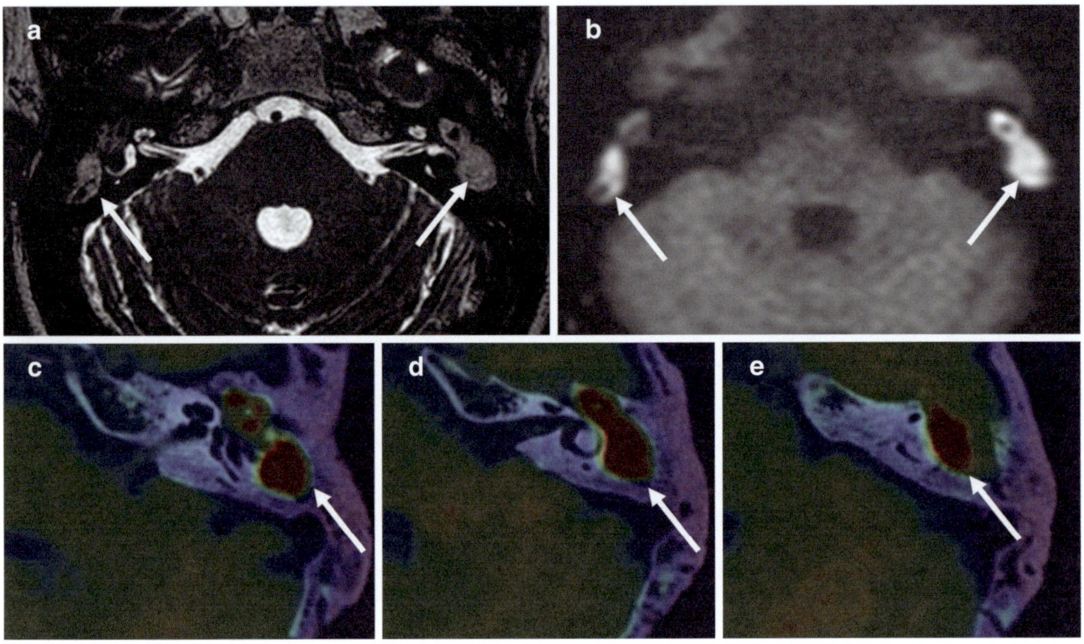

Fig. 7.10 Atticoantral cholesteatoma. MDCT and MRI images can be fused allowing a precise anatomical identification of cholesteatoma within the temporal bone. (**a**) 3D TSE T2W image showing hyperintense tissue in right and left middle ear and antrum (arrows) suspected to be a cholesteatoma. (**b**) Axial DWI image showing that the tissue has diffusion restriction, consistent with cholesteatoma (arrows). (**c**–**e**) Axial images resulting from the fusion of MDCT scan (in grayscale) and DWI non-EPI (TSE) images (in color scale) allow the precise anatomical position of cholesteatomatous tissue shown in red (arrows) in left temporal bone. *MDCT* multidetector computed tomography, *MRI* magnetic resonance imaging, *TSE* turbo spin echo, *DWI* diffusion-weighted imaging, *EPI* echo planar imaging

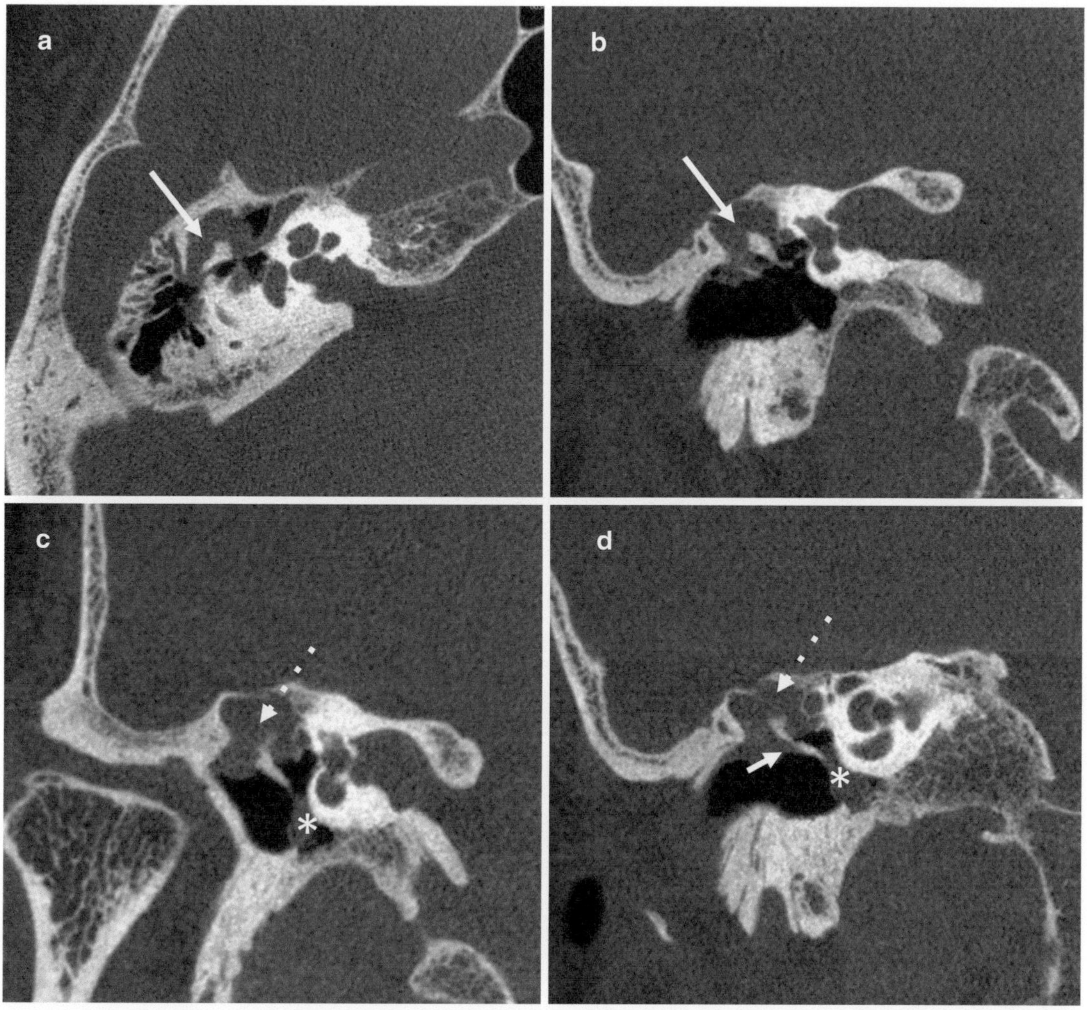

Fig. 7.11 Complications of cholesteatoma: ossicular chain erosion. Ossicular erosion is twice more common in cholesteatoma, in particular in cholesteatoma of pars tensa, than in chronic otitis media. Usually the ossicular chain is spared in less than one third of middle ear cholesteatoma cases. In cholesteatoma arising from the pars tensa, the long process of the incus and the stapes are eroded together with malleus handle. In cholesteatoma arising from the pars flaccida, the long process and body of the incus and the malleus head are typically eroded. Childhood cholesteatoma is more aggressive and causes more frequently ossicular erosion, in particular, of stapes superstructure, compared to adults. (**a**) Axial CBCT image of the right temporal bone in a plane passing through the epitympanum shows a soft-tissue density mass consistent with cholesteatoma surrounding the incus body and the malleus with erosion of both (arrow). (**b**) Coronal CBCT image of the right temporal bone shows a soft-tissue density mass consistent with cholesteatoma in Prussak's space and epitympanum with partial erosion of the body of the incus (arrow). (**c**) Coronal CBCT image of the right temporal bone in a plane passing through the body of the incus shows the presence of a small soft-tissue mass in the meso- and epitympanum consistent with cholesteatoma causing erosion of the head of the malleus (dotted arrow). Aspecific tissue is present into the hypotympanum (asterisk). (**d**) Coronal CBCT image of the right temporal bone in a plane passing through the malleus shows the erosion of the head (dotted arrow) and the handle of the malleus (short arrow). Aspecific tissue is present into the hypotympanum (asterisk). *CBCT* cone beam computed tomography

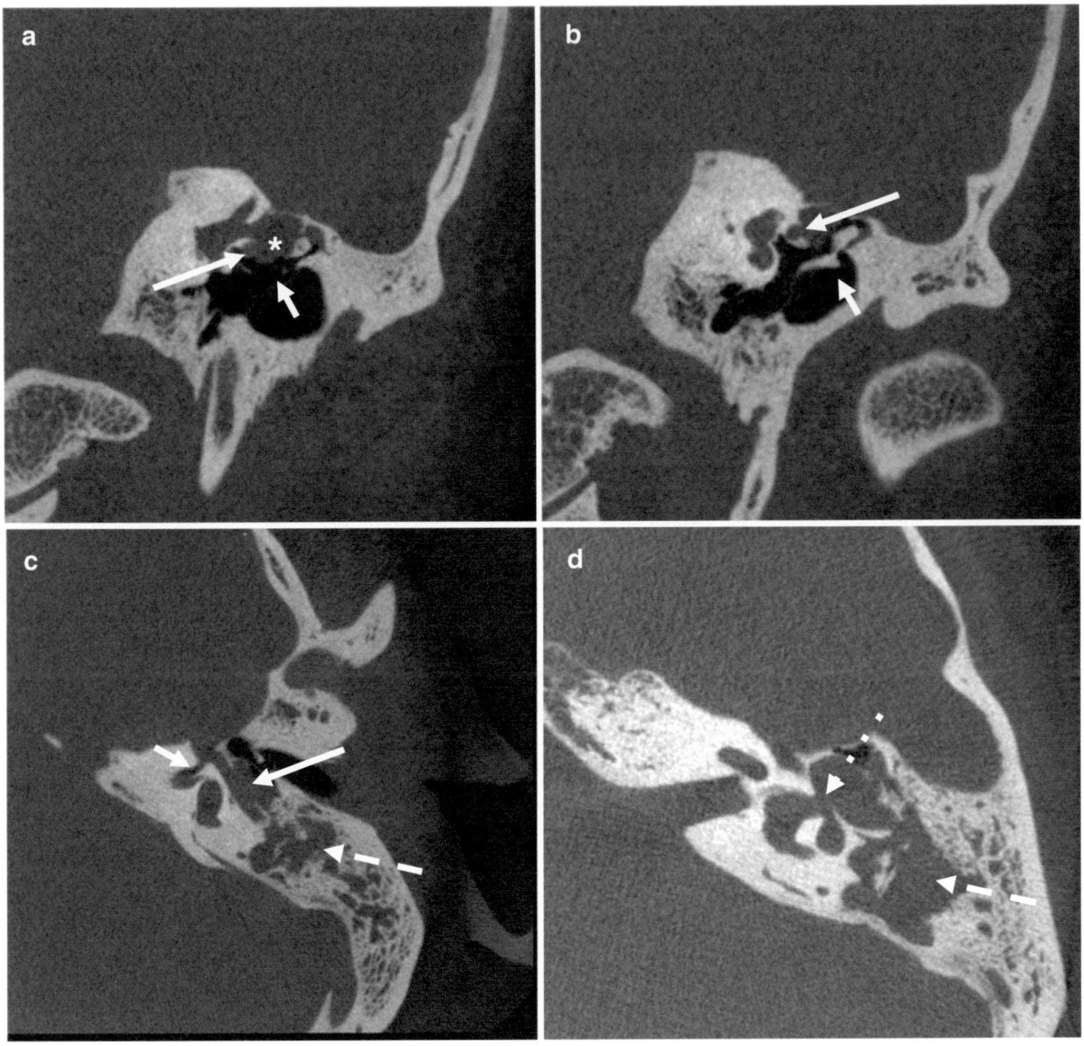

Fig. 7.12 Complications of cholesteatoma: facial nerve canal erosion and labyrinthine fistula. Complications of cholesteatoma are due to bone erosion. Labyrinthine fistula and facial nerve canal erosion are not uncommon. Facial nerve involvement is more often encountered when there is a facial nerve canal erosion, usually occurring at the level of the mid-tympanic segment. It is important to highlight that secondary facial nerve dehiscence may occur after cholesteatoma bone erosion and that it is a predisposing factor to damage of the nerve during surgery. Labyrinthine fistula usually occurs in the lateral semicircular canal, in case of attico-antral cholesteatoma, and less often in the other semicircular canals and cochlea. Cochlea fistula is usually associated with pars tensa cholesteatoma (posterior tympanic) and is usually located in the promontory between the oval and the round window. (**a**) Coronal CBCT image of the left temporal bone in a plane passing through the body of the incus shows the presence of a small soft-tissue mass in the meso- and epitympanum (asterisk) consistent with cholesteatoma. The long process of the incus is absent (short arrow) and probably eroded as well as the tympanic segment of facial nerve canal (arrow). (**b**) Coronal CBCT image of the left temporal bone in a plane passing through the malleus (short arrow) shows the presence of the cholesteatoma that erodes the tympanic segment of facial nerve canal (arrow). (**c**) Axial CBCT image of the left temporal bone in a plane passing through epitympanum shows the cholesteatoma and the erosion of the tympanic segment of facial nerve canal (arrow); the vestibular segment of the facial nerve canal is pointed by the short arrow. Soft-tissue density material is present in the mastoid air cell (dashed arrow). (**d**) Axial CBCT image of the left temporal bone shows the cholesteatoma in the epitympanum and in antrum and the erosion of the wall of ampulla of the lateral semicircular canal consistent with labyrinthine fistula (dotted arrow). Soft-tissue density material is present in the antrum with erosion of the walls of the mastoid air cells (dashed arrow). *CBCT* cone beam computed tomography

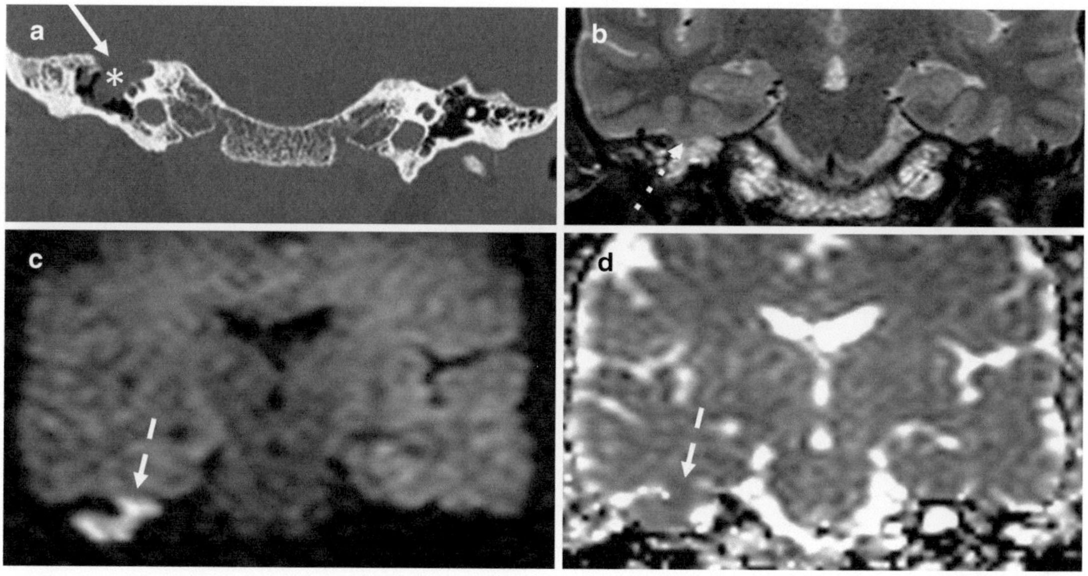

Fig. 7.13 Complications of cholesteatoma: tegmen tympani erosion. The erosion of the tegmen tympani is a complication of cholesteatoma of middle ear and should be always evaluated on coronal images. Through the interruption of the tegmen the cholesteatoma is in direct contact with the meninges of the middle cranial fossa. MRI should be always performed when an erosion of tegmen tympani is detected in order to exclude the presence of meningocele or encephalocele. (**a**) Coronal CT image reveals a soft-tissue mass (asterisk) in middle ear with the erosion of tegmen tympani (arrow). (**b**) T2-weighted coronal image shows hyperintense tissue in middle ear, the interruption of tegmen tympani with the fusiform gyrus (dotted arrow) lying above it. (**c, d**) DWI and ADC images show a diffusion restriction of the tissue consistent with a cholesteatoma (dashed arrow). *MRI* magnetic resonance imaging, *CT* computed tomography, *DWI* diffusion-weighted imaging, *ADC* apparent diffusion coefficient

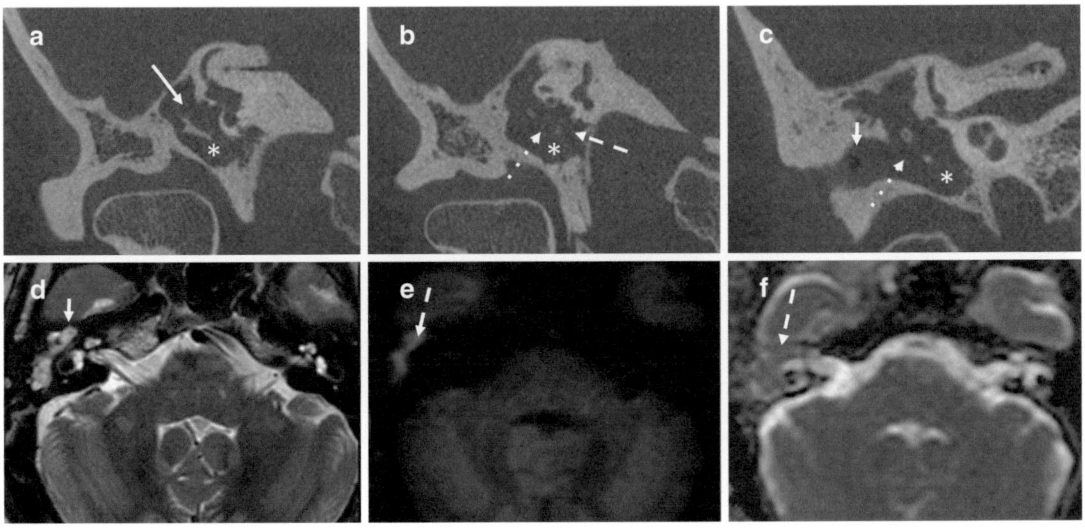

Fig. 7.14 Follow up in postoperative setting after cholesteatoma surgery. MDCT scans do not allow a proper differential diagnosis between different soft-tissue density materials, considering only density characteristics. In post-operative follow-up soft-density tissues can be attributed to inflammation, fibrous and granulation tissue or cholesteatoma. MRI with non-EPI DWI sequences is helpful in the diagnosis of recurrent cholesteatoma, identifying the restriction of the diffusion of water molecules between the keratinous debris of the cholesteatoma content. (**a**) Coronal CBCT image of the right temporal bone in a plane passing through the malleus handle shows soft-tissue density material in the tympanic cavity (asterisk) surrounding the malleus with erosion of the head of malleus (arrow). (**b**) Coronal CBCT image of the right temporal bone in a plane passing through the incudostapedial joint shows soft-tissue density material in the tympanic cavity (asterisk) surrounding the incus and the stapes with erosion of the body of the incus (dotted arrow) and the stapes (dashed arrow). (**c**) Coronal CBCT image of the right temporal bone in a plane passing through the incudostapedial joint shows soft-tissue density material in the EAC (short arrow) and in the tympanic cavity (asterisk) surrounding the incus with erosion of the long process of the incus (dotted arrow). (**d–f**) Axial TSE T2W image, DWI, and ADC axial maps show hyperintense material (short arrow in **a**) in the tympanic cavity and antrum showing diffusion restriction in DWI and ADC images (dashed arrow) consistent with cholesteatoma. *MDCT* multidetector computed tomography, *MRI* magnetic resonance imaging, *EPI* echo planar imaging, *DWI* diffusion-weighted imaging, *CBCT* cone beam computed tomography, *EAC* external auditory canal, *TSE* turbo spin echo, *ADC* apparent diffusion coefficient

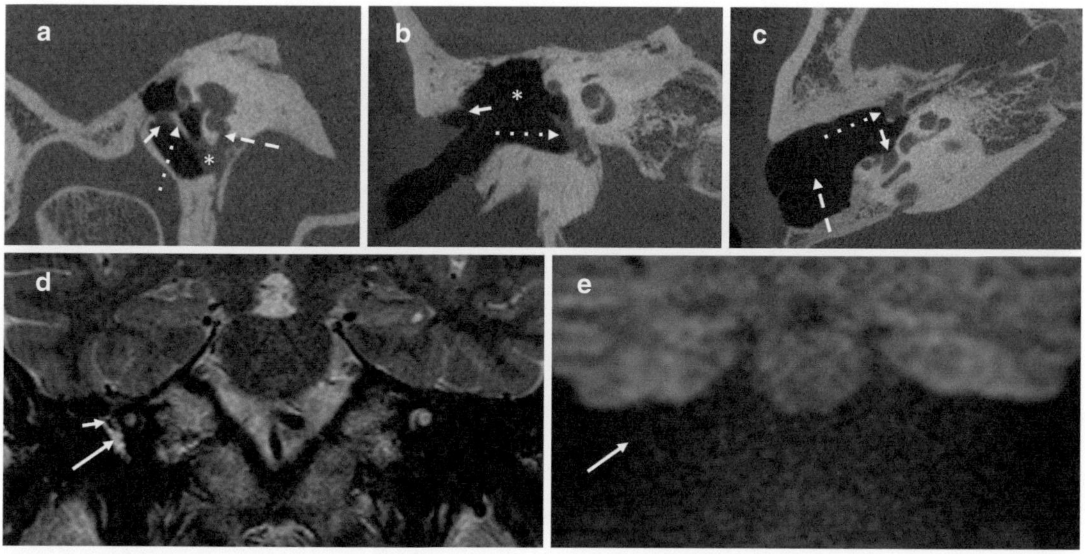

Fig. 7.15 Follow up in postoperative setting after cholesteatoma surgery (continued from Fig. 7.14). CBCT scans of the temporal bone are particularly effective in ruling out the presence of cholesteatoma recurrence. If an abnormal soft-tissue mass is identified, CBCT can raise the suspicion of recurrent cholesteatoma. If the tympanic cavity and mastoid are well ventilated without any tissue, it is unlikely that a recurrence has occurred. Vice versa, diagnosing cholesteatoma recurrence in a patient who has undergone surgery and presents with a poorly aerated middle ear due to extensive soft-tissue opacities poses significant diagnostic challenges. This situation may benefit from performing an MRI with the use of non-EPI DWI sequences, which are helpful in identifying even small areas of diffusion restrictions caused by cholesteatoma recurrences. In this series of images the patient suffering from cholesteatoma described in Fig. 7.13 has undergone a canal wall down mastoidectomy which involves the removal of the mastoid cortex and the air cells and resection of the posterosuperior bony wall of the EAC and the scutum. This type of surgery is more invasive than canal wall up mastoidectomy, which is aimed at preserving the posterosuperior wall of the EAC, but ensures a lower risk of cholesteatoma recurrence. The tympanic membrane was repaired using tissue from temporalis fascia. (**a**) Coronal CBCT reformatted image of the right temporal bone passing through the malleus handle shows the results of partial surgical demolition of the eroded residual ossicular chain, with exclusive sparing of part of the malleus handle (dotted arrow) which is attached to the neomembrane. After surgery the neo-tympanum is partially aerated, and residual soft-tissue density material is recognized laterally to the manubrium of malleus (short arrow) and in the mesial retrotympanum (asterisk) where it obliterates the niche of the round window (dashed arrow). (**b**) Coronal CBCT image of the right temporal bone passing through a more posterior plane shows that the soft-tissue density material also occupies part of the hypotympanum (dotted arrow). The large surgical cavity (asterisk) that remains after the removal of the mastoid cells and the scutum (short arrow) in association with the removal of the cholesteatomatous tissue is depicted. (**c**) Axial CBCT image of the right temporal bone depicts the results of removal of the posterior bony wall of the EAC (dashed arrow). Soft-tissue density material of dubious significance is also recognizable anterior to the manubrium of malleus (dotted arrow) and in the sinus tympani (short arrow). Since the presence of a recurrence of cholesteatoma could not be excluded, an MRI of the temporal bones was performed. (**d, e**) Coronal MR images passing through the malleus handle (short arrow in **d**) which confirm the presence of hyperintense material on TSE T2W image inside the neo-tympanum (arrow in **d**). However, this finding is consistent with the presence of non-cholesteatomatous inflammatory tissue since it is not characterized by pathological restriction of diffusion on TSE DWI (arrow in **e**). A recurrence of cholesteatoma can therefore be excluded. *CBCT* cone bean computed tomography, *EAC* external auditory canal, *MRI* magnetic resonance imaging, *TSE* turbo spin echo, *EPI* echo planar imaging, *DWI* diffusion-weighted imaging, *ADC* apparent diffusion coefficient

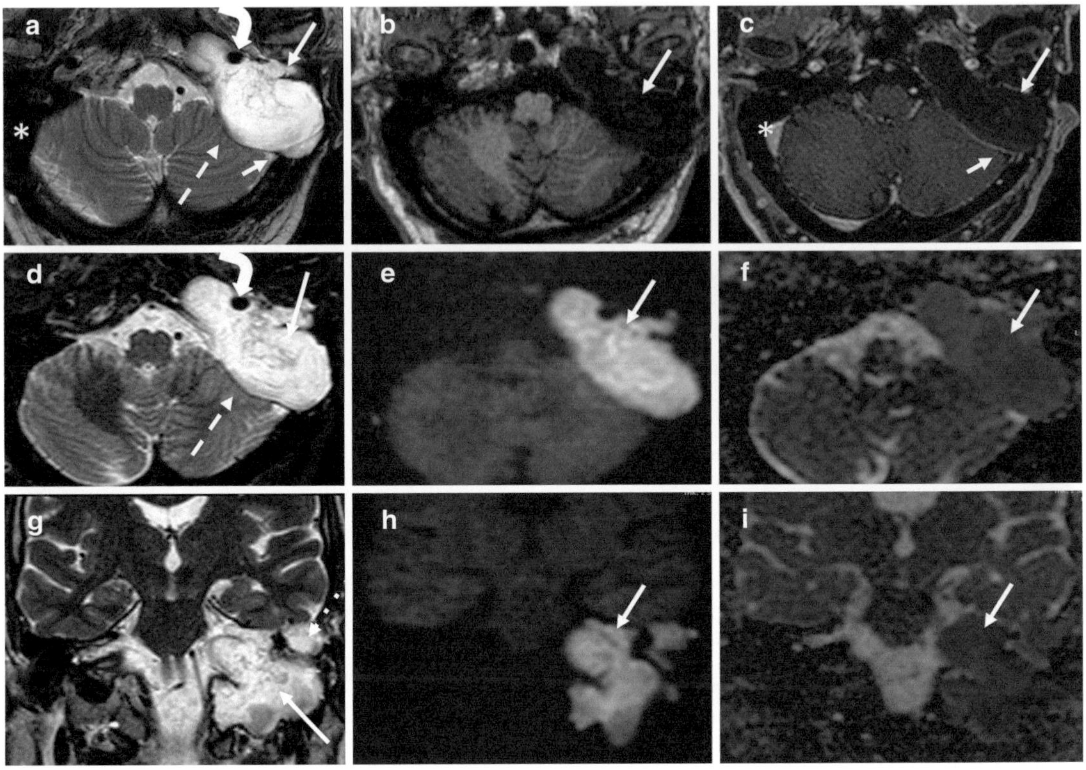

Fig. 7.16 **Invasiveness and recurrence of cholesteatoma**. Cholesteatoma is characterized by bone erosion that leads to remodeling of the temporal bone cavities. Factors involved in bone erosion are several: mechanical, due to the expansion of keratin debris; biochemical, due to endotoxins and inflammation; and cellular, due to osteoclast activity. The bone erosion leads to complicated cholesteatomas with ossicular and facial nerve canal erosion, labyrinthine fistula, and extension to petrous apex and automastoidectomy, when the outer walls of mastoid are involved. Acquired cholesteatoma quite rarely extends to the petrous apex; therefore, alternative diagnoses should be taken into account. Contrast-enhanced MRI may help in the differential diagnosis as aggressive tumors typically enhance while cholesteatoma does not. (**a**–**i**) Axial MRI images of a patient that previously underwent surgical intervention for the removal of left middle ear and mastoid cholesteatoma showing a large recurrence of cholesteatoma invading the petrous bone and the middle and posterior cranial fossae. The TSE T2W axial (**a**, **d**) and coronal (**g**), the unenhanced TSE T1W axial (**b**), and the gadolinium-enhanced TSE T1W axial (**c**) images show the extensive soft-tissue mass (arrow) in the left temporal bone invading the intracranial compartment where the lesion occupies the cerebellopontine angle with compression of cerebellum (dashed arrow in **a**, **d**) as well as the EAC (dotted arrow in **g**). The lesion involves the left internal carotid artery with preserved flow void signal on TSE T2W images (curved arrow in **a**, **d**) and compresses the left transverse dural sinus (short arrow in **a**, **c**). The contralateral normal transverse dural sinus, indicated by the asterisk, is characterized by flow void signal in T2-weighted images (**a**) and contrast medium filling in enhanced T1-weighted images (**c**). The mass shows mixed high signal on T2-weighted images and low signal on T1-weighted images and no gadolinium enhancement. Axial ADC (**f**) and DWI maps (**e**) and coronal ADC (**i**) and DWI (**h**) maps demonstrate high signal on DWI maps (**f**, **h**) and low signal on ADC maps (**e**, **g**) within the mass confirming the suspicion of cholesteatoma recurrence (arrow). *MRI* magnetic resonance imaging, *TSE* turbo spin echo, *EAC* external auditory canal, *ADC* apparent diffusion coefficient, *DWI* diffusion-weighted imaging, *TSE* turbo spin echo

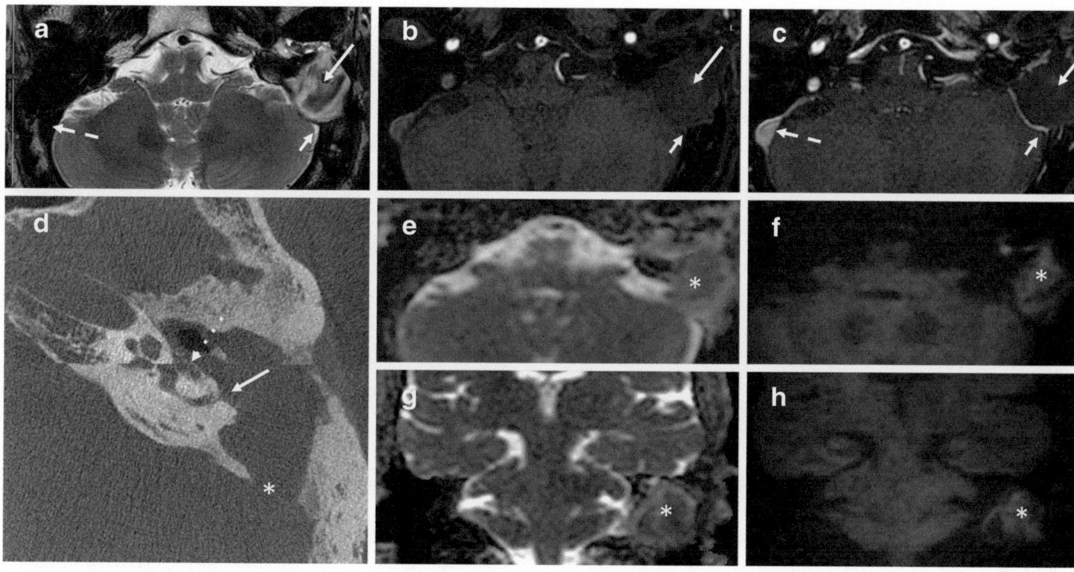

Fig. 7.17 Recurrence of cholesteatoma and intracranial invasion. (**a**–**c**) Axial MRI images of a patient that previously underwent surgical intervention for the removal of left middle ear and mastoid cholesteatoma. The TSE T2W axial (**a**), the unenhanced TSE T1W axial (**b**), and the gadolinium enhanced TSE T1W axial (**c**) images show an extensive soft-tissue mass (arrows in **a**, **b**, and **c**) in the temporal bone surgical cavity with intracranial invasion. The mass compresses the transverse dural sinus (small arrows in **a**, **b**, and **c**). The contralateral normal transverse dural sinus is indicated by dashed arrows and characterized by flow void signal in T2-weighted images (**a**) and contrast medium filling in enhanced T1-weighted images (**c**). The mass shows mixed signal on T2-weighted images and low signal on T1-weighted images and no gadolinium enhancement. (**d**) Axial CBCT image of the left temporal bone in a plane passing through the vestibulum shows the presence of an extensive soft-tissue mass in the surgical cavity eroding the walls of the tympanic cavity, in particular, the tympanic segment of facial nerve canal (dotted arrow) and the lateral semicircular canal (arrow) causing labyrinth fistula and extending in the posterior fossa (asterisk). The mass is suspected to be a recurrence of cholesteatoma. (**e**, **f**, **g**, **h**) Axial ADC (**e**) and DWI maps (**f**) and coronal ADC (**g**) and DWI (**h**) maps from TSE DWI images confirmed the suspicion of cholesteatoma as the mass has high signal on DWI maps (**f**, **h**) and low signal on ADC maps (**e**, **g**) consistent with diffusion restriction (asterisks). *MRI* magnetic resonance imaging, *TSE* turbo spin echo, *CBCT* cone beam computed tomography, *MRI* magnetic resonance imaging, *DWI* diffusion-weighted imaging, *ADC* apparent diffusion coefficient

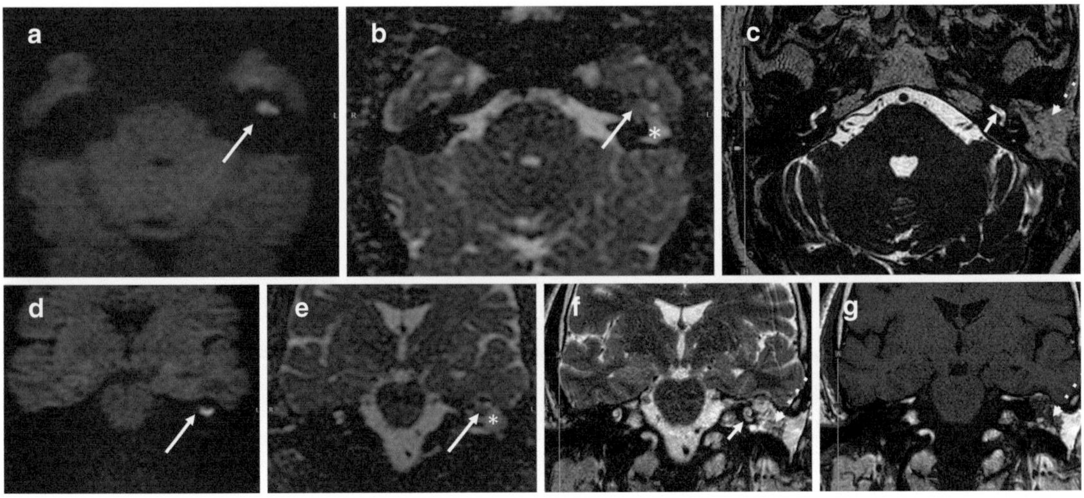

Fig. 7.18 Recurrence of cholesteatoma (continued from Fig. 7.17). MRI images of the same case as that of Fig. 7.17 show the second recurrence of cholesteatoma after second surgery. Diffusion images allow the identification of a small recurrence of cholesteatoma within the inflammatory and postsurgical tissues that occupy the surgical cavity. For this reason MRI with DWI non-EPI sequences is the gold standard imaging technique in the follow-up of patients operated for cholesteatoma. Axial DWI (**a**) and ADC (**b**) maps from TSE DWI images depict the presence of a small lesion with high signal on DWI maps and low signal on ADC maps (arrow in **a**, **b**) consistent with cholesteatoma recurrence within inflammatory tissue that does not show diffusion restriction (asterisk in **b** and **d**). The suspicion of cholesteatoma should be confirmed by the finding of diffusion restriction in both axial and coronal planes (arrows in **d**, **e**). (**c**) Axial 3D TSE T2W image shows the temporal bone surgical cavity filled by inflammatory and postsurgical tissue (dotted arrow). The basal turn of the cochlea is indicated by short arrow. Coronal DWI (**d**) and ADC (**e**) maps from TSE DWI images depict the presence of a small lesion with high signal on DWI maps and low signal on ADC maps (arrow) consistent with cholesteatoma recurrence within inflammatory tissue that does not show diffusion restriction (asterisk in **e**). (**f**, **g**) Coronal TSE T2W and unenhanced TSE T1W images show the temporal bone surgical cavity filled by inflammatory and postsurgical tissue (dotted arrows). The cochlea is indicated by short arrow. *MRI* magnetic resonance imaging, *DWI* diffusion-weighted imaging, *EPI* echo planar imaging, *TSE* turbo spin echo, *ADC* apparent diffusion coefficient

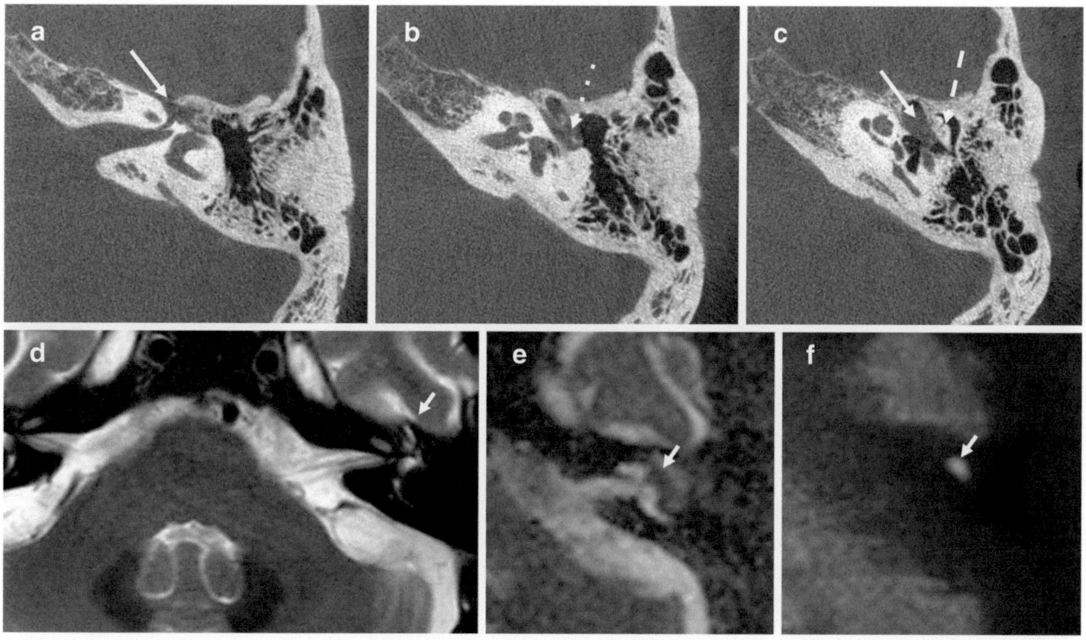

Fig. 7.19 **Geniculate fossa cholesteatoma.** Middle ear cholesteatomas may erode into the facial nerve canal, in particular, the tympanic segment, reaching the geniculate fossa. Rarely cholesteatomas develop in the anterior epitympanic space (the epitympanum anteriorly to the malleus head), and as a consequence the invasion of geniculate fossa and the involvement of the facial nerve at level of the geniculate ganglion are quite common. (**a–c**) Axial CBCT images of the left temporal bone in a plane passing through the epitympanum show the presence of a soft-tissue mass in epitympanum (arrow in **c**) eroding the wall of the tympanic segment of facial nerve canal (dotted arrow in **b**) and extending in the geniculate fossa that is enlarged (arrow in **a**). The mass is located medially to the incudomalleolar joint (dashed arrow in **c**). The mass is suspected to be a cholesteatoma. (**d–f**) Axial MRI images passing through the plane of the internal auditory canal confirm the presence of the soft-tissue mass in the epitympanum. The TSE T2W axial image (**d**) shows the small mass close to geniculate fossa (**d**, short arrow), and the TSE DWI images (**e, f**) confirmed the suspicion of cholesteatoma showing high signal on DWI (**f**) and low signal on ADC maps (**e**) consistent with diffusion restriction. (short arrows in **e, f**). *CBCT* cone beam computed tomography, *MRI* magnetic resonance imaging, *TSE* turbo spin echo, *DWI* diffusion-weighted imaging, *ADC* apparent diffusion coefficient

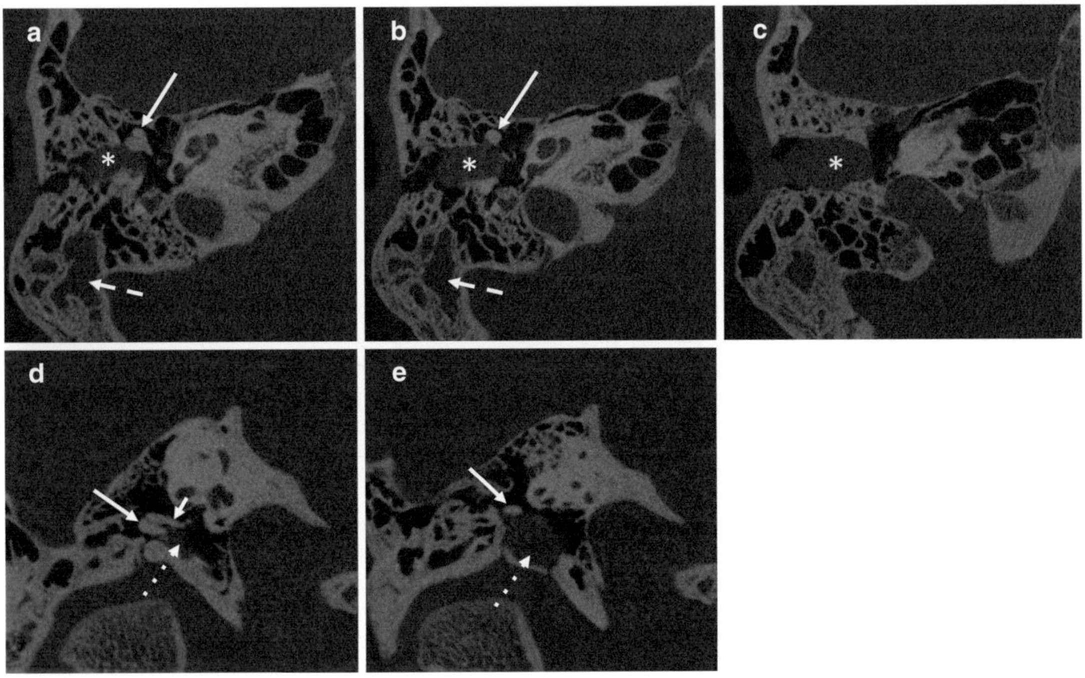

Fig. 7.20 Incomplete external auditory canal atresia and recurrence of external auditory canal cholesteatoma. EAC atresia or congenital aural atresia is a complete or incomplete narrowing of bony EAC. It is often isolated but can be depicted in syndromic cases. In case of incomplete bony atresia, the EAC may be further narrowed by soft tissue (membranous EAC atresia). EAC atresia can be complicated by the formation of a congenital cholesteatoma behind the atresia plate. EAC atresia or congenital aural atresia is a complete or incomplete narrowing of bony EAC. It is more often monolateral but can be bilateral. It is often isolated but can be depicted in syndromic cases (Crouzon, Goldenhar, Pierre Robin, and Treacher Collins syndromes) in which the malformation is more severe than in isolated cases. In case of incomplete bony atresia, the EAC may be further narrowed by soft tissue (membranous EAC atresia). EAC atresia is often associated with a dysplastic auricle and malformation of middle ear cavity and ossicles due to common embryologic origin of the external and middle ear. On the contrary the internal ear and the internal auditory canal are usually normal because of their earlier embryological formation. EAC atresia can be complicated by the formation of a congenital cholesteatoma behind the atresia plate. (**a**–**c**) Axial CBCT image of the right temporal bone passing through the mesotympanum shows a case of incomplete bony atresia of EAC that was previously surgically reconstructed with the formation of a new EAC and a new tympanic membrane. In the new EAC a mass with ovalar shape is depicted (asterisk), suspected to be a cholesteatoma. The mass displaces the ossicle, in particular, the incus, medially and anteriorly (arrow). The incus and the malleus are dysmorphic. Some mastoid air cells are obliterated by inflammatory soft-tissue material (dashed arrow). (**d**, **e**) Coronal CBCT image of the right temporal bone passing through the tympanic cavity shows the small mass with ovalar shape (dotted arrow) in the EAC that protrudes in the middle ear close to the head of the malleus (arrow) and the long process and the body of the incus (short arrow). The suspicion about the presence of an underlying cholesteatoma should lead to consider further investigation with MRI to confirm the diagnosis (see Fig. 7.21). *EAC* external auditory canal, *CBCT* cone beam computed tomography, *MRI* magnetic resonance imaging

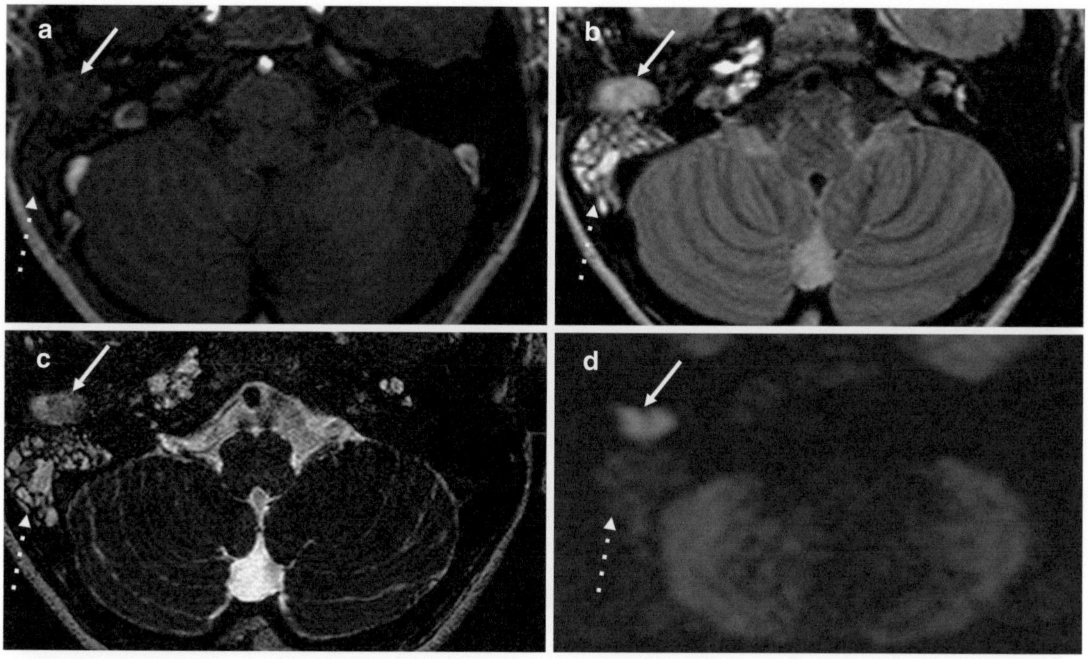

Fig. 7.21 Incomplete external auditory canal atresia and recurrence of external auditory canal cholesteatoma. Continues from Fig. 7.20. (**a–d**) Axial MRI images passing through the plane of EAC show a case of incomplete bony atresia of EAC that was previously surgically reconstructed and complicated by the recurrence of a cholesteatoma in the EAC. In TSE T1W (**a**), TSE T2W (**b**), and 3D TSE T2W (**c**) axial images, a T2 hyperintense and T1 hypointense mass with ovalar shape is depicted (arrow). The TSE DWI image (**d**) confirms the suspicion of cholesteatoma showing high signal consistent with diffusion restriction due to the keratinous debris of the cholesteatoma contents. MRI images confirmed the presence of inflammatory soft-tissue material (dotted arrow) in mastoid air cells; inflammatory tissue is hyperintense in T2-weighted images but does not show diffusion restriction in DWI images. *EAC* external auditory canal, *MRI* magnetic resonance imaging, *TSE* turbo spin echo, *DWI* diffusion-weighted imaging, *ADC* apparent diffusion coefficient

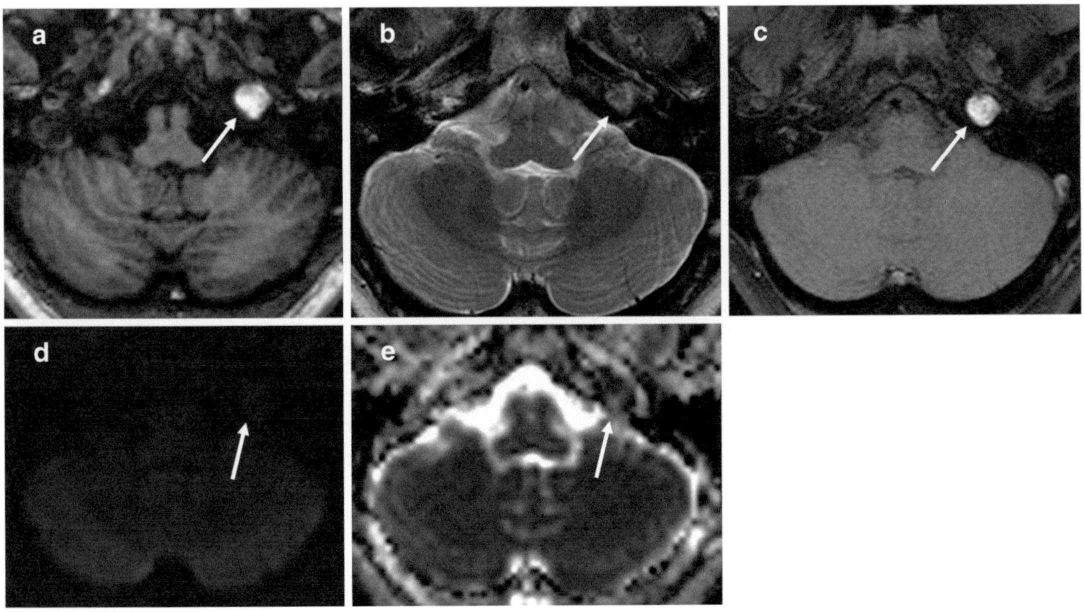

Fig. 7.22 Temporal bone cholesterol granuloma. On CT images the differential diagnosis between cholesteatoma, typical inflammatory granulomatous tissue and CG is not possible. MRI may help in the diagnosis as CG is typically hyperintense in T1 images, also with fat suppression, while typical granulomatous tissue and cholesteatoma are not. Usually CG does not show diffusion restriction. (**a**–**e**) Axial MR images of CG of left petrous apex. Axial unenhanced TSE T1W image (**a**), TSE T2W image (**b**), unenhanced TSE T1W image with fat suppression (**c**), DWI (**d**), and ADC axial images (**e**). On T1-weighted unenhanced images (**a** and **c**) a small hyperintense mass is depicted in petrous apex, consistent with CG (arrows). The CG has mixed signal in T2 with some hypointense components due to hemosiderin content (**b**). On DWI images no signs of diffusion restriction are depicted (isointense signal on DWI maps (**d**) and predominantly hyperintense signal in ADC maps (**e**). *CG* cholesterol granuloma, *MRI* magnetic resonance imaging, *TSE* turbo spin echo, *DWI* diffusion-weighted imaging, *ADC* apparent diffusion coefficient

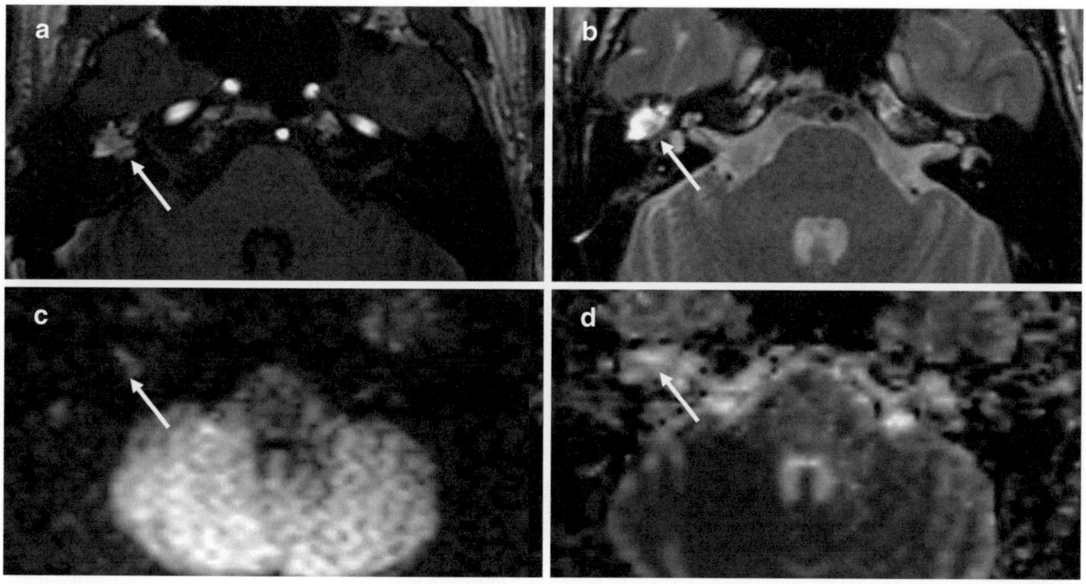

Fig. 7.23 Temporal bone cholesterol granuloma. Another case of temporal bone cholesterol granuloma. (**a–d**) Axial MRI images of CG of right petrous apex. Axial unenhanced TSE T1W image (**a**), TSE T2W image (**b**), TSE DWI (**c**), and ADC axial images (**d**). On T1-weighted unenhanced image (**a**) a small hyperintense mass is depicted in petrous apex, consistent with CG (arrow). The CG has mixed signal in T2 mainly hyperintense (**b**). On DWI images no signs of diffusion restriction are depicted (**c**) and predominantly hyperintense signal in ADC maps (**d**). *CG* cholesterol granuloma, *MRI* magnetic resonance imaging, *TSE* turbo spin echo, *DWI* diffusion-weighted imaging, *ADC* apparent diffusion coefficient

References

Lemmerling MM, De Foer B, Verbist BM, VandeVyver V. Imaging of inflammatory and infectious diseases in the temporal bone. Neuroimaging Clin N Am. 2009;19(3):321–37. https://doi.org/10.1016/j.nic.2009.06.006.

Campion T, Taranath A, Pinelli L, Ugga L, Nash R, Talenti G, Dahmoush H, D'Arco F. Imaging of temporal bone inflammations in children: a pictorial review. Neuroradiology. 2019;61(9):959–70. https://doi.org/10.1007/s00234-019-02258-1. Epub 2019 Jul 18. PMID: 31321462.

Bauer PW, Brown KR, Jones DT. Mastoid subperiosteal abscess management in children. Int J Pediatr Otorhinolaryngol. 2002;63(3):185–8. https://doi.org/10.1016/s0165-5876(02)00006-x.

Swartz JD, Wolfson RJ, Marlowe FI, Popky GL. Postinflammatory ossicular fixation: CT analysis with surgical correlation. Radiology. 1985;154(3):697–700. https://doi.org/10.1148/radiology.154.3.3918333.

Swartz JD. Cholesteatomas of the middle ear. Diagnosis, etiology, and complications. Radiol Clin North Am. 1984;22(1):15–35.

Baráth K, Huber AM, Stämpfli P, Varga Z, Kollias S. Neuroradiology of cholesteatomas. AJNR Am J Neuroradiol. 2011;32(2):221–9. https://doi.org/10.3174/ajnr.A2052. Epub 2010 Apr 1. PMID: 20360335; PMCID: PMC7965719

Lingam RK, Nash R, Majithia A, Kalan A, Singh A. Non-echoplanar diffusion weighted imaging in the detection of post-operative middle ear cholesteatoma: navigating beyond the pitfalls to find the pearl. Insights Imaging. 2016;7(5):669–78. https://doi.org/10.1007/s13244-016-0516-3. Epub 2016 Aug 24. PMID: 27558789; PMCID: PMC5028345.

Gulati M, Gupta S, Prakash A, Garg A, Dixit R. HRCT imaging of acquired cholesteatoma: a pictorial review. Insights Imaging. 2019;10(1):92. https://doi.org/10.1186/s13244-019-0782-y. PMID: 31578644; PMCID: PMC6775179.

Pisaneschi MJ, Langer B. Congenital cholesteatoma and cholesterol granuloma of the temporal bone: role of magnetic resonance imaging. Top Magn Reson Imaging. 2000;11(2):87–97. https://doi.org/10.1097/00002142-200004000-00004.

Razek AA, Huang BY. Lesions of the petrous apex: classification and findings at CT and MR imaging. Radiographics. 2012;32(1):151–73. https://doi.org/10.1148/rg.321105758.

Jackson R, Addison AB, Prinsley PR. Cholesteatoma in children and adults: are there really any differences? J Laryngol Otol. 2018;132(7):575–8. https://doi.org/10.1017/S0022215118000890. Epub 2018 Jun 18. PMID: 29909808.

Otosclerosis

8

Guido Del Vecchio, Luca Caschera,
Giorgia Schiraldi, Roberto Cintioli, Giorgio Conte,
Antonia Valentina Genovese, Fabio Triulzi,
Diego Zanetti, Lorenzo Maria Gaini, and Elisa Scola

Otosclerosis (OS) is a primary disease of the otic capsule bone that leads to progressive conductive hearing loss, despite a normal tympanic membrane and no evidence of middle ear inflammation [1]. It is more commonly bilateral and typically occurs between the second and fourth decades of life [2].

The main symptom is conductive hearing loss, which can progress to mixed or sensorineural hearing loss (SNHL) as the disease advances.

The diagnosis of OS is traditionally based on clinical grounds and is often supported by audiometric findings [3]. High-resolution CT is the imaging modality of choice for the diagnosis. It is essential for preoperative evaluation, as it helps define the extent of bone involvement and prevent surgical complications.

OS involves the middle layer of the otic capsule and progresses through two phases [3]:

1. In the vascular phase (i.e., otospongiosis), the dense middle layer of endochondral bone is resorbed and replaced by spongy, vascular bone, seen as areas of reduced bone density.
2. In the sclerotic phase, as the disease progresses or becomes inactive, the "spongy" areas recalcify, becoming less vascular and more dense and sclerotic. This phase could be misinterpreted, and irregular bone contours are key to making an accurate diagnosis.

G. Del Vecchio (✉) · L. Caschera · A. V. Genovese
E. Scola
Neuroradiology Unit, Fondazione IRCCS Ca' Granda
Ospedale Maggiore Policlinico, Milan, Italy
e-mail: guido.delvecchio@policlinico.mi.it;
luca.caschera@policlinico.mi.it;
valentina.genovese@policlinico.mi.it;
elisa.scola@policlinico.mi.it

G. Schiraldi · R. Cintioli
Postgraduate School in Radiodiagnostics, Università
degli Studi di Milano, Milan, Italy
e-mail: giorgia.schiraldi@unimi.it;
roberto.cintioli@unimi.it

G. Conte · F. Triulzi
Neuroradiology Unit, Fondazione IRCCS Ca' Granda
Ospedale Maggiore Policlinico, Milan, Italy

Department of Pathophysiology and Transplantation,
University of Milan, Milan, Italy
e-mail: giorgio.conte@policlinico.mi.it;
fabio.triulzi@policlinico.mi.it

D. Zanetti
Audiology Unit, Fondazione IRCCS Ca' Granda
Ospedale Maggiore Policlinico, Milan, Italy

Department of Clinical Sciences and Community
Health University of Milan, Milan, Italy
e-mail: diego.zanetti@policlinico.mi.it

L. M. Gaini
Department of Otolaryngology and Head and Neck
Surgery, Fondazione IRCCS Ca' Granda Ospedale
Maggiore Policlinico, Milan, Italy
e-mail: lorenzo.gaini@policlinico.mi.it

G. Conte et al. (eds.), *Atlas of Normal and Pathological Findings in Otoneuroradiology*,
https://doi.org/10.1007/978-3-032-08232-9_8

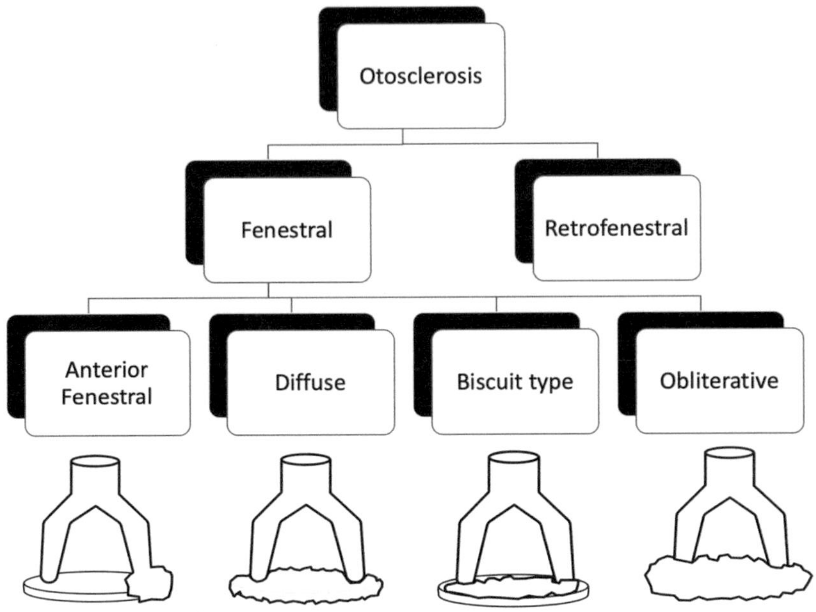

Fig. 8.1 Otosclerosis classification. OS can be divided in fenestral OS which is the most prevalent form, primarily affecting the stapes footplate and leading to conductive hearing loss, and retrofenestral (or cochlear) OS which is less common and usually associated with fenestral OS. Fenestral OS based on extension of the disease can be divided in anterior fenestral, diffuse, biscuit type, and obliterative OS. *Abbreviation:* OS = otosclerosis

The disease initially involves the embryologic *fissula ante fenestram*, a thin fold located just anterior to the oval window, composed of embryonic cartilage and connective tissue.

OS can be categorized in [3, 4] (Fig. 8.1):

- *Fenestral Otosclerosis:* it is the most prevalent form, primarily affecting the stapes footplate and leading to conductive hearing loss. HRCT shows either hypodense (spongiotic) or hyperdense (sclerotic) changes surrounding the oval window, typically located in the *fissula ante fenestram* region. These changes may result in thickening of the stapes footplate or alterations in the round or oval windows, such as decalcification, narrowing or enlargement. In 2% of cases, thickened bony plaques can completely close the oval window, a condition known as obliterative fenestral otosclerosis. These findings must be mentioned in the report because they may reduce the efficacy of stapedectomy (Figs. 8.2, 8.3, 8.4, 8.5, 8.6).
- *Retrofenestral* (or Cochlear) *Otosclerosis*: it is less common and rarely occurs as an isolated entity; it is often associated with fenestral OS [2] (Fig. 8.7). It manifests as SNHL or mixed hearing loss (MHL), with some patients also experiencing vestibular symptoms [2]. CT reveals hypoattenuating spongiotic bone in the endochondral layer of the otic capsule, particularly in the pericochlear region, characterized by a hypodense double ring or "halo" around the cochlea (also known as the fourth ring of Valvassori) [5]. The disease may extend to involve the vestibule, semicircular canals and internal auditory canal. Additionally, demineralization can affect the round window, tympanic canal of the facial nerve and cochlear promontory. The promontory may appear pink when observed through the tympanic membrane, referred to as the Schwartze sign (Figs. 8.8, 8.9, 8.10, 8.11, 8.12, 8.13, 8.14, 8.15).

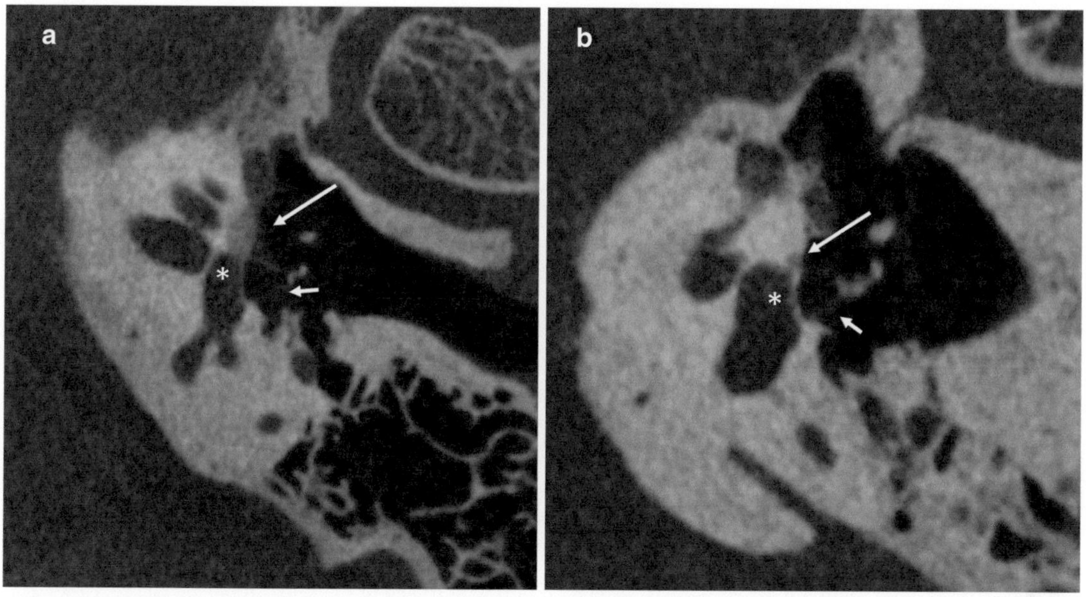

Fig. 8.2 **Fenestral otosclerosis.** Fenestral otosclerosis is the most prevalent form. It is typically located in the fissula ante fenestram region. (**a** and **b**) Demineralized otosclerotic foci are best seen on axial CBCT because of the anteroposterior orientation of the oval window (asterisk) and stapes crura (short arrow). Axial reformatted CBCT images from two different cases showing a hypodense demineralized plaque (arrow) in the region of the fissula ante fenestram. *Abbreviation:* CBCT = cone beam computed tomography

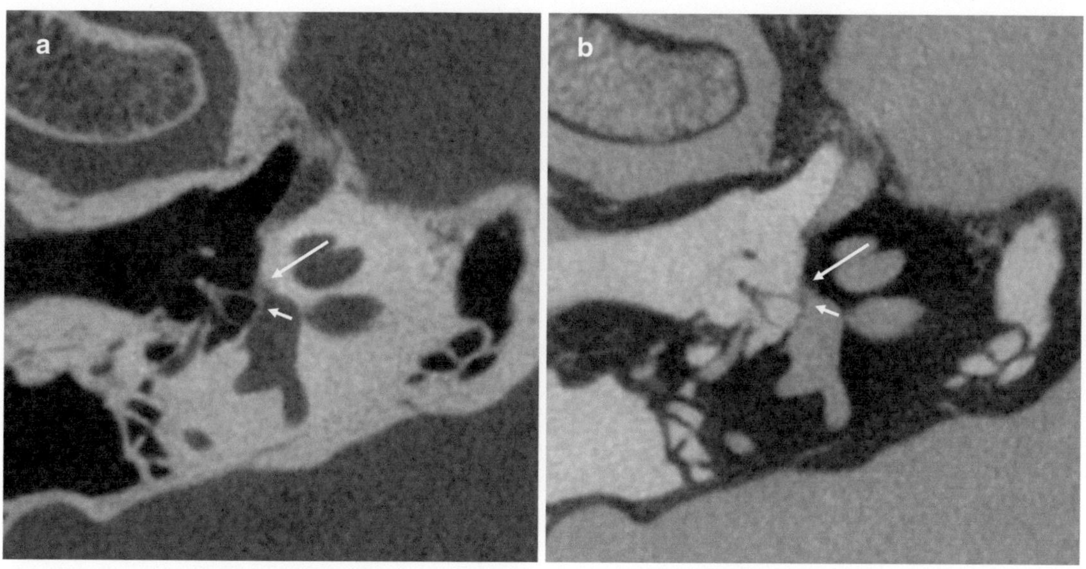

Fig. 8.3 **Anterior fenestral otosclerosis.** The anterior fenestral otosclerosis is characterized by the unique involvement of the anterior footplate rim of the oval window. (**a**) Axial reformatted CBCT shows a hypodense demineralized plaque (arrow) involving the fissula ante fenestram and the anterior stapedio-oval joint. The anterior portion of the footplate is thickened and hypodense (short arrow). (**b**) Axial reformatted CBCT with inverted grayscale allows a better detection of the demineralized plaque. *Abbreviation:* CBCT = cone beam computed tomography

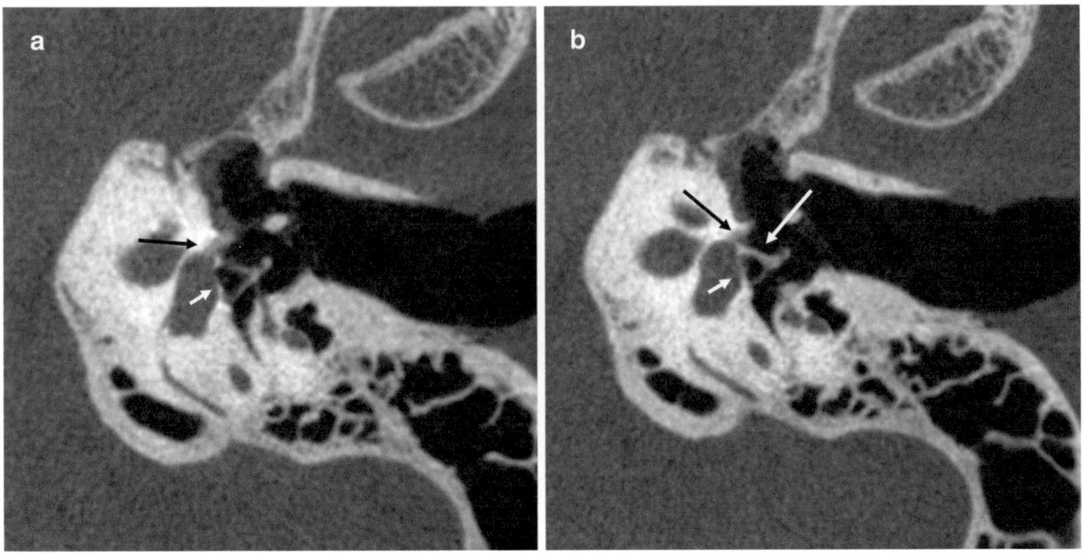

Fig. 8.4 **Biscuit-type footplate osteosclerosis.** It represents the involvement of the stapes footplate with a well-delimited rim. (**a** and **b**) Axial reformatted CBCT images show the thickening of the anterior stapedial crura (white arrow in **b**) and of the stapes footplate (short arrow). It is also noted a focus of demineralized otosclerosis in the fissula ante fenestram (black arrow). *Abbreviation:* CBCT = cone beam computed tomography

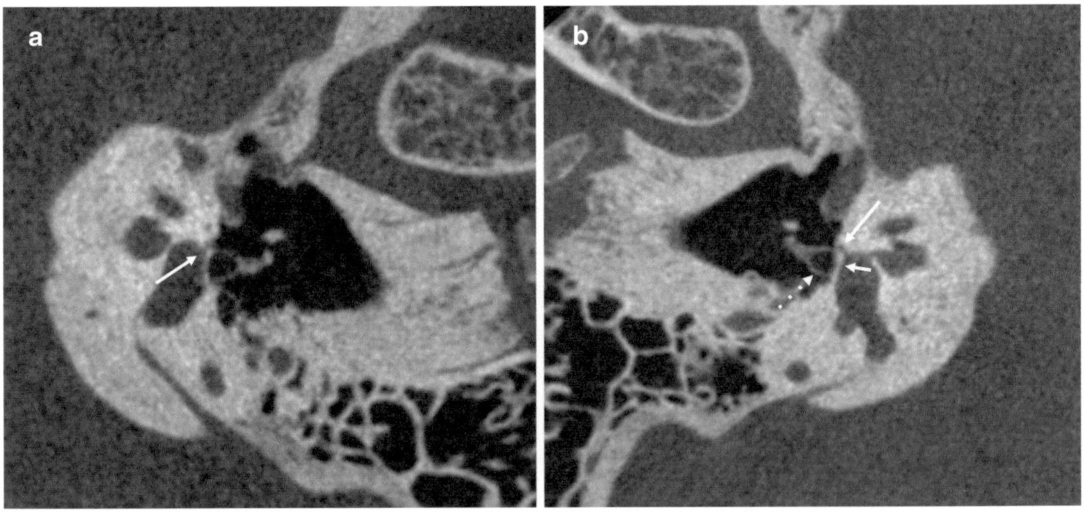

Fig. 8.5 **Diffuse fenestral otosclerosis.** It represents the involvement of the stapes footplate, of the anterior crura and posterior crura. (**a**) Axial reformatted CBCT image shows a "dot-like" area of demineralized otosclerosis in the region of the fissula ante fenestram (arrow). (**b**) Axial reformatted CBCT image shows thickening and sclerosis of the stapes footplate (short arrow) and of the anterior and posterior crura (dotted arrow). A small area of demineralized otosclerosis is evident in the region of the fissula ante fenestram, adjacent to the anterior portion of the stapes footplate (arrow). *Abbreviation:* CBCT = cone beam computed tomography

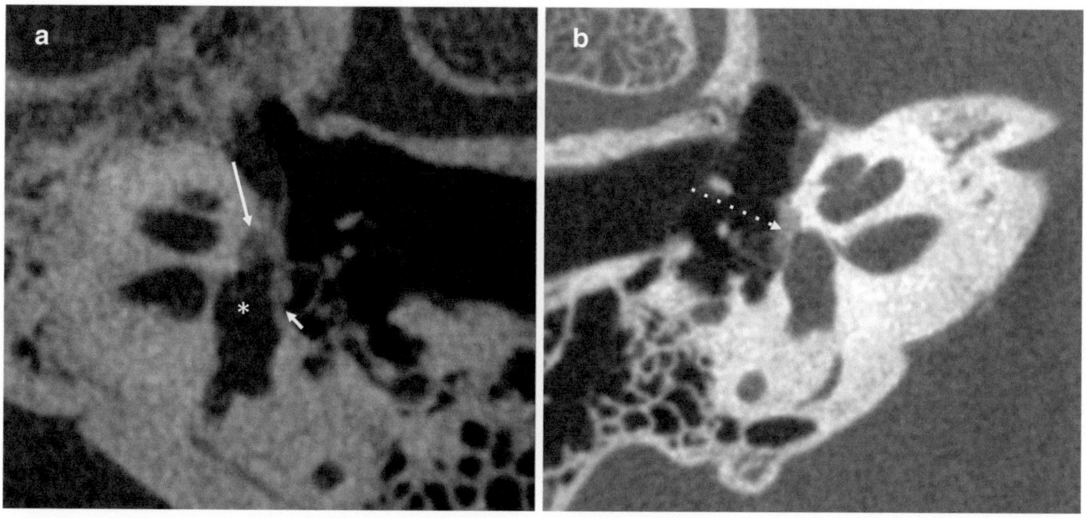

Fig. 8.6 Obliterative otosclerosis. Massive otospongiotic focus covers the footplate and completely close the oval window. (**a**) Axial reformatted CBCT image shows an area of demineralized otosclerosis in the fissula ante fenestram region (arrow) disrupting the normal density of the otic capsule bone near the stapedial attachment and extending to the vestibular surface (asterisk). A thick irregular bone plaque replaces the stapes footplate, near the oval window (short arrow). (**b**) Axial reformatted CBCT image shows an analogous area of otospongiosis (dotted arrow), involving the stapedial-ovalar surface. *Abbreviation:* CBCT = cone beam computed tomography

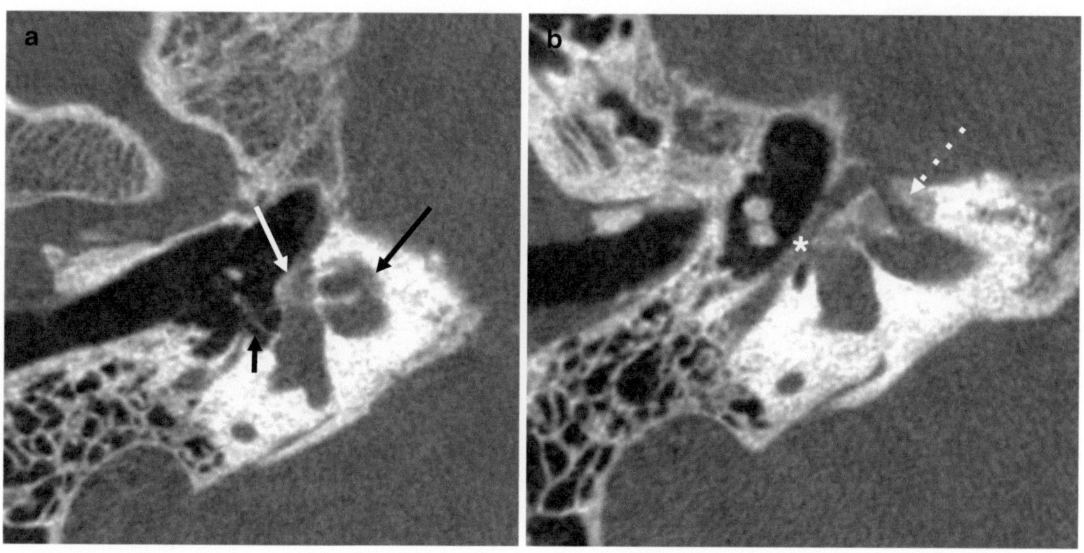

Fig. 8.7 Fenestral and retrofenestral otosclerosis involving the facial nerve canal. Axial (**a** and **b**) reformatted CBCT images show an area of lucency involving the otic capsule near the oval window surface, extending along the posterior bony wall of the tympanic part (asterisk in **b**), the labyrinthine segment of the facial nerve (dotted arrow in **b**), and the pericochlear region (black arrow in **a**). Reabsorption of the stapedial crus is also evident (short black arrow in **a**). *Abbreviation:* CBCT, cone beam computed tomography

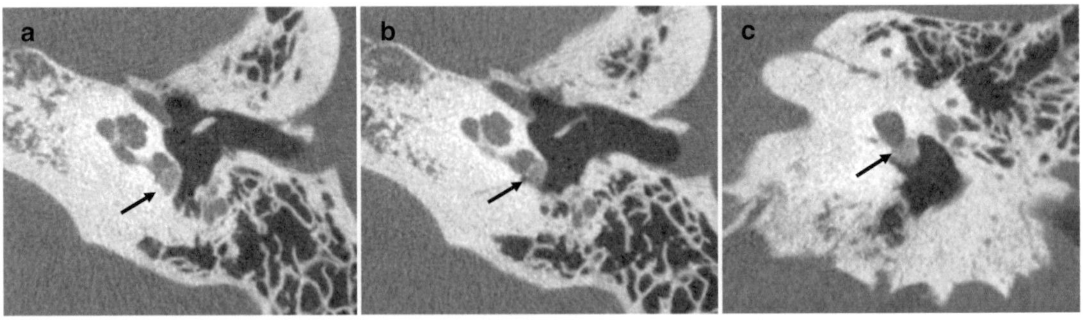

Fig. 8.8 **Retrofenestral otosclerosis with involvement of round window.** (**a** and **b**) Axial reformatted CBCT images and (**c**) coronal reformatted CBCT images show otosclerotic plaques (black arrow) causing nearly complete obliteration of the round window (asterisk in **c**). *Abbreviation:* CBCT = cone beam computed tomography

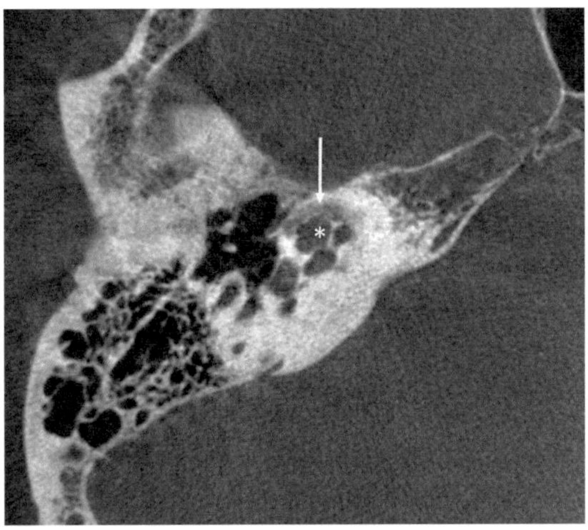

Fig. 8.9 **Anterior pericochlear otosclerosis.** Cochlear involvement with demineralization of the otic capsule causing hypodense double ring or "halo" around the cochlea, also known as the fourth ring of Valvassori. (**a**) Axial reformatted CBCT image shows hypoattenuating spongiotic bone (arrow) in the anterior pericochlear region near the middle and apical cochlear turns (asterisk). *Abbreviation:* CBCT = cone beam computed tomography

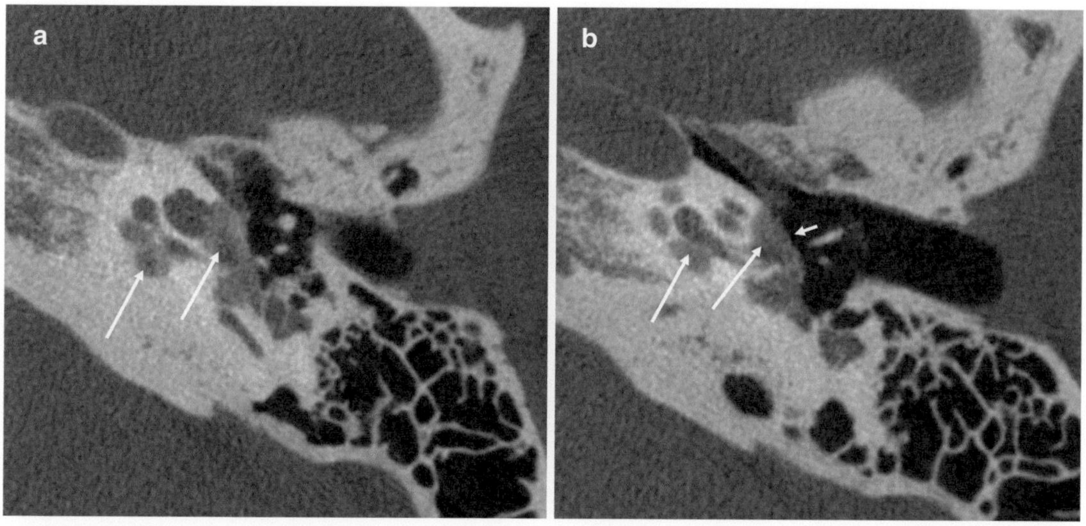

Fig. 8.10 **Retrofenestral otosclerosis.** (**a** and **b**) Axial reformatted CBCT images show an extensive hypodense area of reabsorption in the pericochlear otic capsule (arrows), extending to the cochlear promontory (short arrow). *Abbreviation:* CBCT = cone beam computed tomography

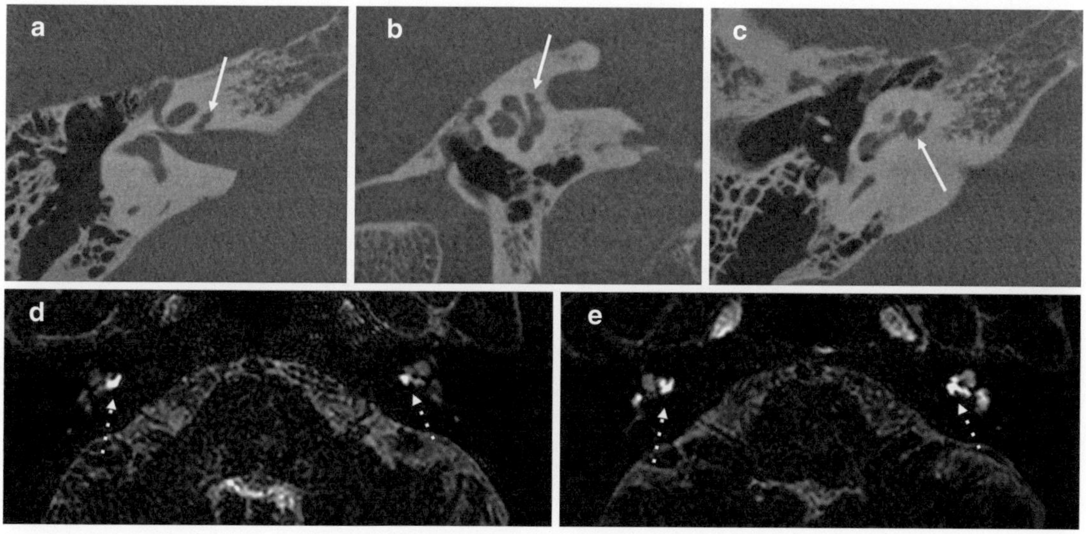

Fig. 8.11 **MR imaging in retrofenestral otosclerosis.** In retrofenestral otosclerosis, the use of the 3D-FLAIR sequence with gadolinium contrast agent is effective in evaluating cochlear damage. 3D-FLAIR contrast enhancement indicate changes in the permeability of the BLB and are good predictors of disease progression. (**a** and **c**) axial and (**b**) oblique reformatted CBCT images show the demineralized otospongiotic foci (arrow). (**d** and **e**) MR 3D-FLAIR sequence acquired 4 h after gadolinium injection shows the accumulation of gadolinium in otospongiotic foci indicating a communication between otosclerotic foci and perilymphatic spaces (dotted arrow). *Abbreviations:* BLB = blood-labyrinth barrier; CBCT = cone beam computed tomography; FLAIR = fluid-attenuated inversion recovery; MR = magnetic resonance

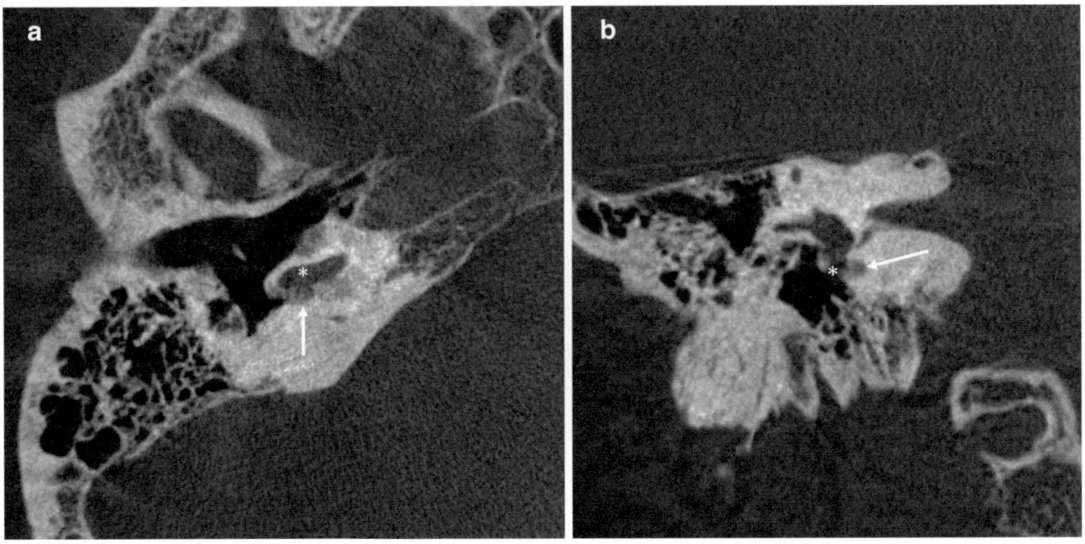

Fig. 8.12 **Cochlear and round window otosclerosis.** (**a**) Axial reformatted CBCT image shows the typical pericochlear "halo" consistent with a wide area of otosclerosis (arrow), posterior to the basal turn of the cochlea (asterisk). (**b**) Coronal reformatted CBCT image shows a focal area of otosclerosis (arrow) medially to the round window niche (asterisk). *Abbreviation:* CBCT = cone beam computed tomography

Some authors correlate the frequency of hearing loss with the part of the cochlear capsule that is affected: low-frequency sounds are best detected at the apical turn, and high-frequency sounds are best detected at the basilar turn, where the basilar membrane is thinner [1].

Magnetic resonance imaging (MRI): contrast enhancement in the region of the oval window or round window should raise suspicion for OS. In cases of retrofenestral OS, a ring of isointense T1-weighted signal in the pericochlear and perilabyrinthine regions accompanied by mild to moderate contrast enhancement related to hypervascularity and inflammatory response can be observed [3, 5].

In retrofenestral OS, the use of the 3D-FLAIR sequence with gadolinium contrast agent is effective in evaluating cochlear damage. 3D-FLAIR hyperintensity and contrast enhancement indicate changes in the permeability of the blood-labyrinth barrier (BLB) and are good predictors of disease progression.

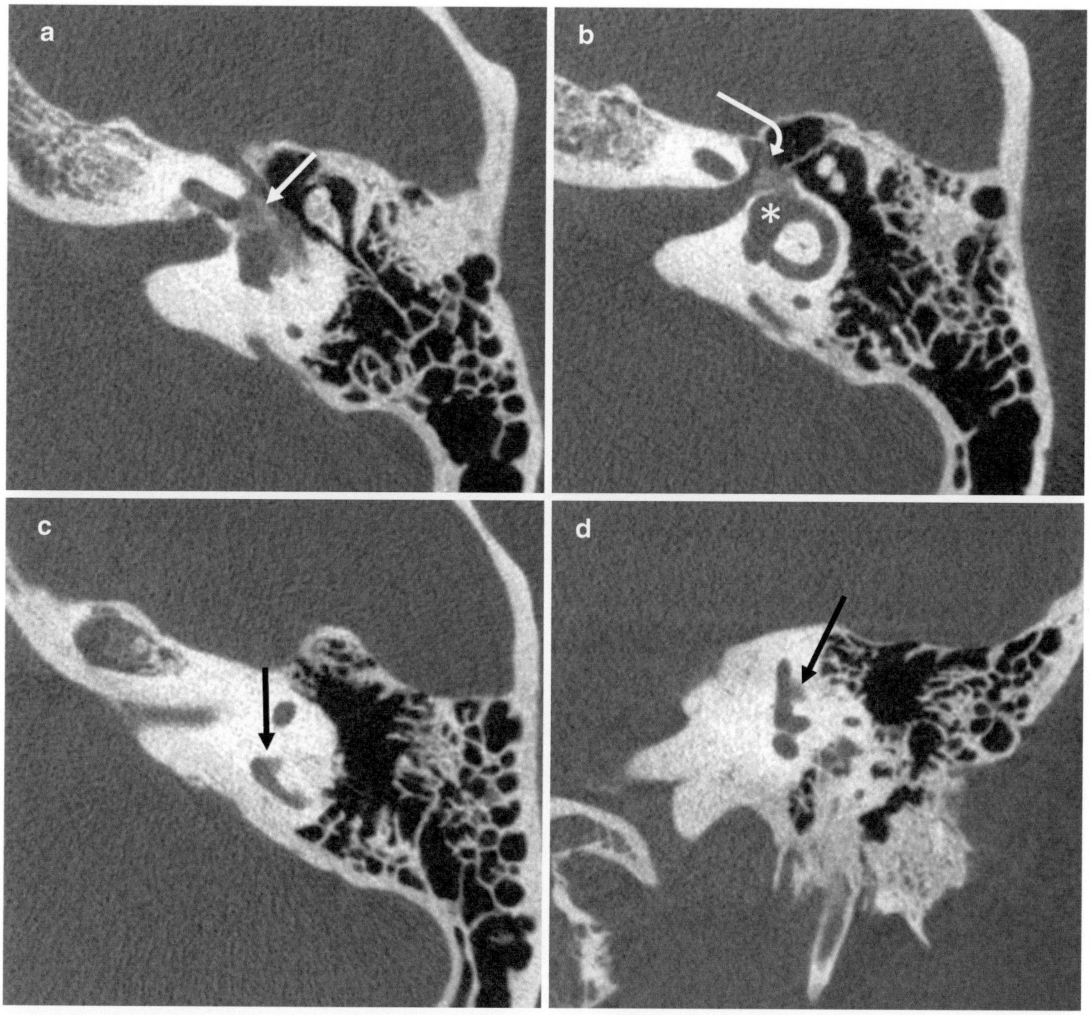

Fig. 8.13 Retrofenestral otosclerosis, with involvement of the semicircular canals and vestibule. (a, b) Axial reformatted CBCT images show a hypodense area of otosclerosis (arrow in **a**) in the anterolateral part of the vestibule (astesisk in **b**) involving the bony canal of labyrinthine segment of the facial nerve (VII cranial nerve) (curved arrow). (**c**) Axial reformatted CBCT image and (**d**) coronal reformatted CBCT image show a focal area of otosclerosis involving the posterior semicircular canal (black arrow). *Abbreviaton:* CBCT = cone beam computed tomography

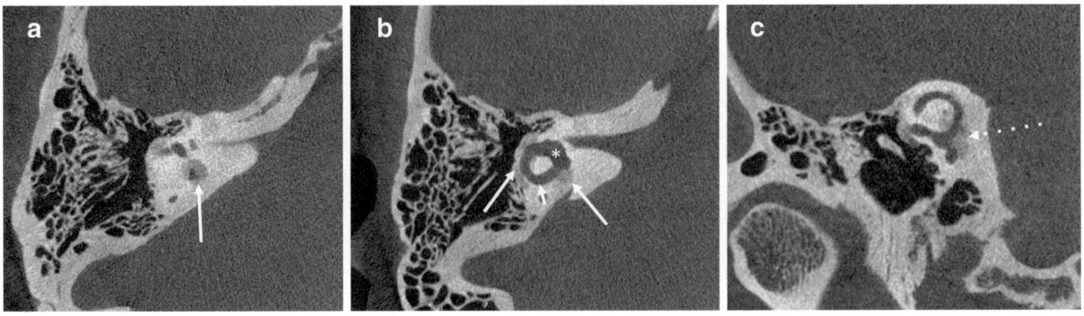

Fig. 8.14 Retrofenestral otosclerosis with semicircular canal involvement. (**a**) Axial reformatted CBCT image shows patchy hypodense plaque near the superior semicircular canal (arrow). (**b**) Axial reformatted CBCT image shows an hypodense otosclerotic foci (arrow) near the vestibule (asterisk) and lateral semicircular canal (short arrow). (**c**) Coronal reformatted CBCT image shows the hypodense otosclerotic foci along the surface of the vestibule and the superior semicircular canal (dotted arrow). *Abbreviation:* CBCT = cone beam computed tomography

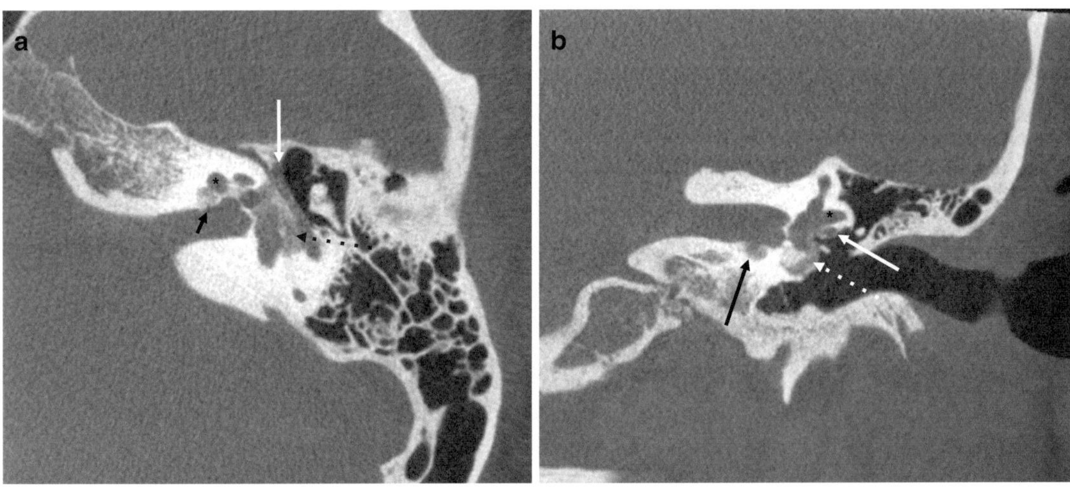

Fig. 8.15 Severe fenestral and retrofenestral otosclerosis. (**a**) Axial reformatted CBCT image shows diffuse hypodense otosclerotic alterations involving the anterolateral portion of the vestibule (dotted black arrow), the tympanic canal of the facial nerve (white arrow), the middle and the basal turn of cochlea (black asterisk), and the anterior surface of the internal auditory canal (black arrowhead). (**b**) Coronal reformatted CBCT image shows diffuse hypodense otosclerotic alterations involving the lateral semicircular canal (black asterisk), the inferolateral portion of the vestibule (dotted arrow), the tympanic segment of the facial nerve (arrow), and the fundus of the internal acoustic meatus (black arrow). *Abbreviation:* CBCT = cone beam computed tomography

8.1 Grading System

Several CT grading systems were proposed according to the location and stage of OS.

The Symons and Fanning classification grades OS based on location and appearance [1] (Fig. 8.16):

- Grade 1: Solely fenestral, with either spongiotic or sclerotic lesions
- Grade 2: Patchy localized cochlear disease (Figs. 8.17, 8.18, 8.19)
  - 2A: basal cochlear turn
  - 2B: middle/apical turns
  - 2C: both basal and middle/apical turns

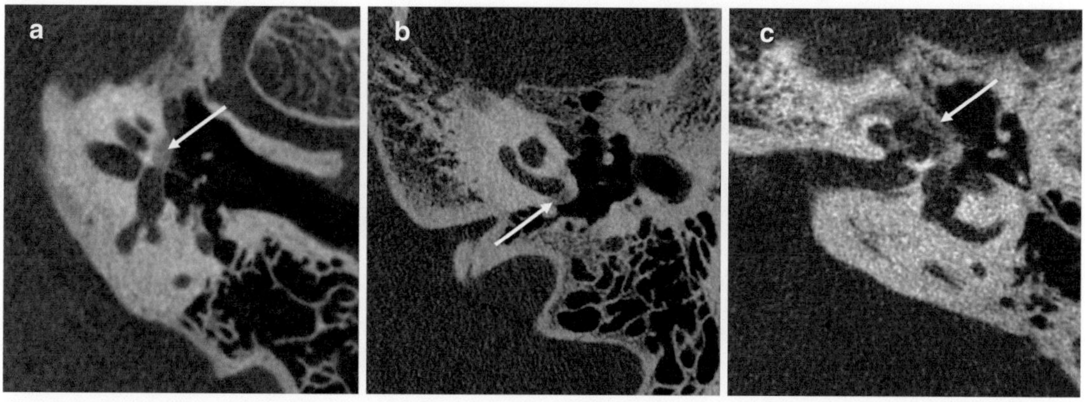

Fig. 8.16 Symons and Fanning classification. (**a**) Grade 1: Solely fenestral, with either spongiotic or sclerotic lesions (arrow). (**b**) Grade 2: Patchy localized cochlear disease (arrow). (**c**) Grade 3: Diffuse confluent cochlear involvement (arrow)

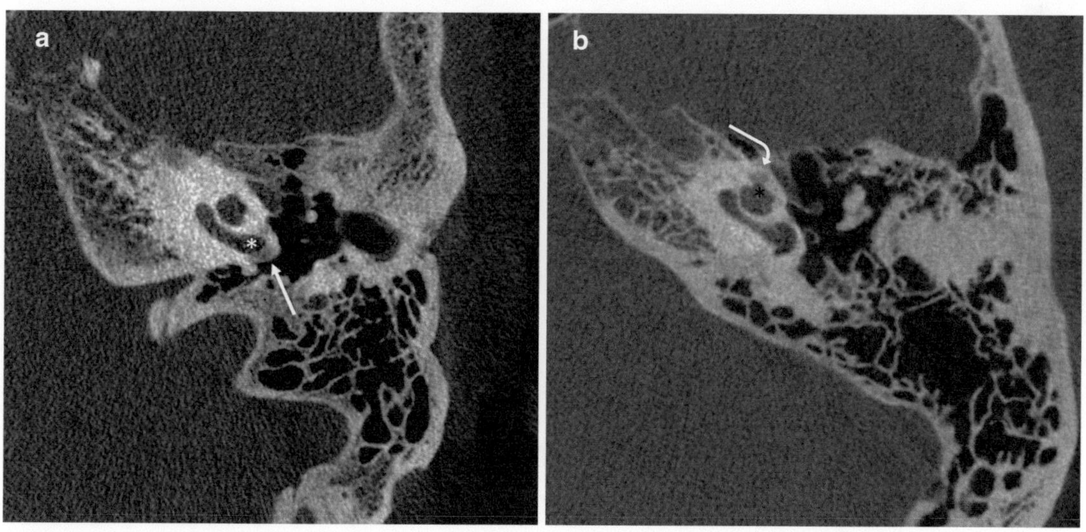

Fig. 8.17 Symons and Fanning Grade 2a and 2b. Grade 2 is divided in 2a (patchy localized cochlear disease, at the basal cochlear turn) and 2b (involvement of the middle/apical cochlear turns) and 2c. (**a**) Axial reformatted CBCT image shows a hypodense plaque (arrow) near the basal turn of the cochlea (asterisk) consistent with grade 2a of Symons and Fanning classification. (**b**) Axial reformatted CBCT image shows a hypodense plaque (curved arrow) near the apical turn of the cochlea (black asterisk) consistent with grade 2b of Symons and Fanning classification. *Abbreviation:* CBCT = cone beam computed tomography

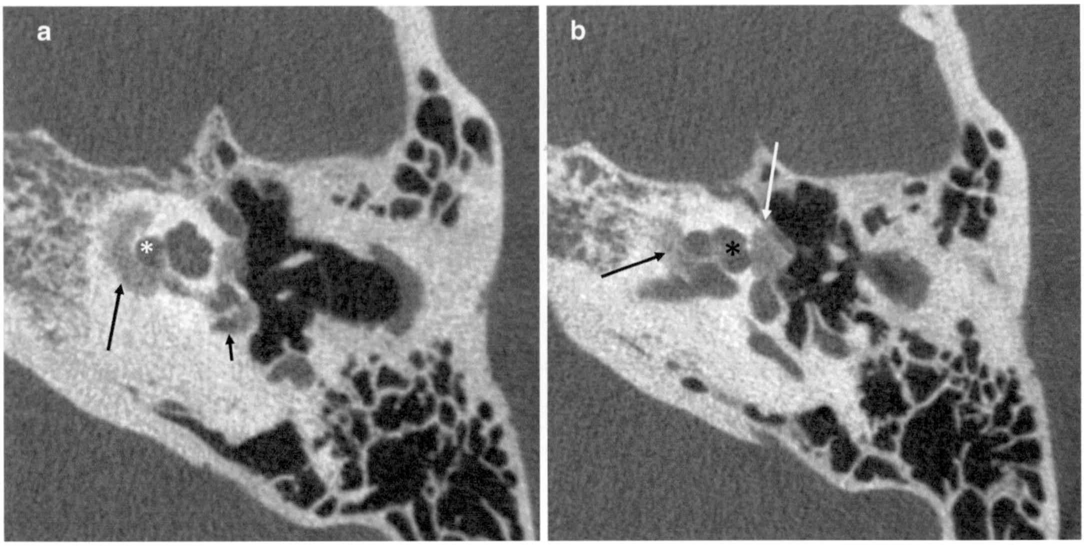

Fig. 8.18 Symons and Fanning Grade 2c. Patchy localized cochlear disease involving both basal and middle/apical turns. (**a** and **b**) Axial reformatted CBCT images show a hypodense plaque in the otic capsule (black arrow) surrounding the basal turn (white asterisk in **a**) and the middle apical turns of the cochlea (black asterisk in **b**). Of note, otosclerotic foci are also observed close to the surface of a semicircular canal (black short arrow in **a**) and along the tympanic tract of the canal of the VII cranial nerve (white arrow in **b**). *Abbreviation:* CBCT = cone beam computed tomography

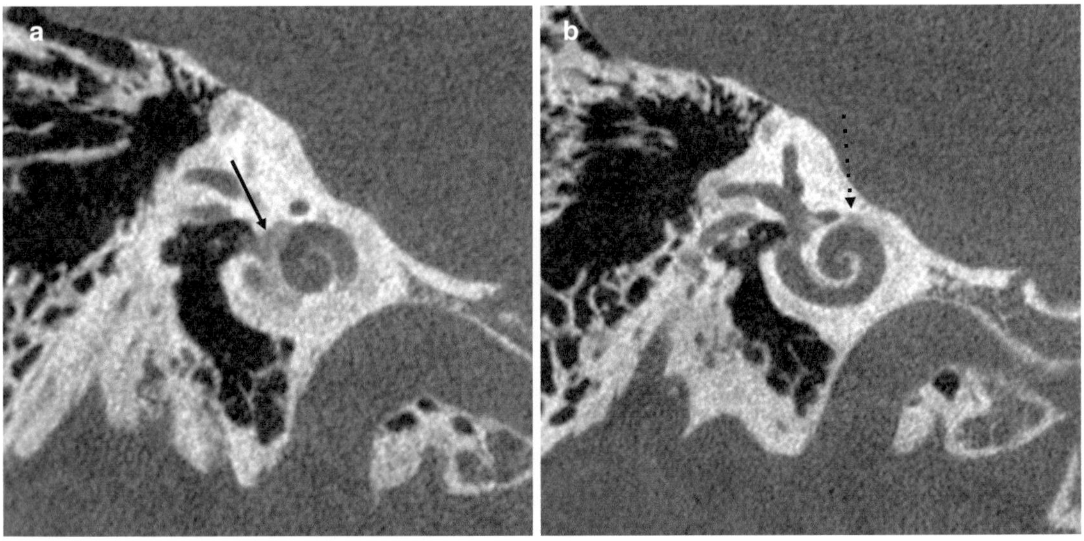

Fig. 8.19 Otosclerosis grade 2c. (**a** and **b**) Coronal reformatted CBCT image shows patchy hypodense otosclerotic alterations with involvement of both the basal (black arrow in **a**) and middle/apical (black dotted arrow in **b**) cochlear turns. *Abbreviation:* CBCT = cone beam computed tomography

- Grade 3: Diffuse confluent cochlear involvement (Fig. 8.20)

The Veillon system stages otosclerosis in four levels based on the location of otosclerotic foci within the labyrinthine capsule [3, 6]:

- Type 1: divided into
  - 1A: isolated thickened and hypodense stapes footplate (thickness >0.6 mm)
  - 1B: anterior fenestral hypodensity, less than or equal to 1 mm in diameter, without extension to the anterior middle labyrinthine layer
- Type 2: anterior fenestral hypodensity greater than 1 mm, not in contact with the cochlear lumen
- Type 3: anterior fenestral hypodensity greater than 1 mm, in contact with the cochlear lumen
- Type 4: divided into
  - 4A: hypodensities located anteriorly, medially, or below the cochlea, in the middle layer of the labyrinthine capsule (anterior labyrinth)
  - 4B: hypodensities in the labyrinthine layers, posteriorly around the lumen of the semicircular canals or vestibule (posterior labyrinth)

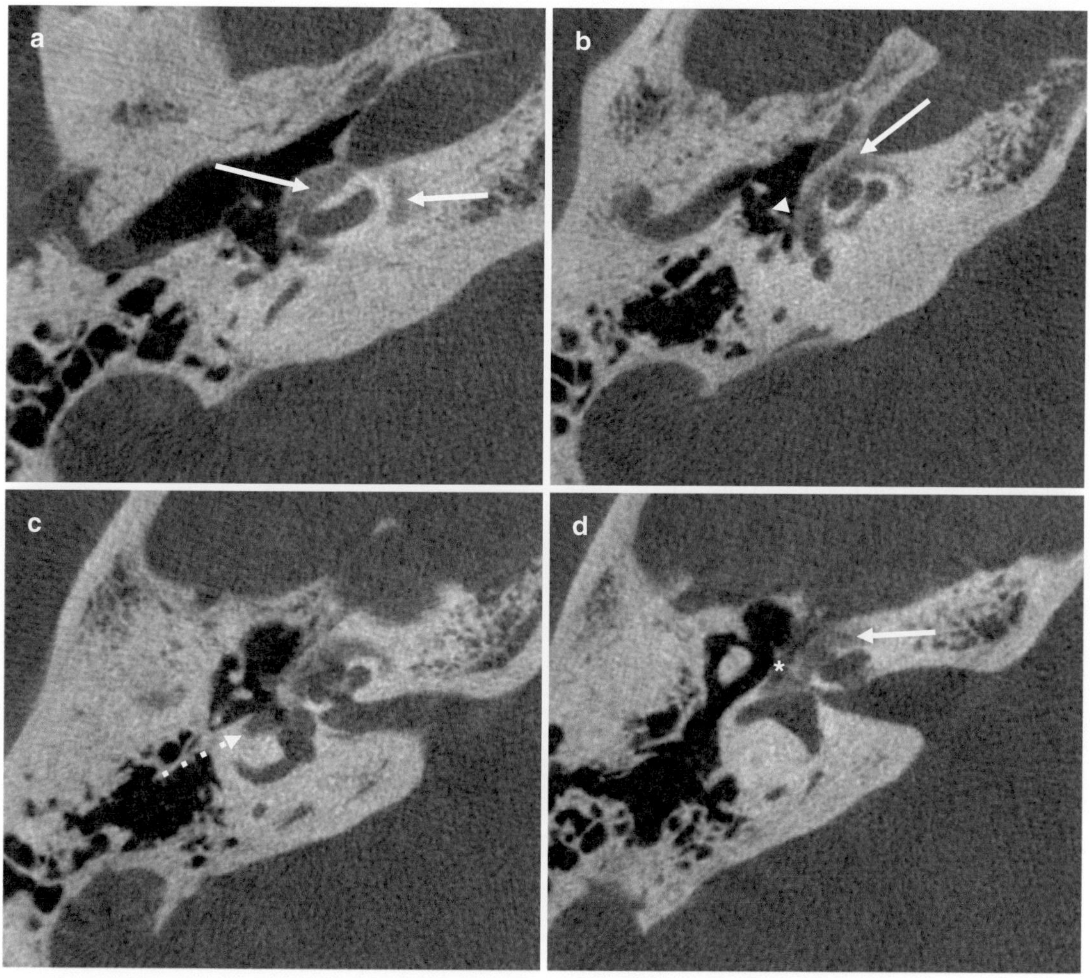

Fig. 8.20 Otosclerosis grade 3. Diffuse confluent cochlear involvement. (**a–d**) Axial reformatted CBCT images show extensive areas of otospongiosis involving the otic capsule surrounding the cochlea (arrows), the oval window (arrowhead in **b**), the tympanic tract of the facial nerve (asterisk in **d**) and the semicircular canals (dotted arrow in **c**). *Abbreviation:* CBCT = cone beam computed tomography

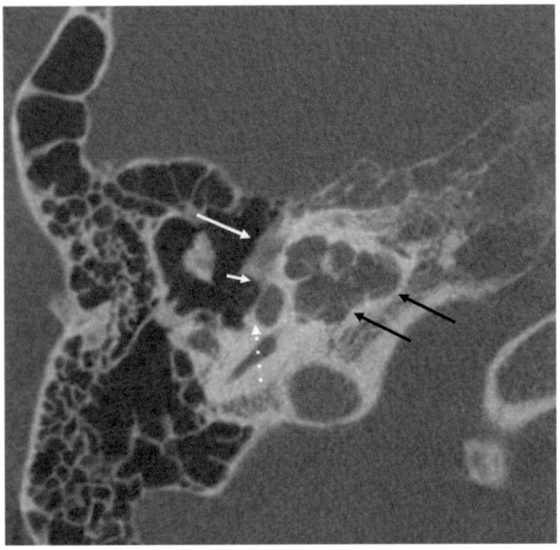

Fig. 8.21 **Osteogenesis imperfecta.** (**a**) Axial reformatted CBCT images show hypodense area involving the fissula ante fenestram (short arrow), along the cochlear promontory (arrow) and also pericochlear region (black arrow). Note also thickening of the footplate (dotted arrow). *Abbreviation:* CBCT = cone beam computed tomography

Imaging may help in the differential diagnosis between OS and other causes of conductive or mixed hearing loss, excluding malformations of middle ear, ossicular chain fixation, post-traumatic ossicular dislocationt, Minor syndrome and bone disease such as Paget disease or osteogenesis imperfecta (Fig. 8.21).

8.2 Treatment

8.2.1 Fenestral Otosclerosis

Treatment involves surgery, with stapedotomy or, more rarely, complete or partial stapedectomy, followed by placement of a stapes prosthesis in order to restore ossicular chain mobility [2, 5]. CT is helpful in surgical planning and in identifying causes of post-stapedectomy complications. A meticulous and systematic assessment of pre-operative images prevents misdiagnoses and potential intraoperative complications [5].

Preoperative MRI may also be considered in patients with suspected OS and symptoms associated with endolymphatic hydrops [5]. One of the most common post-surgery complications is the migration or dislocation of the prosthesis, with the more common issue being "lateralized piston syndrome". This condition refers to the lateral migration of the implant out of the oval window, often due to incus necrosis, or to the conflict between the utricle and saccule and the medial end of the implant entering the vestibule when the implant is too long, causing vertigo. Other common complications are perilymphatic fistula (it is a pathological communication between the air-filled space of the middle ear and the fluid-filled space of the inner ear, typically occurring at the level of the round or oval window) and intralabyrinthine hemorrhage. Pneumolabyrinth may indicate the presence of a perilymphatic fistula: patients may experience sensorineural hearing loss or vertigo [3]. Reparative granuloma is a rare complication that causes hearing loss 1–2 weeks post-surgery due to severe inflammation near the vestibule. It can be identified by MRI with gadolinium, which shows enhancement of the otic capsule and middle ear, and by CT, which reveals bony erosion in the middle ear [5].

8.2.2 Retrofenestral Otosclerosis

Treatment is medical, aimed at limiting the growth of otosclerotic foci and promoting remineralization of the otosclerotic plaque. In cases of severe bilateral sensorineural hearing loss, cochlear implantation may be considered.

Cochlear OS on CT can be rarely mimicked by other diseases that demineralize the otic capsule, such as osteogenesis imperfecta and Paget's disease. However, the clinical symptoms and involvement of other bones help distinguish these conditions from cochlear OS [4].

Preoperative Checklist for Assessment of Otologic Structures [5]

Structure	Action
Temporal bone	Signs of fractures;
	Rule out minor syndrome;
	Presence of lesions or metabolic/infectious/neoplastic bone disease
Mastoid	Rule out chronic otitis media;
	Rule out bony erosion (cholesteatoma)
Middle ear	Rule out inflammatory disease;
	Abnormal vascular structures (high-riding jugular bulb, persistence of stapedial artery)
Ossicular chain	Integrity; morphology; fixation, dislocation; fractures; erosion; esostosis
Stapes	Position; morphology; adjacent structures
Oval window	Thickness and level of obliteration (drilling needed?)
Round window	Obliteration
Facial nerve	Overhanging of tympanic segment; Abnormal position of mastoid segment (might influence choice of approach)
Inner ear	Malformation; Enlarged vestibular or cochlear aqueduct; Enlarged Rosenthal canal; Obliterated cochlea; Acoustic schwannoma
Otosclerotic lesions	Grading and location
Opposite ear	Disease is bilateral in 80–85% of cases

References

1. Lee TC, Aviv RI, Chen JM, Nedzelski JM, Fox AJ, Symons SP. CT grading of otosclerosis. AJNR Am J Neuroradiol. 2009;30(7):1435–9. https://doi.org/10.3174/ajnr.A1558.
2. Juliano AF, Ginat DT, Moonis G. Imaging review of the temporal bone: part II. Traumatic, postoperative, and noninflammatory non neoplastic conditions. Radiology. 2015;276(3):655–72. https://doi.org/10.1148/radiol.2015140800.
3. Mangia LRL, Coelho LOM, Carvalho B, de Oliveira AKP, Hamerschmidt R. Imaging studies in otosclerosis: an up-to-date comprehensive review. Int. Arch Otorhinolaryngol. 2021;25(2). https://doi.org/10.1055/s-0040-1715149.
4. Purohit B, Hermans R, Op de Beeck K. Imaging in otosclerosis: a pictorial review. Insights Imaging. 2014;5(2):245–52. https://doi.org/10.1007/s13244-014-0313-9.
5. Wolfovitz A, Luntz M. Impact of imaging in management of otosclerosis. Otolaryngol Clin N Am. 2018;51(2):343–55. https://doi.org/10.1016/j.otc.2017.11.005.
6. Veillon F, Stierle JL, Dussaix J, Ramos-Taboada L, Riehm S. Imagerie de l'otospongiose: confrontation clinique et imagerie. J Radiol. 2006;87(11 Pt 2):1756–64. https://doi.org/10.1016/S0221-0363(06)74157-9.

Pathology of the Inner Ear

9

Computed Tomography (CT) and Magnetic Resonance (MR) Imaging Findings in Inner Ear Pathology

Elisa Massullo, Antonia Valentina Genovese, Federica Di Berardino, Diego Zanetti, Stefania Barozzi, Elisa Scola, Silvia Casale, Fabio Triulzi, and Giorgio Conte

9.1 Introduction

Acquired inner ear pathologies encompass a wide range of etiologies and clinical presentations. These conditions may arise from infectious or inflammatory processes, autoimmune diseases, vascular events, trauma, or neoplastic involvement. Clinically, patients often present with sensorineural hearing loss, tinnitus, vertigo, or imbalance—symptoms that may be acute or progressive, unilateral or bilateral. Some disorders, such as sudden sensorineural hearing loss (SSHL), manifest abruptly and unpredictably, whereas others, like endolymphatic hydrops (EH), tend to follow a more chronic or episodic course.

9.2 Sudden Sensorineural Hearing Loss

SSHL is defined as a rapid-onset sensorineural hearing loss of at least 30 dB across three contiguous frequencies, occurring within 72 h [1] (Figs. 9.1, 9.2, 9.3, 9.4, 9.5, 9.6, 9.7, 9.8, 9.9, 9.10, 9.11, and 9.12). Its incidence is estimated at 5–27 cases per 100,000 individuals annually, though underreporting and misdiagnosis may obscure the true prevalence [2]. Various etiological factors have been proposed [3, 4]; however, in 71–85% of cases, no definitive cause is identified, and the condition is classified as idiopathic [5].

E. Massullo (✉) · A. V. Genovese · E. Scola
S. Casale
Neuroradiology Unit, Fondazione IRCCS Ca' Granda Ospedale Maggiore Policlinico, Milan, Italy
e-mail: elisa.massullo@policlinico.mi.it; valentina.genovese@policlinico.mi.it; elisa.scola@policlinico.mi.it; silvia.casale@policlinico.mi.it

F. Di Berardino · D. Zanetti
Audiology Unit, Fondazione IRCCS Ca' Granda Ospedale Maggiore Policlinico, Milan, Italy

Department of Clinical Sciences and Community Health, Università Degli Studi Di Milano, Milan, Italy
e-mail: federica.diberardino@policlinico.mi.it; diego.zanetti@policlinico.mi.ti

S. Barozzi
Department of Clinical Sciences and Community Health, Università Degli Studi Di Milano, Milan, Italy
e-mail: stefania.barozzi@unimi.it

F. Triulzi · G. Conte
Neuroradiology Unit, Fondazione IRCCS Ca' Granda Ospedale Maggiore Policlinico, Milan, Italy

Department of Pathophysiology and Transplantation, University of Milan, Milan, Italy
e-mail: fabio.triulzi@policlinico.mi.it; giorgio.conte@policlinico.mi.it

G. Conte et al. (eds.), *Atlas of Normal and Pathological Findings in Otoneuroradiology*,
https://doi.org/10.1007/978-3-032-08232-9_9

Table 9.1 Four primary MRI patterns of sudden sensorineural hearing loss

Pattern	T1w	3D-FLAIR	CE 3D-FLAIR	4 h CE 3D-FLAIR
Negative	–	–	–	–
Hemorrhagic	+	+	–/+	–/+
Inflammatory	–	+	–/+	–/+
Isolated BLB breakdown	–	–	–	+
Hydrops	–	–	–	Hydrops

Magnetic resonance imaging (MRI) plays a central role in the diagnostic workup of SSHL. It is essential for excluding central and retrocochlear causes—particularly vestibular schwannomas or metastasis (Fig. 9.12)—and for detecting subtle inner ear abnormalities. High-resolution MRI, particularly with 3 T scanners, has improved our understanding of SSHL pathophysiology due to its superior spatial resolution and signal-to-noise ratio compared to 1.5 T systems.

A standard MRI protocol for temporal bone assessment should include axial pre-contrast 3D turbo spin echo (TSE) T2-weighted imaging, pre- and post-contrast TSE T1-weighted imaging, pre- and post-contrast 3D-FLAIR, and a 4-h delayed post-contrast 3D-FLAIR [6]. Diffusion-weighted imaging (DWI) and 3D-FLAIR sequences of the brain are also recommended to exclude ischemic lesions.

Four primary MRI patterns of SSHL have been described [7] and are summarized in Table 9.1:

- *Hemorrhagic pattern*: High signal intensity on both T1-weighted and 3D-FLAIR sequences due to the presence of methemoglobin; enhancement on contrast-enhanced 3D-FLAIR may indicate disruption of the blood-labyrinth barrier (BLB).
- *Inflammatory pattern*: Normal signal on T1-weighted imaging and high signal on 3D-FLAIR sequences due to proteinaceous exudate; enhancement on contrast-enhanced 3D-FLAIR may indicate disruption of the BLB.
- *Isolated BLB breakdown*: No signal alterations on pre-contrast sequences; enhancement visible only on 4-h delayed post-contrast 3D-FLAIR, indicating mild BLB dysfunction.
- *Hydropic pattern*: Dilatation of the endolymphatic spaces, especially within the cochlea or vestibule, visible on 4-h delayed contrast-enhanced 3D-FLAIR, typically associated with low-frequency sensorineural hearing loss and consistent with endolymphatic hydrops (EH).

Treatment options for SSHL include oral corticosteroids, hyperbaric oxygen therapy, and intratympanic steroid injections as salvage therapy. In infectious, inflammatory, or autoimmune SSHL, the condition may progress to irreversible inner ear damage, potentially leading to labyrinthitis ossificans (Fig. 9.10).

9.3 Labyrinthitis Ossificans

Labyrinthitis is an acute or subacute inflammation of the membranous labyrinth, typically affecting both cochlear and vestibular structures (Figs. 9.10, 9.13, 9.14, and 9.15). It presents with vertigo, imbalance, ingravescent sensorineural hearing loss, and often tinnitus. The condition is most commonly related to infections or autoimmune diseases. Differential diagnoses include vestibular neuritis (without cochlear symptoms), Ménière's disease, stroke, and acoustic schwannoma. The disease progresses in three stages:

- Acute phase: initial inflammation with labyrinthine cellular infiltration and proteinaceous exudate. MRI shows normal signal on TSE T2-weighted images, high signal on pre-contrast 3D-FLAIR sequence with or without enhancement on post-contrast 3D-FLAIR.

Table 9.2 Phases of pathological process of labyrinthitis ossificans

Stage	Pathological features	MRI sequences			CBCT
		3D-DRIVE	3D-FLAIR	CE T1w	
Early stage (inflammation)	Acute inflammation, with proteinaceuos exudate in the membranous labyrinth	–	+	–	–
Intermediate stage (fibrosis)	Replacement of labyrinthine fluid with fibrous tissue	+	+	+	–
Advanced stage (fibro-ossification)	Fibrous tissue begins to ossified	+	–/+	–/+	+
Late stage (complete ossification)	Complete obliteration of labyrinthine spaces by bone	+	–	–	+

- Fibrotic phase: replacement of normal structures with fibrous tissue with consequent decreased signal on TSE T2-weighted images, high signal in 3D-FLAIR, and enhancement on contrast-enhanced T1-weighted and 3D-FLAIR sequences.
- Ossification phase: labyrinthine bone deposition determining decreased signal on all MRI sequences; contrast-enhancement could disappear.

Note that CBCT results are positive only in the ossification phase, thus not resulting diagnostic in the early phase of the pathological process.

Ossification usually begins in the basal turn of the cochlea, progressing apically and sometimes involving the semicircular canals and vestibule [8]. The progression of the pathological process of labyrinthitis ossificans is summarized in Table 9.2.

9.4 Endolymphatic Hydrops

EH is the pathological accumulation of endolymph within the membranous labyrinth, leading to distension of endolymphatic spaces and disruption of auditory and vestibular function [9]. Impaired absorption by the endolymphatic sac causes elevated inner ear pressure, potentially leading to membrane distension or microruptures, particularly of Reissner's membrane, further altering inner ear fluid balance. MRI has become essential for visualizing membranous labyrinth in vivo (Figs. 9.16, 9.17, 9.18, 9.19, 9.20, 9.21, 9.22, 9.23, 9.24, 9.25, 9.26, 9.27, 9.28, 9.29, and 9.30). Specific sequences such as 3D inversion recovery T1-weighted and 4-h delayed 3D-FLAIR, after intratympanic or intravenous gadolinium administration, respectively, allow differentiation between endolymph and perilymph [10]. With intratympanic administration, gadolinium diffuses through the round window into the perilymph only. However, it is invasive, allows only a unilateral ear assessment, and requires a 24-h delay for optimal uptake. In contrast, intravenous administration allows gadolinium to enter the perilymph via the blood-labyrinth barrier, with imaging performed at 4 h. Though contrast resolution is lower, this method enables bilateral assessment and is less invasive. MRI protocol for EH should include pre- and post-contrast T1-TSE, 3D-FLAIR, 3D T2-TSE, and 4-h delayed 3D-FLAIR. In our institution we assess hydrops severity on delayed 3D-FLAIR using the Bernaerts classification [11], which grades separately cochlear hydrops into three degrees of severity (0,1,2) and vestibular hydrops into four degrees of severity (0, 1, 2, 3). Other pathologies that can mimic endolymphatic hydrops symptomatology are atelectasis of the sacculus and utriculus (Figs. 9.25, 9.26, and 9.27), which can also be demonstrated on the 4-h delayed 3D-FLAIR.

9.5 Inner Ear Dehiscence Syndrome

Inner ear dehiscence syndrome refers to a group of disorders caused by an abnormal opening in the bony structures of the inner ear, particularly the superior semicircular canal (most common), but it may also involve the posterior semicircular canal, cochlea, or vestibule (Figs. 9.31, 9.32, 9.33, 9.34, 9.35 and 9.36). Normally, the inner ear has two "windows" (oval and round) that help transmit sound and pressure. A third abnormal opening (the dehiscence) leads to abnormal transmission of pressure and sound between the intracranial cavity and the inner ear.

Superior semicircular canal dehiscence syndrome (Minor syndrome) is a vestibular disorder caused by a dehiscence of the bony roof of the superior semicircular canal. It typically manifests with Tullio phenomenon: vertigo and nystagmus induced by loud noises or by sudden changes in pressure (Valsalva maneuver). Other symptoms include disequilibrium, conductive hearing loss (mimicking otospongiosis), autophony, and pulsatile tinnitus.

9.6 Perilymphatic Fistula

A perilymphatic fistula (PLF) is a leak of perilymphatic liquid from the inner to the middle ear via the oval or round window (Fig. 9.37). Barotrauma, head injury, congenital disease, and prior surgery are well-known causative factors. PLF may also be present without any known etiology, especially in patients with chronic and fluctuating cochleovestibular symptoms like probable Menière's disease. PLF can be assessed with 4-h delayed contrast-enhanced 3D-FLAIR sequence demonstrating the leakage of contrast medium from the perilymphatic space to middle ear.

9.7 Intralabyrinthine Schwannomas

Intralabyrinthine schwannomas are rare, benign tumors arising from the Schwann cells of the cochlear or vestibular nerves within the membranous labyrinth (Figs. 9.38, 9.39, and 9.40). Unlike classic vestibular schwannomas, which develop in the internal auditory canal or cerebellopontine angle, these tumors are confined to the cochlea, vestibule, or semicircular canals. Cochlear schwannomas typically present with progressive or sudden sensorineural hearing loss and tinnitus, usually without vertigo. In contrast, vestibular schwannomas commonly cause vertigo, imbalance, and positional dizziness, while hearing is often initially preserved.

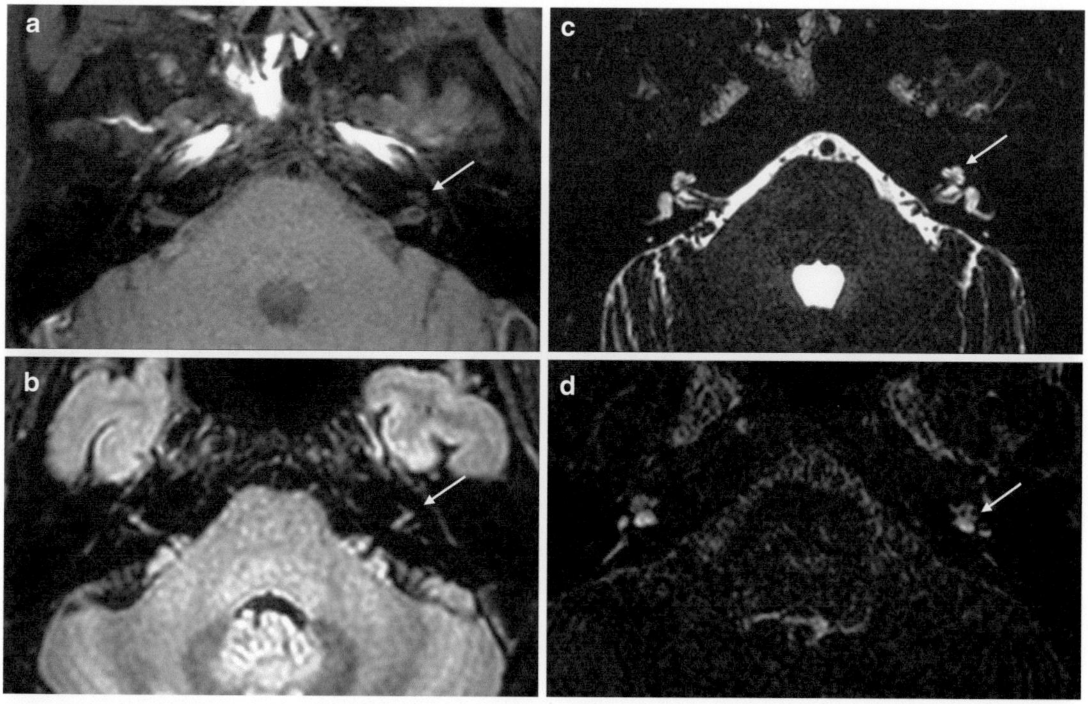

Fig. 9.1 24-year-old male patient who has been complaining of left low-tone sudden hearing loss for 2 days showing left grade 2 cochlear hydrops (according to Bernaerts's score). (**a**) Axial FSE-T1W, (**b**) Axial 3D-FLAIR, (**c**) Axial 3D TSE-T2W, (**d**) Axial 4-h delayed contrast-enhanced 3D-FLAIR. Normal signal of the left cochlea in **a–c** (arrow). In (**d**) we can see cochlear hydrops grade 2 with enlargement of the cochlear duct (arrow). The imaging characteristics are consistent with an SSHL due to membranous labyrinth hydrops. *Abbreviations*: FSE = fast spin echo; FLAIR = fluid-attenuated inversion recovery; TSE = turbo spin echo; SSHL = sudden sensorineural hearing loss

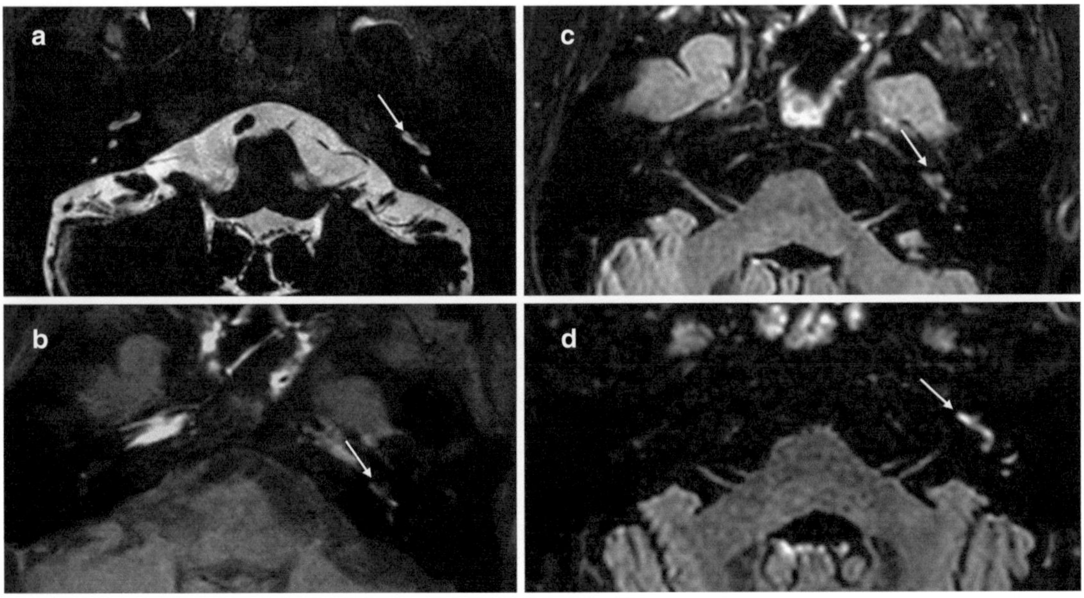

Fig. 9.2 36-year-old male patient with left pantonal sudden hearing loss after COVID-19 ChAdOx1-S vaccine (day 4) showing left cochlear hemorrhagic pattern. (**a**) Axial 3D TSE-T2W, (**b**) axial FSE-T1W, (**c**) axial 3D-FLAIR, (**d**) axial 4-h delayed contrast-enhanced 3D-FLAIR. There is a high signal in the left cochlea on FSE-T1W sequence, particularly in the basal turn (arrow in **b**), suggestive of methemoglobin. This corresponds to high signal on the 3D-FLAIR sequence (arrow in **c**) and contrast enhancement in the left basal turn of the cochlea (arrow in **d**). The signal of the left basal turn of the cochlea appears normal on 3D TSE-T2W (arrow in **a**). The imaging characteristics are consistent with a hemorrhagic pattern of SSHL. *Abbreviations*: TSE = turbo spin echo; FSE = fast spin echo; FLAIR = fluid-attenuated inversion recovery; SSHL = sudden sensorineural hearing loss

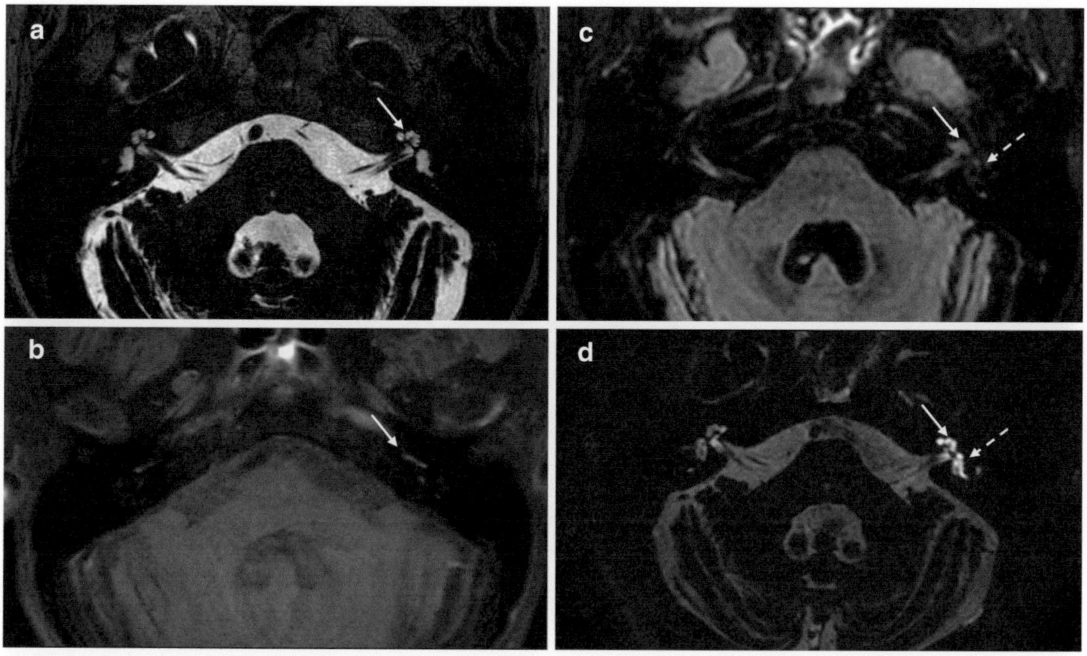

Fig. 9.3 **75-year-old male patient with central vertigo and sudden left sensorineural hearing loss after COVID-19 ChAdOx1-S vaccine showing left cochlear hemorrhagic pattern.** (**a**) Axial 3D TSE-T2W, (**b**) Axial FSE-T1W, (**c**) Axial 3D-FLAIR, (**d**) Axial 4-h delayed contrast-enhanced 3D-FLAIR. There is a high signal in the left cochlea, particularly in the basal turn (arrow in **b**), indicative of methemoglobin. Corresponding high signal is observed on the 3D-FLAIR sequence in both the left cochlea (arrow in **c**) and vestibule (dashed arrow in **c**). The delayed post-contrast 3D-FLAIR images show enhancement in the cochlea (arrow in **d**) and vestibule (dashed arrow in **d**), suggestive of the blood-labyrinth barrier breakdown. On 3D TSE T2W sequence, the inner ear structures appear normal in signal (arrow in **a**). The imaging characteristics are consistent with a hemorrhagic pattern of SSHL. *Abbreviations*: TSE = turbo spin echo; FSE = fast spin echo; FLAIR = fluid-attenuated inversion recovery; SSHL = sudden sensorineural hearing loss

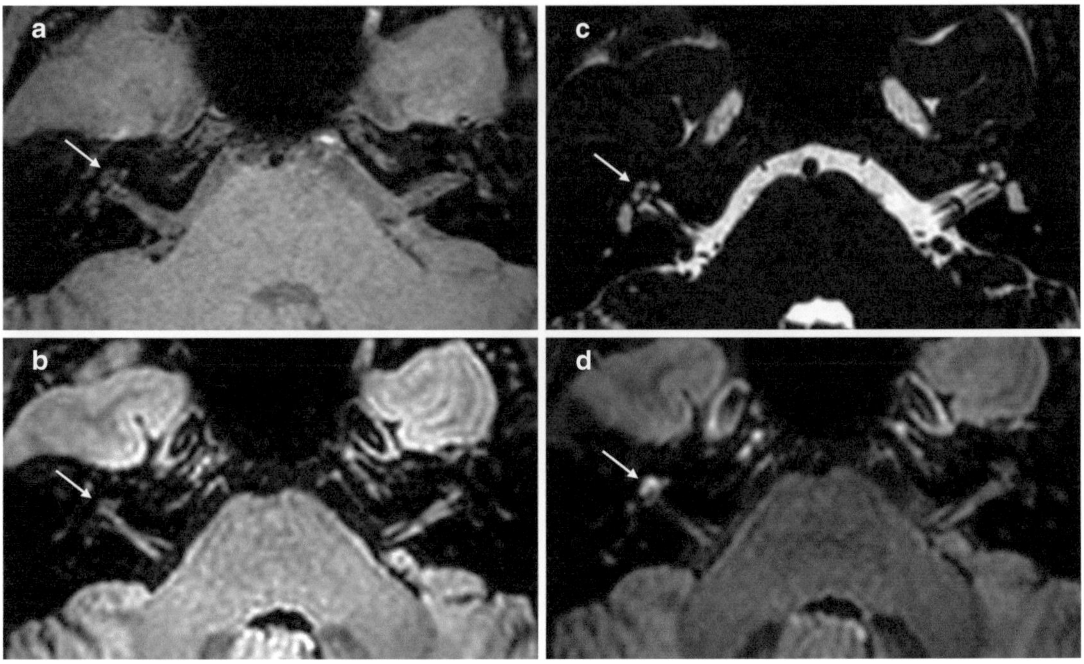

Fig. 9.4 **36-year-old male patient who has been complaining of right low-tone sudden hearing loss for 5 days showing right isolated blood-labyrinth barrier breakdown**. (**a**) Axial FSE-T1W, (**b**) Axial 3D-FLAIR, (**c**) Axial 3D TSE-T2W, (**d**) Axial 4-h delayed contrast-enhanced 3D-FLAIR. Normal T2, T1 and FLAIR signal of the right cochlea in **a**–**c** (arrow). In image **d** there is an abnormal enhancement in the medio-apical turns of the right cochlea (arrow), suggestive of blood-labyrinth barrier breakdown. The imaging characteristics are consistent with an isolated blood-labyrinth barrier breakdown pattern of SSHL. *Abbreviations*: FSE = fast spin echo; FLAIR = fluid-attenuated inversion recovery; TSE = turbo spin echo; SSHL = sudden sensorineural hearing loss

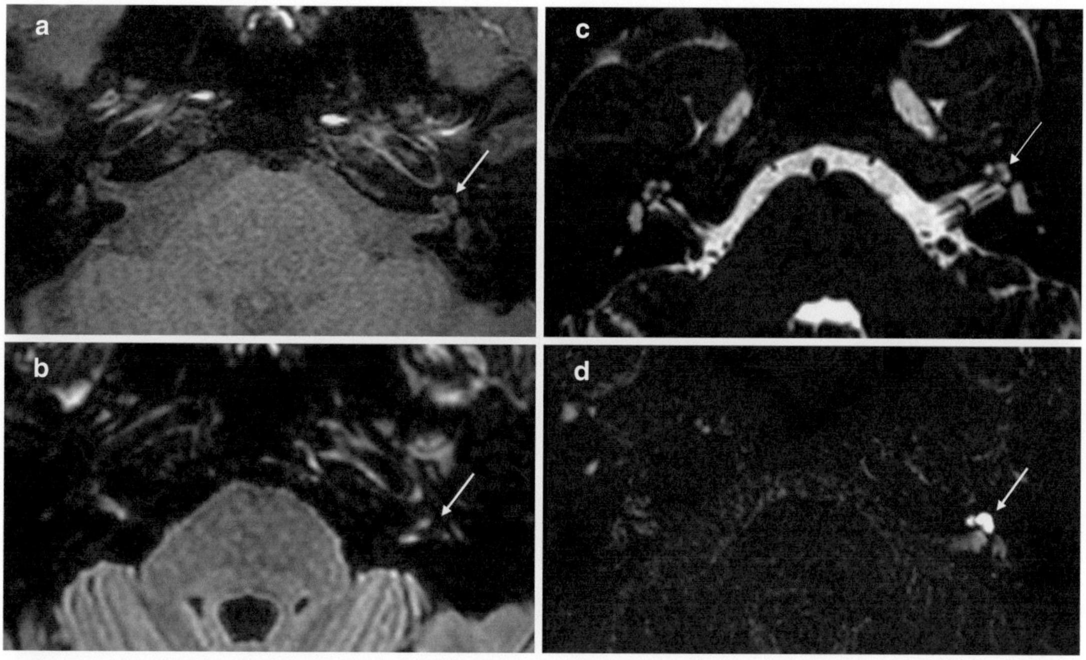

Fig. 9.5 36-year-old male patient who has been complaining of left low-tone sudden hearing loss for 5 days showing left isolated blood-labyrinth barrier breakdown. (**a**) Axial FSE-T1W, (**b**) Axial 3D-FLAIR, (**c**) Axial 3D TSE-T2W, (**d**) Axial 4-h delayed contrast-enhanced 3D-FLAIR. Normal signal of the inner ear structures in **a**–**c** (arrows). Image **d** demonstrates abnormal delayed enhancement in the left cochlea (arrow). The imaging characteristics are consistent with an isolated blood-labyrinth barrier breakdown pattern of SSHL. *Abbreviations*: FSE = fast spin echo; FLAIR = fluid-attenuated inversion recovery; TSE = turbo spin echo; SSHL = sudden sensorineural hearing loss

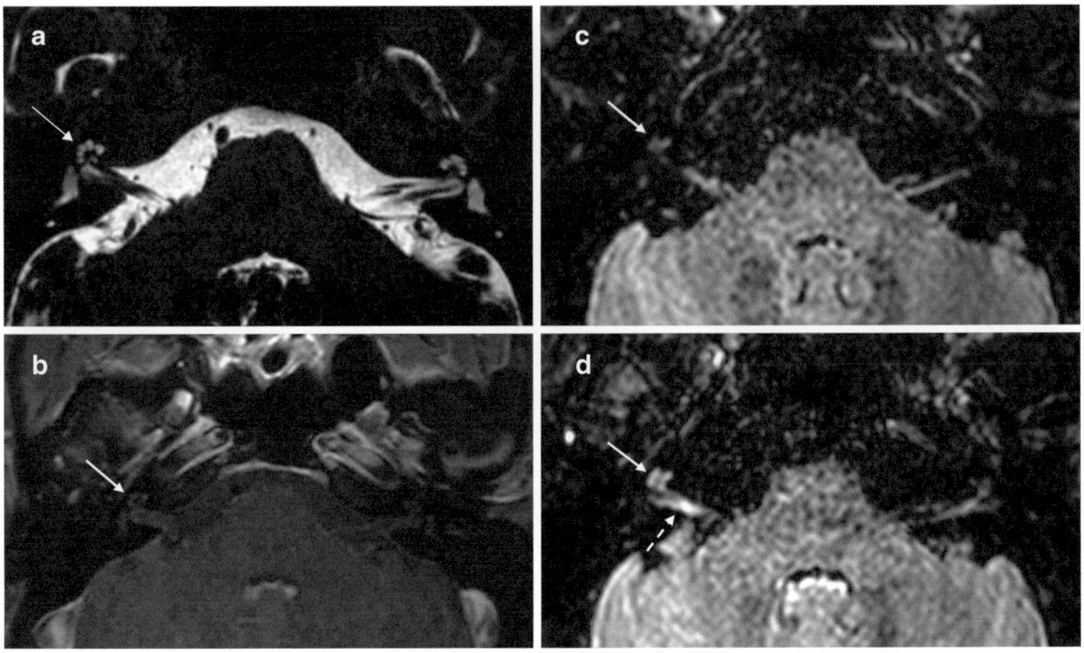

Fig. 9.6 **55-year-old male patient with right pantonal sudden hearing loss for 5 days with a positive blood test of CMV infection showing right cochlear inflammation pattern**. (**a**) Axial 3D TSE-T2W, (**b**) Axial FSE-T1W show normal signal in the inner ear structures (arrows). (**c**) Axial 3D-FLAIR shows high signal in the right cochlea (arrow), suggestive of proteinaceous exudate. (**d**) Contrast-enhanced 3D-FLAIR shows abnormal delayed enhancement of the right cochlea (arrow) and of the facial and vestibulocochlear nerves (dashed arrow), suggestive of active inflammation and neuritis. The imaging characteristics are consistent with an inflammatory pattern of SSHL. *Abbreviations*: CMV = cytomegalovirus; TSE = turbo spin echo; *FSE* = fast spin echo; FLAIR = fluid-attenuated inversion recovery; SSHL = sudden sensorineural hearing loss

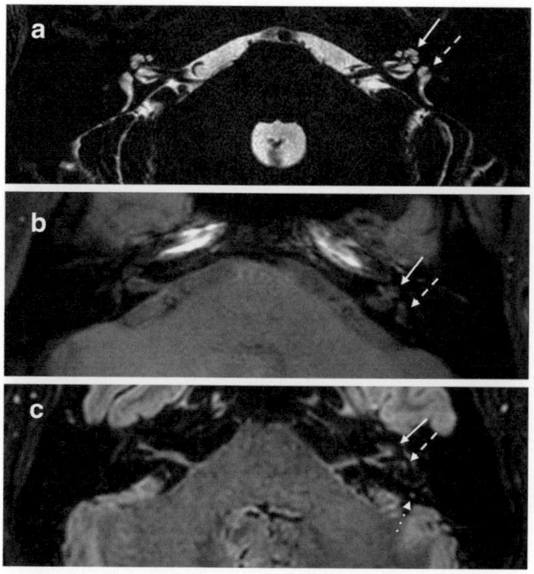

Fig. 9.7 26-year-old male patient with left-sudden sensorineural hearing loss showing ischemic pattern of SSHL in the territory of the left vestibulocochlear artery. (**a**) Axial 3D TSE-T2W, (**b**) Axial FSE-T1W show normal T2 and T1 signal in the left cochlea (arrow) and vestibule (dashed arrow). (**c**) Axial 3D-FLAIR shows high signal in the left cochlea (arrow), vestibule (dashed arrow), and posterior semicircular canal (dotted arrow), due to proteinaceous exudate. *Abbreviations*: SSHL = sudden sensorineural hearing loss; TSE = turbo spin echo; FSE = fast spin echo; FLAIR = fluid-attenuated inversion recovery

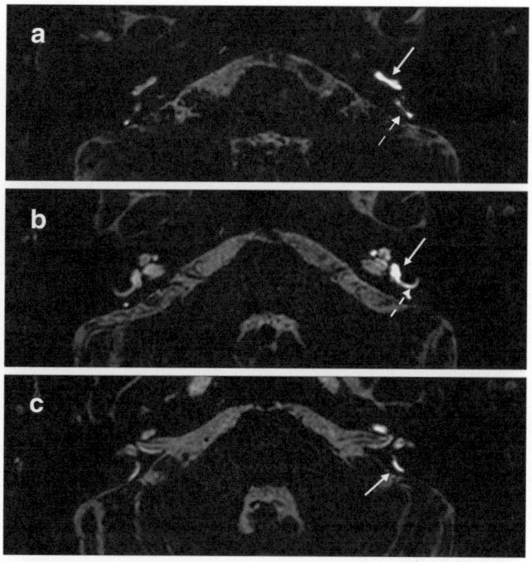

Fig. 9.8 26-year-old male patient with sudden left sensorineural hearing loss showing ischemic pattern of SSHL in the territory of the left vestibulocochlear artery (continues from Fig. 9.7). (**a–c**) Axial 4-h delayed contrast-enhanced 3D-FLAIR images show abnormal enhancement in the basal turn of the cochlea (arrow in **a**), in the posterior semicircular canal (dashed arrow in **a**), in the inferior portion of the vestibule (arrow in **b**), in the non-ampullary segment of the lateral semicircular canal (dashed arrow in **b and arrow in c**). These findings indicate blood-labyrinth barrier breakdown corresponding to the vascular territories of the left vestibulocochlear artery. The imaging characteristics are consistent with an ischemic pattern of SSHL. *Abbreviations*: SSHL = sudden sensorineural hearing loss; FLAIR = fluid-attenuated inversion recovery

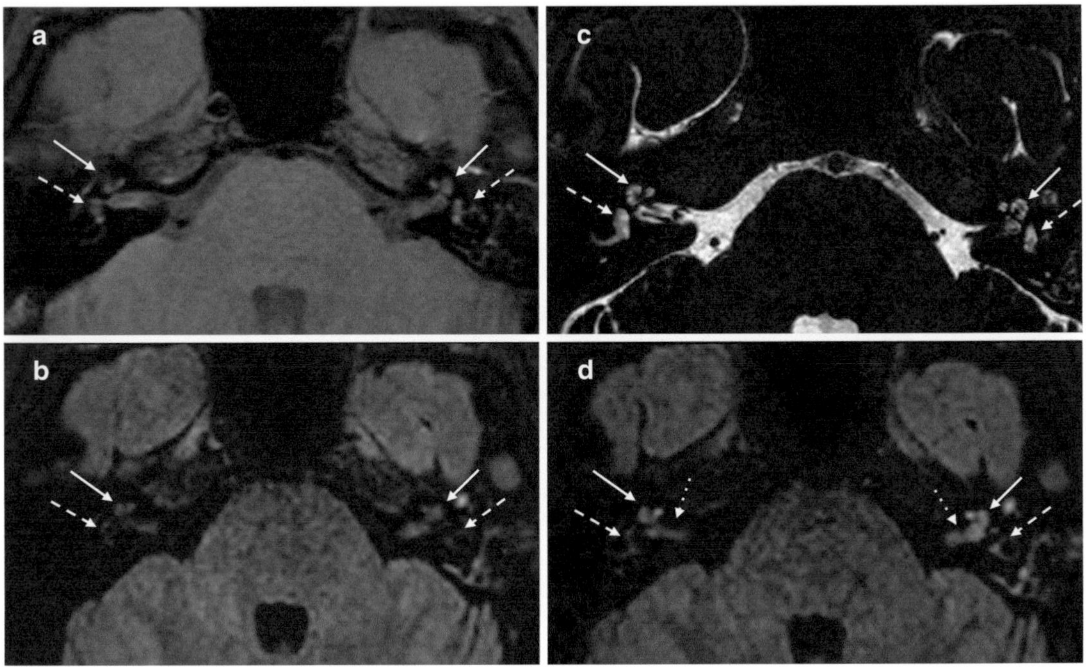

Fig. 9.9 **A 26-year-old female patient with bilateral profound hearing loss for 32 days, diagnosed with Cogan syndrome, demonstrates a bilateral inflammatory pattern of SSHL**. Cogan syndrome is an autoimmune vasculitis primarily affecting young adults. It classically involves the eyes—most commonly presenting with interstitial keratitis—and the inner ears, causing audio-vestibular symptoms that resemble Menière's disease.

There are two clinical forms.

Typical Cogan Syndrome: Characterized by interstitial keratitis and audiovestibular symptoms similar to Menière's disease. These symptoms may precede or follow the ocular findings, typically within a 2-year window.

Atypical Cogan Syndrome: Presents with other forms of ocular inflammation (like uveitis) and audiovestibular symptoms that do not resemble Menière's disease.

A minority of patients may develop systemic vasculitis with multi-organ involvement. (**a**) Axial FSE-T1W and (**c**) Axial 3D TSE-T2W sequences show normal T1 and T2 signal intensity of the inner ear structures; cochlea (arrows) and vestibule (dashed arrows). (**b**) Axial 3D-FLAIR demonstrates high signal in the bilateral inner ear structures—cochleae (arrows) and vestibules (dashed arrows), consistent with proteinaceous exudate. (**d**) Axial contrast-enhanced 3D-FLAIR reveals enhancement of the bilateral cochleae (arrows), vestibules (dashed arrows), and internal auditory canals (dotted arrows), indicating active inflammation. The imaging features are consistent with a bilateral inflammatory inner ear pattern of SSHL, suggestive of autoimmune disorders. *Abbeviations*: SSHL = sudden sensorineural hearing loss; FSE = fast spin echo; TSE = turbo spin echo; FLAIR = fluid-attenuated inversion recovery

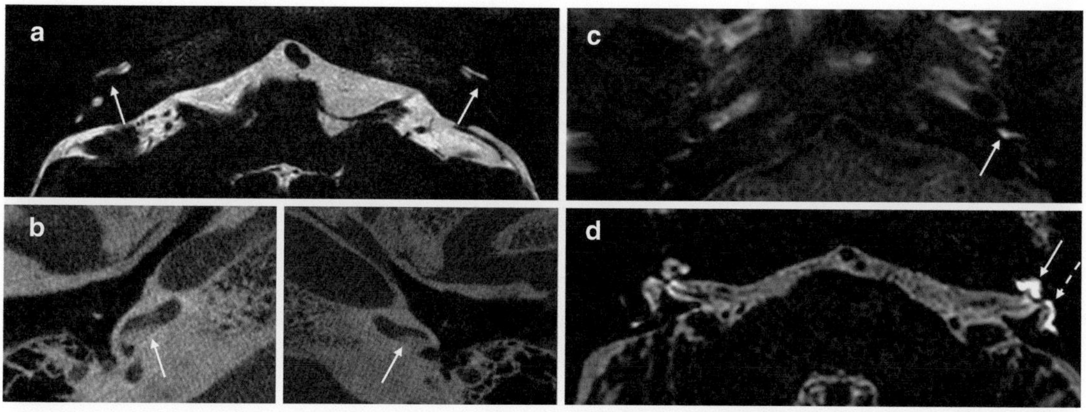

Fig. 9.10 Patient with Cogan syndrome progressed to labyrinthitis ossificans. In infectious, inflammatory, or autoimmune SSHL, the condition may progress to irreversible inner ear damage, potentially leading to labyrinthitis ossificans. (**a**) Axial 3D TSE-T2W shows absence of the normal T2 signal in the basal turn of the cochlea bilaterally (arrows). (**b**) Axial CBCT shows bilateral ossification of part of the basal turn of the cochlea bilaterally (arrows), consistent with ossificans labyrinthitis. (**c**) Axial contrast-enhanced FSE-T1W shows enhancement of the non-ossified portion of the basal turn of the left cochlea (arrow), in keeping with the inflammatory stage. (**d**) Axial 4-h delayed contrast-enhanced 3D-FLAIR shows blood-labyrinth barrier breakdown in the left cochlea (arrow) and vestibule (dashed arrow). *Abbreviations*: SSHL = sudden sensorineural hearing loss; TSE = turbo spin echo; CBCT = cone-beam computed tomography; FSE = fast spin echo; FLAIR = fluid-attenuated inversion recovery

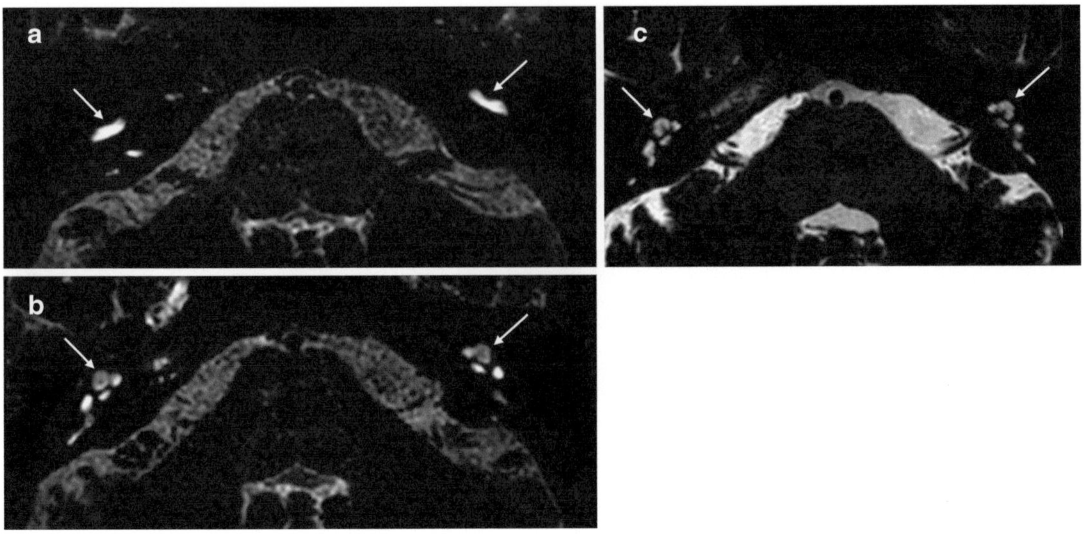

Fig. 9.11 **Inflammatory pattern of SSHL in a 40-year-old female presenting with bilateral low-frequency hearing loss, later diagnosed with bilateral inner ear sarcoidosis.** Sarcoidosis is a multisystem inflammatory disease of unknown cause, characterized by non-caseating granulomas. These lesions typically lack necrosis, except in rare variants such as necrotizing sarcoid granulomatosis. Granulomas may resolve spontaneously or progress to fibrosis. The disease most commonly involves: the lungs and mediastinum (hilar lymphadenopathy, interstitial lung disease), the heart (arrhythmias, conduction defects, heart failure), the muscles and joints (arthritis, myopathy), the head and neck region (salivary and lacrimal gland enlargement, lymphadenopathy), the abdomen (hepatic, splenic, renal, or nodal involvement), the skin (erythema nodosum, lupus pernio, skin nodules), and the central nervous system (cranial neuropathies, meningitis, brain and spinal cord lesions). A rare involvement of sarcoidosis is the inner ear, which can cause hearing loss and vestibular dysfunction. It involves the formation of granulomas within the cochlea and/or vestibular system, potentially disrupting both auditory and vestibular functions. (**a**–**b**) Axial 4-h delayed contrast-enhanced 3D-FLAIR sequences shows normal signal intensity in the basal turn of the cochlea bilaterally (arrows in **a**), and low signal intensity in the medio-apical turn of the cochlea bilaterally (arrow in b) probably due to initial deposition of granulomatous tissue. (**c**) Axial 3D TSE-T2W sequence shows normal T2 signal intensity in the cochlea bilaterally (arrows). *Abbreviations*: SSHL = sudden sensorineural hearing loss; FLAIR = fluid-attenuated inversion recovery; TSE = turbo spin echo

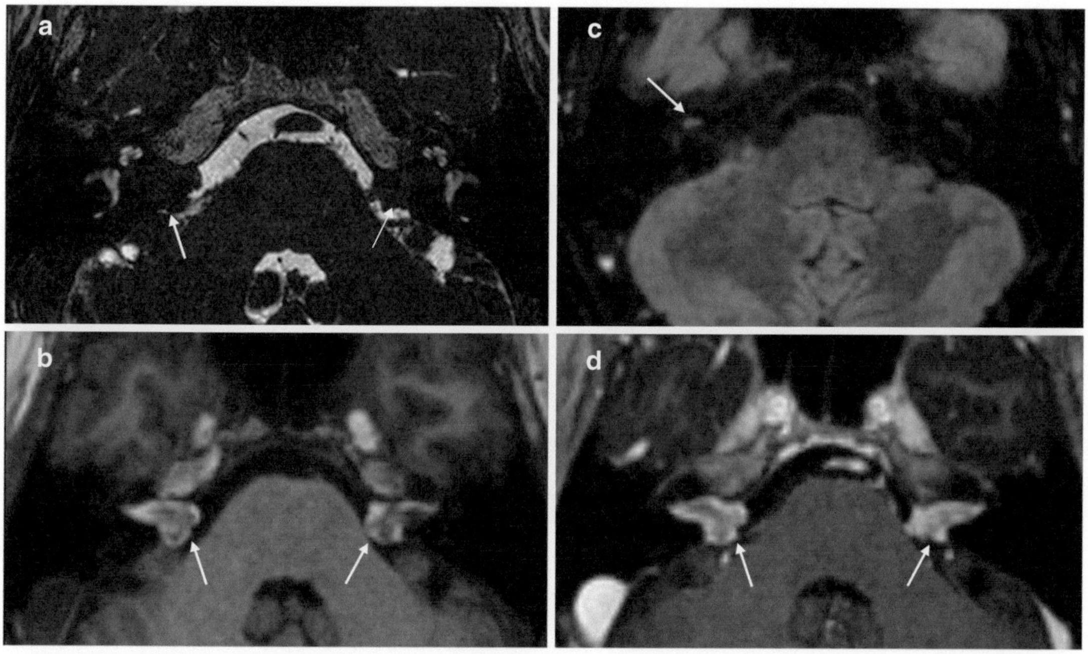

Fig. 9.12 64-years-old male with known bilateral internal acoustic metastasis from melanoma presenting with right anacusis for 3 days with right indirect cochlear damage. MRI is essential for excluding retrocochlear causes (e.g. space-occupying lesions) of SSHL. (**a**) Axial 3D TSE-T2W, (**b**) Axial FSE-T1W, and (**d**) Axial contrast-enhanced FSE-T1W show bilateral internal auditory canal masses (arrows in **a**), which demonstrates high signal on FSE-T1W (arrows in **b**), likely due to melanin content. Post-contrast image shows mild enhancement of the lesions (arrows in **d**) consistent with metastases from metastatic melanoma. (**c**) Axial 3D-FLAIR reveals high signal in the right cochlea (arrow), probably due to proteinaceous exudate, indicative of indirect cochlear damage. *Abbreviations*: MRI = magnetic resonance imaging; SSHL = sudden sensorineural hearing loss; TSE = turbo spin echo; FSE = fast spin echo; FLAIR = fluid-attenuated inversion recovery

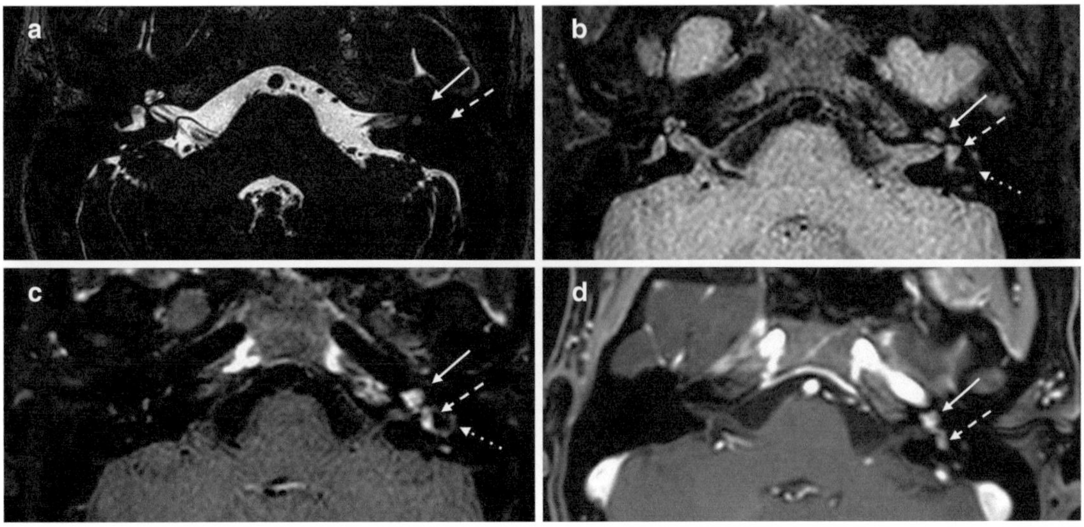

Fig. 9.13 **Left vestibulocochlear labyrinthitis — fibro-osseous stage.** (**a**) Axial 3D TSE-T2W shows absence of the normal T2 signal in the left inner ear structures: cochlea (arrow) and vestibule (dashed arrow). (**b**) Axial 3D-FLAIR demonstrates high signal in the cochlea (arrow) and vestibule (dashed arrow), but absence of signal in the lateral semicircular canal (dotted arrow). (**c**) Axial contrast-enhanced 3D TSE-T1W BB and (**d**) Axial contrast-enhanced 3D FFE-T1W with fat suppression sequences show enhancement of the left cochlea (arrow) and vestibule (dashed arrow), and faint enhancement in the lateral semicircular canal (dotted arrow in **c**) consistent with active fibrosis. *Abbreviations*: TSE = turbo spin echo; FLAIR = fluid-attenuated inversion recovery; BB = black blood; FFE = fast field echo

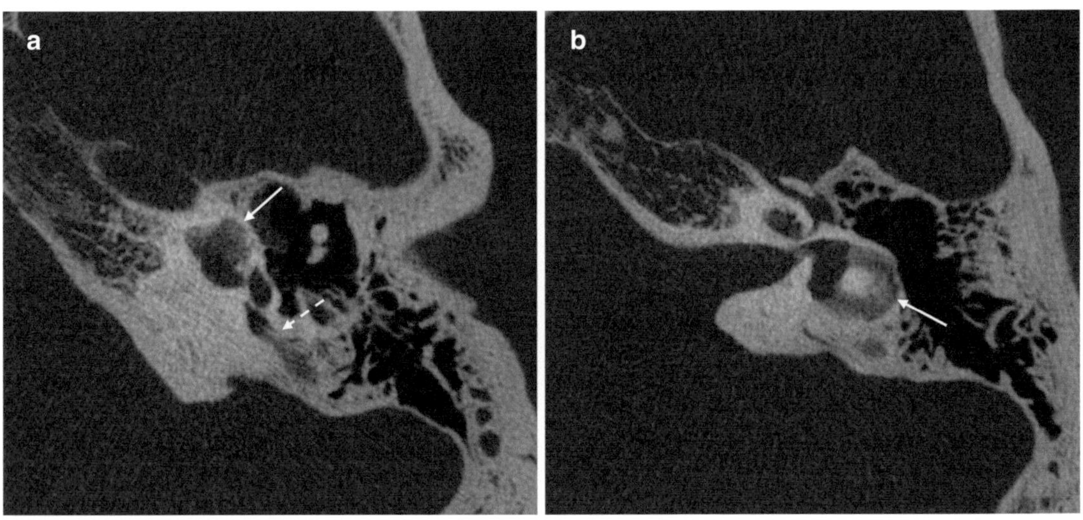

Fig. 9.14 **Left vestibulocochlear labyrinthitis — fibro-osseous stage (continues from Fig.** 9.13). (**a** and **b**) Axial CBCT show initial ossification of the cochlea (arrow in **a**), posterior semicircular canal (dashed arrow in **a**) and lateral semicircular canal (arrow in **b**). *Abbreviation*: CBCT = cone-beam computed tomography

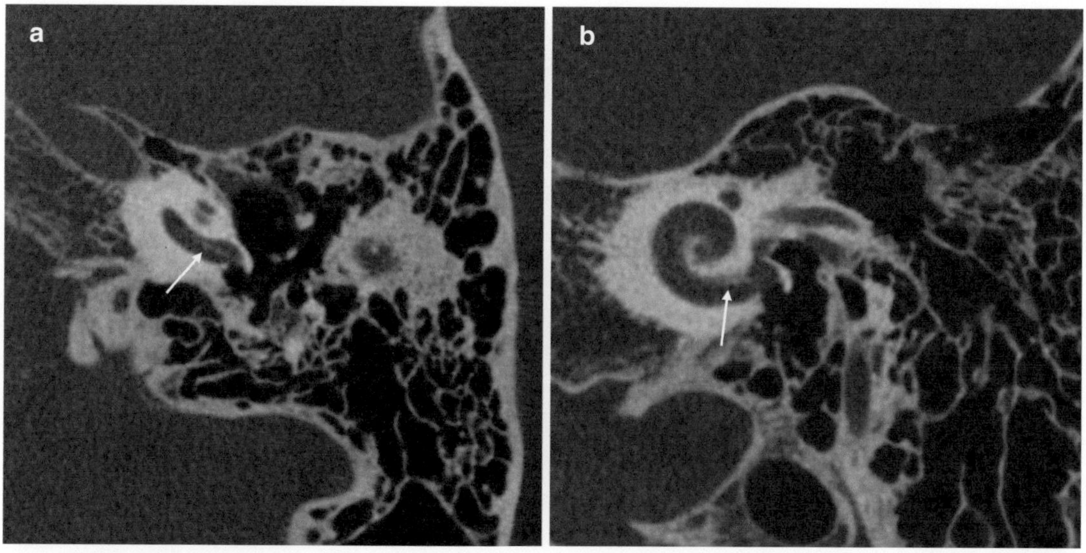

Fig. 9.15 Left labyrinthitis — Subtle left spiral lamina thickening. (**a**) Axial, (**b**) Coronal CBCT images show subtle spiral lamina thickening (arrow), an early sign of labyrinthine ossification. *Abbreviation*: CBCT = cone-beam computed tomography

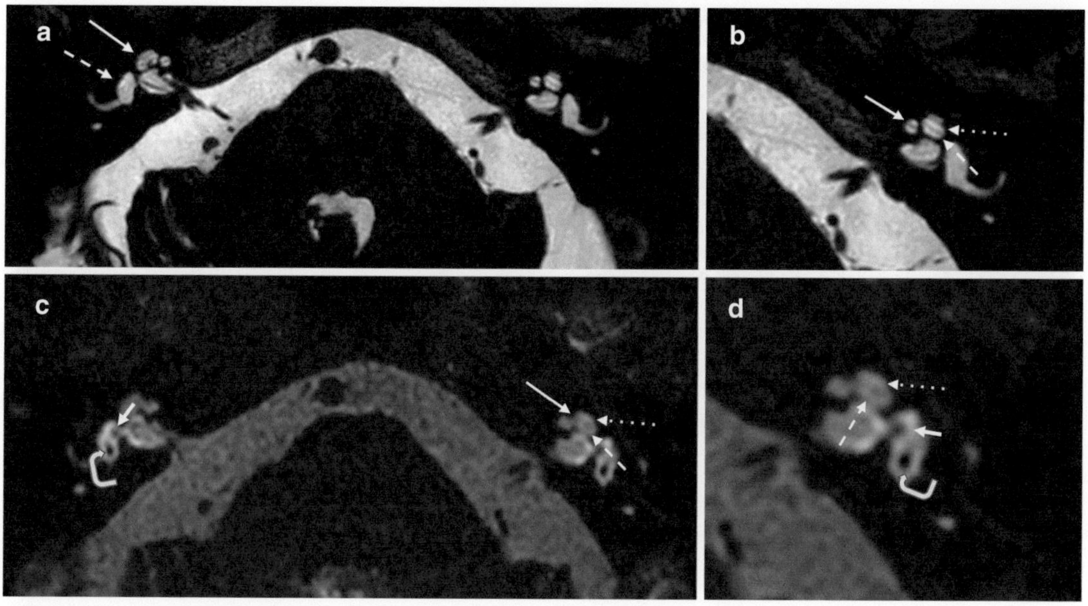

Fig. 9.16 Normal aspect of the membranous labyrinth (Bernaerts classification grade 0). (**a**) Axial 3D TSE-T2W shows normal T2 signal in the cochlea (arrow) and vestibule (dotted arrow). (**b**) Magnified view of (**a**) demonstrates the osseous spiral lamina, visible as a dark tiny linear structure (arrow), which separates the scala tympani inferiorly (dashed arrow) from the scala vestibuli superiorly (dotted arrow). (**c**) Axial 4-h delayed contrast-enhanced 3D-FLAIR demonstrates a normal membranous labyrinth, corresponding to grade 0 according to the Bernaerts classification. Within the normal cochlea, the osseous spiral lamina (arrow), scala tympani (dashed arrow), and scala vestibuli (dotted arrow) are visible, while the scala media is either minimally visible or not visible, as expected. In the vestibule, both the saccule (small arrow) and the utricle (curved arrow) are identifiable, appearing as distinct structures, with the saccule slightly smaller than the utricle. (**d**) Magnified view of (**c**) further highlights the saccule (small arrow), the utricle (curved arrow), the scala tympani inferiorly (dashed arrow), and the scala vestibuli superiorly (dotted arrow). *Abbreviations*: TSE = turbo spin echo; FLAIR = fluid-attenuated inversion recovery

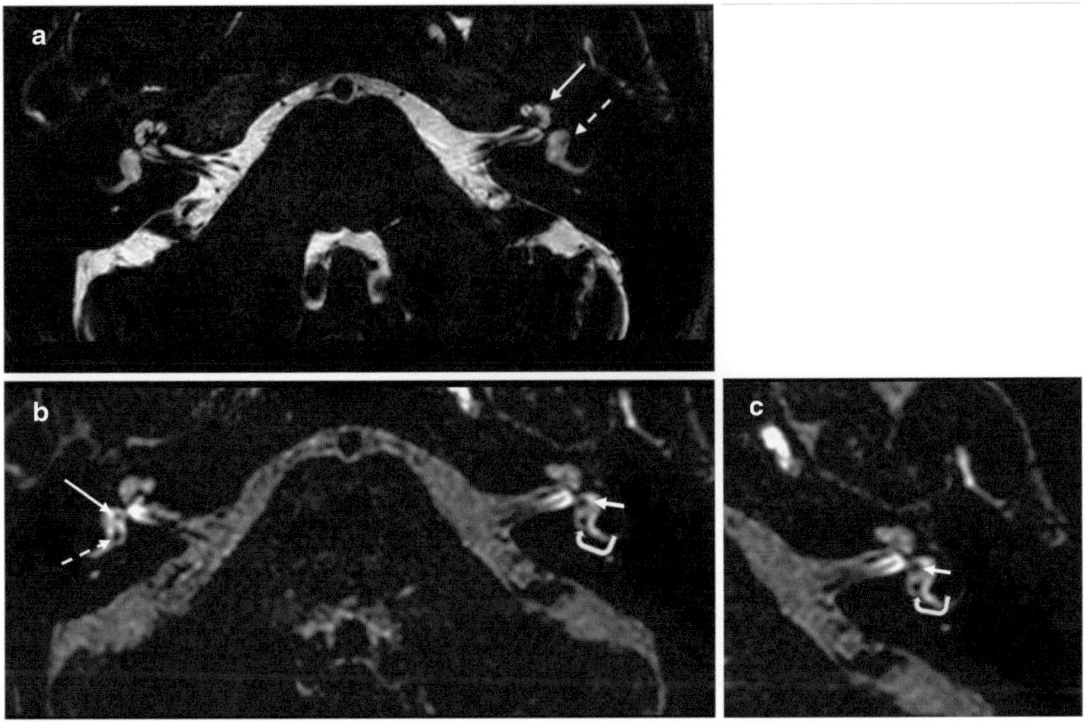

Fig. 9.17 **Grade 1 left vestibular hydrops (according to Bernaerts) in patient with Menière disease**. Menière's disease is a chronic inner ear disorder characterized by fluctuating sensorineural hearing loss, episodic vertigo, tinnitus, and aural fullness. The hallmark pathological feature is endolymphatic hydrops, an excessive accumulation of endolymph within the membranous labyrinth. In grade 1 vestibular hydrops, the saccule becomes equal to or slightly larger than the utricle, but they remain distinct and do not merge together. (**a**) Axial 3D TSE-T2W shows normal T2 signal in the left inner ear structures; cochlea (arrow) and vestibule (dashed arrow). (**b**) Axial 4-h delayed contrast-enhanced 3D-FLAIR demonstrates mild vestibular endolymphatic hydrops on the left: the saccule (small arrow) appears slightly larger than the utricle (curved arrow), but the two structures are still clearly separated. The right vestibule appears normal, with the saccule (arrow) smaller than the utricle (dashed arrow). (**c**) Magnified view of image (**b**) provides clearer visualization of the saccule (small arrow) and the utricle (curved arrow). *Abbreviations*: TSE = turbo spin echo; FLAIR = fluid-attenuated inversion recovery

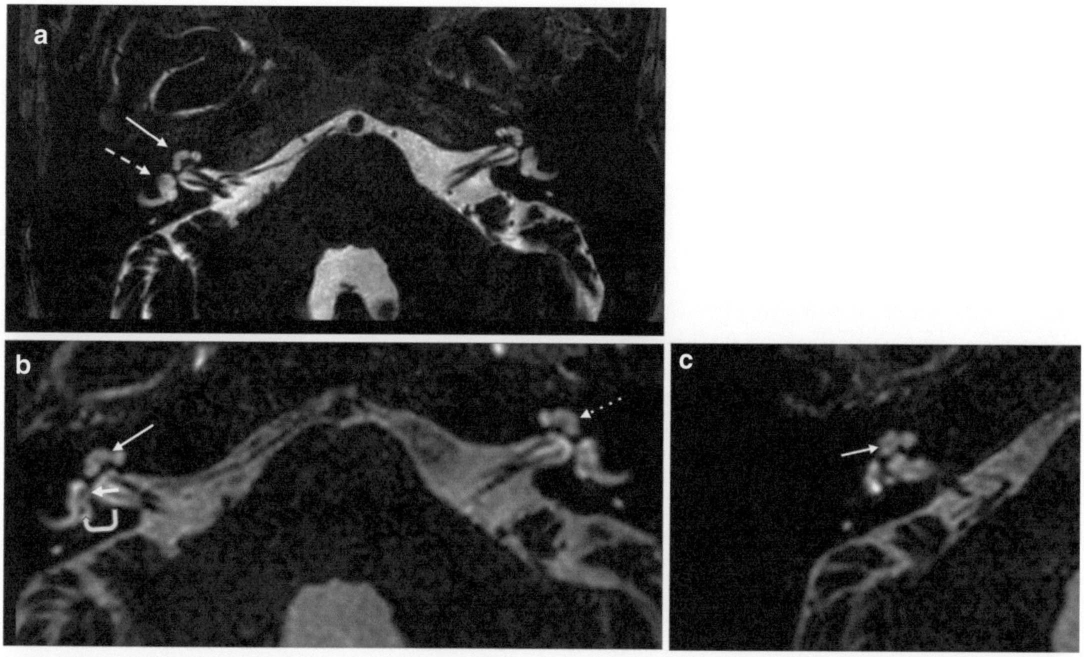

Fig. 9.18 Grade 1 right medio-apical cochlear hydrops (according to Bernaerts) in patient with Menière disease. In grade 1 cochlear hydrops, the scala media becomes slightly visible as a nodular black signal void within the scala vestibuli. (**a**) Axial 3D TSE-T2W shows normal T2 signal of the right inner ear structure; cochlea (arrow) and vestibule (dashed arrow). (**b**) Axial 4-h delayed contrast-enhanced 3D-FLAIR demonstrates slight enlargement of the scala media, visible as a tiny signal void in the medio-apical turns of the right cochlea (arrow). Additionally, grade 1 vestibular hydrops is present on the same side, with the saccule enlarged (small arrow). The left cochlea appears normal (dotted arrow). (**c**) Magnified view of image (**b**) better depicts the slight enlargement of the scala media (arrow). *Abbreviations*: TSE = turbo spin echo; FLAIR = fluid-attenuated inversion recovery

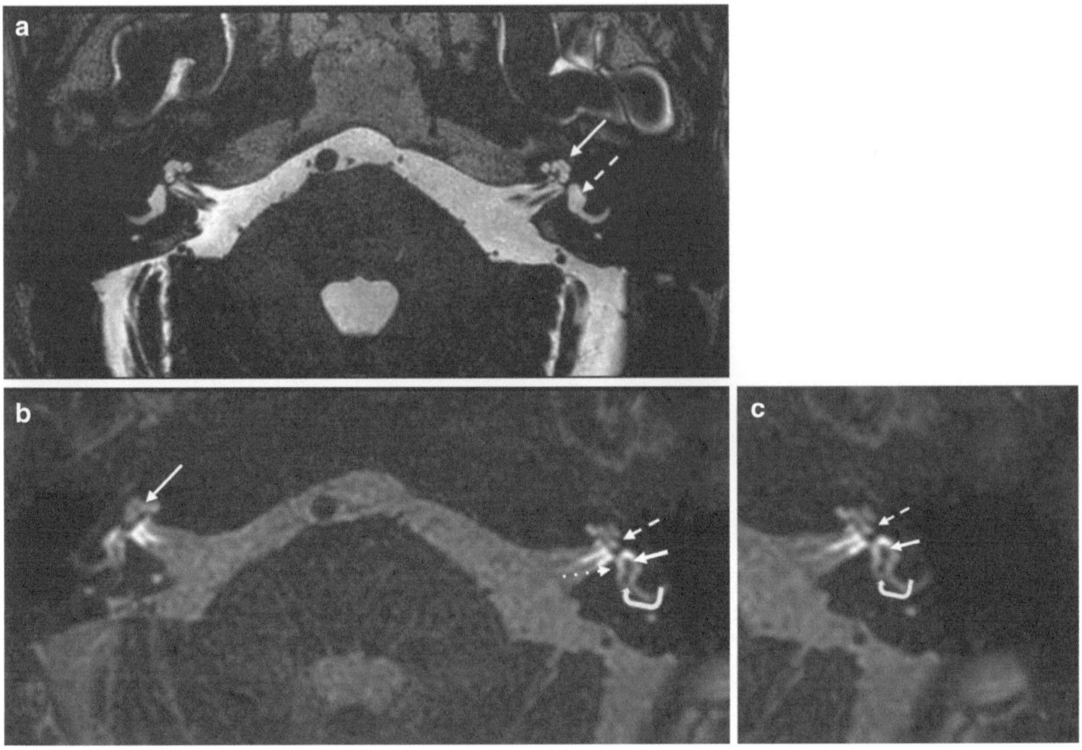

Fig. 9.19 Grade 2 left cochleo-vestibular hydrops (according to Bernaerts) in patient with Menière disease. In grade 2 vestibular hydrops, the saccule is larger than the utricle, with a confluence between the two structures; however, the perilymphatic space remains visible as peripheral enhancement. In grade 2 cochlear hydrops, the scala vestibuli is completely obliterated due to an enlarged cochlear duct. (**a**) Axial 3D TSE-T2W sequence demonstrates normal T2 signal intensity of the inner ear structures; cochlea (arrow) and vestibule (dashed arrow). (**b**) Axial 4-h delayed contrast-enhanced 3D-FLAIR: on the left side, the saccule (small arrow) appears enlarged relative to the utricle (curved arrow), with initial confluence between the two. The perilymphatic space remains visible as peripheral enhancement (dotted arrow), consistent with grade 2 vestibular hydrops. The left scala vestibuli is no longer visible, fully obliterated by the enlarged cochlear duct (dashed arrow), consistent with grade 2 cochlear hydrops. On the right side, there is mild enlargement of the cochlear duct (arrow), indicative of grade 1 cochlear hydrops. (**c**) Magnified view of image **b** provides better visualization of: the enlarged saccule (small arrow) confluent with the utricle (curved arrow), and the enlarged cochlear duct (dashed arrow). *Abbreviations*: TSE = turbo spin echo; FLAIR = fluid-attenuated inversion recovery

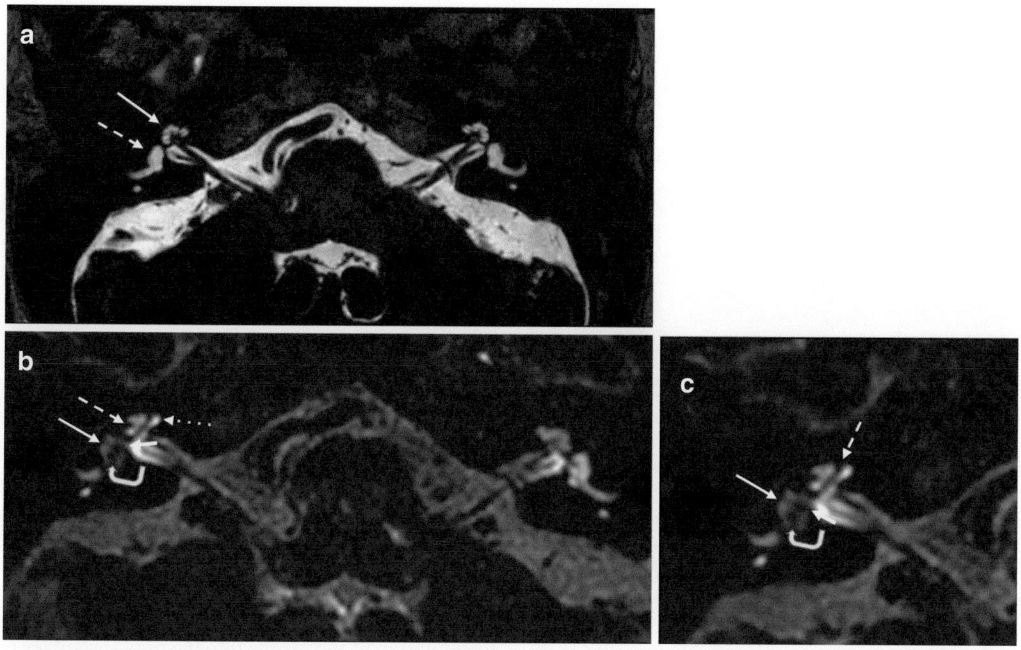

Fig. 9.20 Grade 3 right vestibular hydrops and grade 2 right cochlear hydrops (according to Bernaerts) in patient with Menière disease. In grade 3 vestibular hydrops, the vestibule is completely obliterated by the enlarged saccule and utricle, and perilymphatic enhancement is no longer visible. (**a**) Axial 3D TSE-T2W sequence shows normal T2 signal intensity of the right inner ear structures; the cochlea (arrow) and vestibule (dashed arrow). (**b**) Axial 4-h delayed contrast-enhanced 3D-FLAIR sequence shows enlargement of the saccule (small arrow) and utricle (curved arrow), with absence of enhancement in the perilymphatic space (arrow), consistent with grade 3 vestibular hydrops. The image also demonstrates grade 2 cochlear hydrops (dashed arrow) and breakdown of the blood-labyrinth barrier, with increased enhancement in the medial turn of the cochlea (dotted arrow). (**c**) Magnified view of image b better shows the enlarged saccule (small arrow), enlarged utricle (curved arrow), non-enhanced perilymphatic space (arrow), and the enlarged cochlear duct (dashed arrow). *Abbreviations*: TSE = turbo spin echo; FLAIR = fluid-attenuated inversion recovery

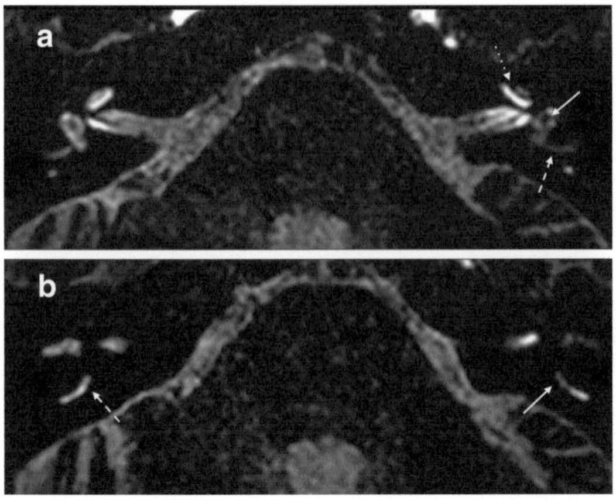

Fig. 9.21 **Grade 3 left vestibular hydrops and grade 2 left cochlear hydrops (according to Bernaerts), with invagination of the utricle into the non-ampullary tract of the lateral semicircular canal and hydrops of the ampulla of the posterior semicircular canal. Patient with Menière disease**. (**a**) Axial 4 h delayed contrast-enhanced 3D-FLAIR sequence demonstrates grade 3 vestibular hydrops on the left. The ampulla of the lateral semicircular canal is positioned supero-laterally than the saccule and is clearly visualized (arrow) on a more cranial axial plane than the plane where the saccule is usually visualized, the utricle is not well defined and is invaginated into the non-ampullary tract of the lateral semicircular canal (dashed arrow), which also lacks normal perilymphatic enhancement, indicating hydrops. There is also evidence of grade 2 cochlear hydrops (dotted arrow). (**b**) Axial 4-h delayed contrast-enhanced 3D-FLAIR (same sequence as in a, at a lower axial plane) demonstrates hydrops of the ampulla of the left posterior semicircular canal (arrow), which is characterized by absence of normal perilymphatic enhancement. The contralateral posterior semicircular canal ampulla appears normal (dashed arrow), showing intact perilymphatic enhancement. *Abbreviation*: FLAIR = fluid-attenuated inversion recovery

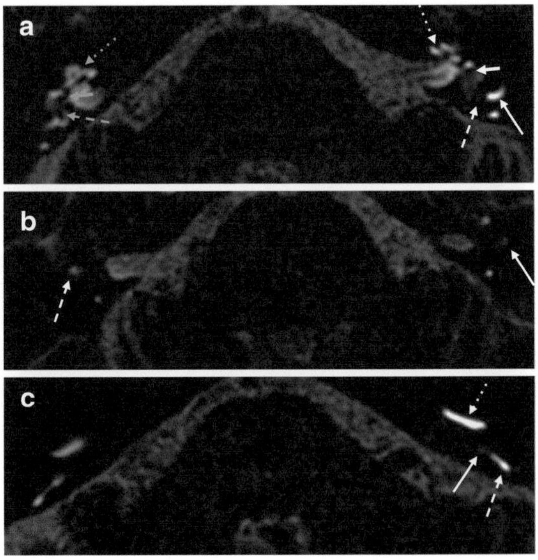

Fig. 9.22 **Grade 3 left vestibular hydrops and grade 2 left cochlear hydrops (according to Bernaerts), with invagination of the utricle into the non-ampullary tract of the lateral semicircular canal, and hydrops of the ampullae of all three semicircular canals. On the right, there is grade 2 vestibular hydrops and grade 1 cochlear hydrops (according to Bernaerts). Patient with Menière disease**. (**a**) Axial 4-h delayed contrast-enhanced 3D-FLAIR sequence shows grade 3 vestibular hydrops on the left (arrow). The saccule is visible within the vestibule (small arrow), but the utricle is not well delineated, it is invaginated into the non-ampullary tract of the lateral semicircular canal (dashed arrow), which lacks the normal perilymphatic enhancement. There is also evidence of abnormal contrast-enhancement in the remaining segment of the lateral semicircular canal (arrow), compatible with blood-labyrinth barrier breakdown. Grade 2 cochlear hydrops is noted (dotted arrow). On the right, a grade 1 cochlear hydrops is observed (grey dotted arrow), along with grade 2 vestibular hydrops, characterized by confluence of the saccule (grey small arrow) and utricle (gray dotted arrow) while perilymphatic space remains visible. (**b**) Axial 4-h delayed contrast-enhanced 3D-FLAIR (same sequence as in **a**, at a lower axial plane) demonstrates hydrops of the ampulla of the left superior semicircular canal (arrow), which lacks normal perilymphatic enhancement. The contralateral ampullary tract of the right superior semicircular canal appears normal (dashed arrow). (**c**) Axial 4-h delayed contrast-enhanced 3D-FLAIR (same sequence as in **a**, at a lower axial plane) shows hydrops of the ampulla of the left posterior semicircular canal (arrow), with absence of normal perilymphatic enhancement. Additionally, there is abnormal contrast enhancement in the remaining segment of the posterior semicircular canal (dashed arrow) and in the basal turn of the cochlea (dotted arrow), indicating blood-labyrinth barrier breakdown. *Abbreviation*: FLAIR = fluid-attenuated inversion recovery

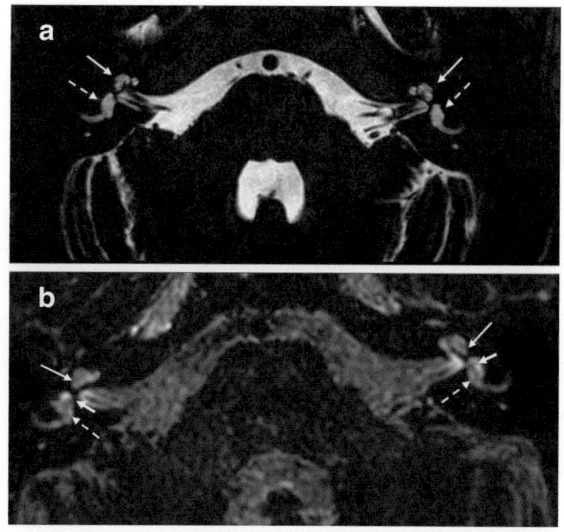

Fig. 9.23 Grade 2 bilateral vestibular hydrops "faint" aspect and grade 1 bilateral cochlear hydrops (according to Bernaerts) in patient with Menière disease. (**a**) Axial 3D TSE-T2W sequence shows normal T2 signal intensity of the bilateral inner ear structures; the cochlea (arrows) and vestibule (dashed arrows). (**b**) Axial 4-h delayed contrast-enhanced 3D-FLAIR sequence: the saccule (small arrow) and the utricle (dashed arrow) are barely visible and appear confluent. The perilymphatic space in the vestibule is normally visualized bilaterally. There is also mild bilateral enlargement of the cochlear duct (arrow), consistent with grade 1 cochlear hydrops. *Abbreviations*: TSE = turbo spin echo; FLAIR = fluid-attenuated inversion recovery

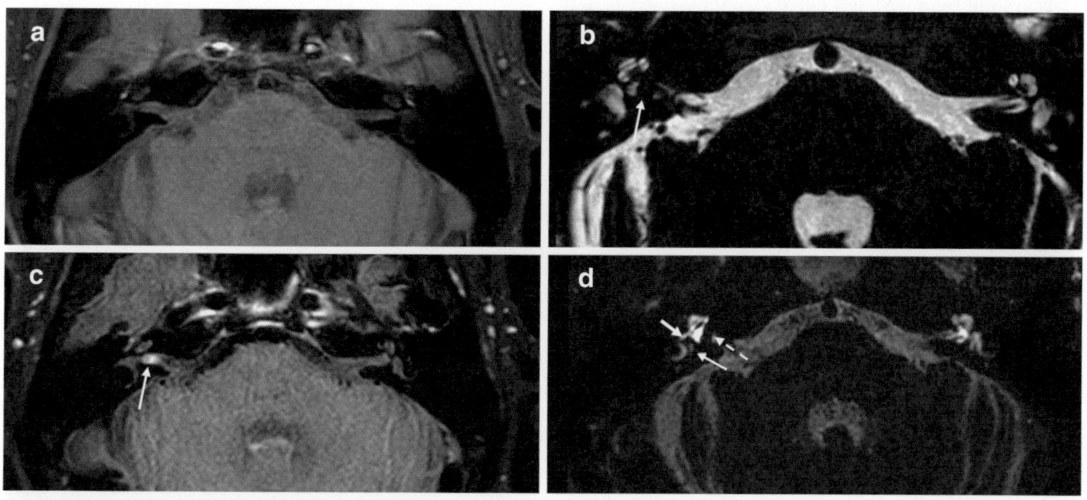

Fig. 9.24 Right cochleo-vestibular schwannoma causing grade 2 right vestibular hydrops (according to Bernaerts). (**a**) Axial FSE-T1W, (**b**) Axial 3D TSE-T2W, (**c**) Axial contrast-enhanced 3D TSE-T1W show a right intracanal cochleo-vestibular schwannoma (arrow in **b** and **c**). (**d**) Axial 4-h delayed contrast-enhanced 3D-FLAIR shows a grade 2 vestibular hydrops (saccule, small arrow; utricle, arrow) caused by the cochleovestibular schwannoma (dashed arrow). Abbreviations: FSE = fast field echo; TSE = turbo spin echo; FLAIR = fluid-attenuated inversion recovery

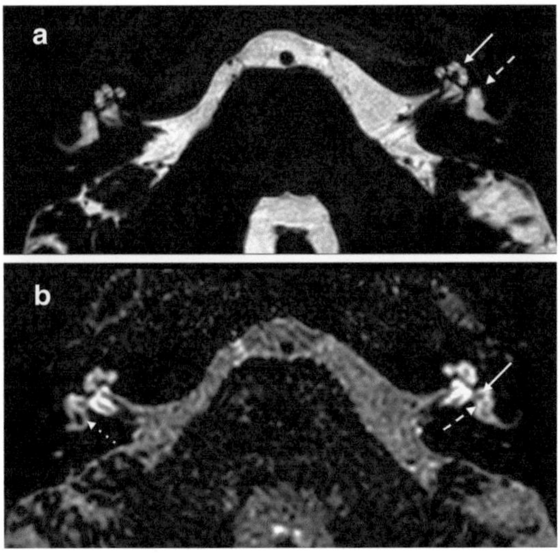

Fig. 9.25 Complete left utricle atelectasis in a 32-years-old man with left paroxysmal nystagmus and low-pitched hearing loss. (**a**) Axial 3D TSE-T2W shows normal T2 signal of the left inner ear structure (cochlea, arrow and vestibule, dashed arrow). (**b**) Axial 4-h delayed contrast-enhanced 3D-FLAIR. In the left vestibule the saccule is normal (arrow), while the utricle (dashed arrow) is barely seen and much smaller than the contralateral one (dotted arrow). *Abbreviations*: TSE = turbo spin echo; FLAIR = fluid-attenuated inversion recovery

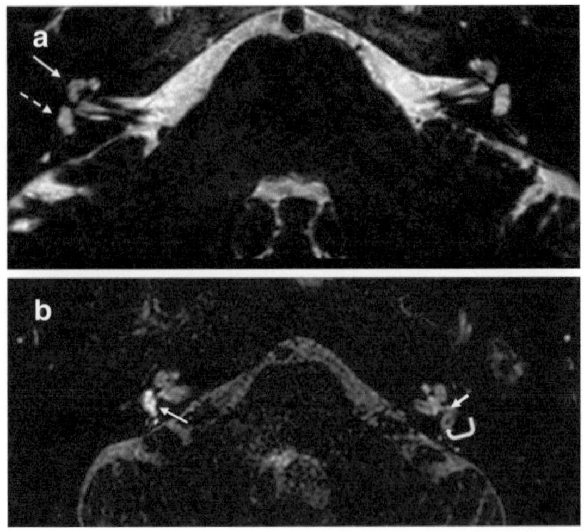

Fig. 9.26 Complete right vestibule atelectasis in a 33-years-old man with right sensorineural hearing loss. (**a**) Axial 3D TSE-T2W shows normal T2 signal of the right inner ear structure: cochlea (arrow) and vestibule (dashed arrow). (**b**) Axial 4-h delayed contrast-enhanced 3D-FLAIR sequence: in the right vestibule the saccule and utricle are no longer visible, consistent with atelectasis; there is also evidence of abnormal contrast-enhancement suggestive for blood-labyrinth barrier breakdown (arrow). For comparison, note the normal appearance of the saccule (small arrow) and the utricle (curved arrow) in the left vestibule. *Abbreviations*: TSE = turbo spin echo; FLAIR = fluid-attenuated inversion recovery

Fig. 9.27 Complete right saccule atelectasis in a patient with right sensorineural hearing loss and bilateral tinnitus. (**a**) Axial 3D TSE-T2W sequence shows normal T2 signal intensity of the right inner ear structures: the cochlea (arrow) and vestibule (dashed arrow). (**b**) Axial 4-h delayed contrast-enhanced 3D-FLAIR sequence: in the right vestibule, the saccule is no longer visible (arrow), consistent with atelectasis, while the utricle appears normal (dashed arrow). Note the normal saccule in the left vestibule (small arrow). *Abbreviations*: TSE = turbo spin echo; FLAIR = fluid-attenuated inversion recovery

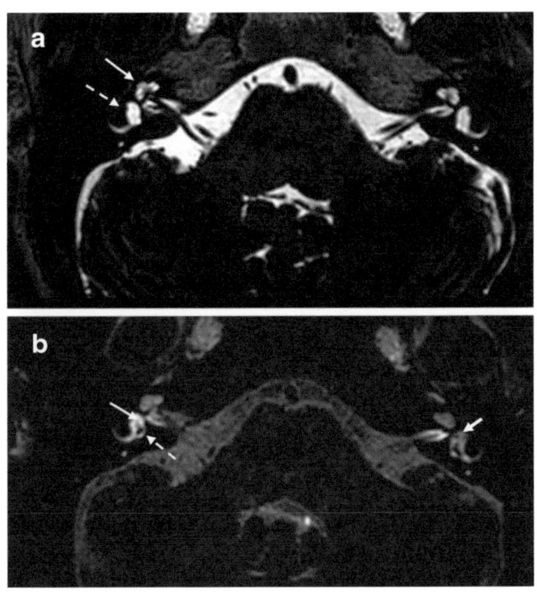

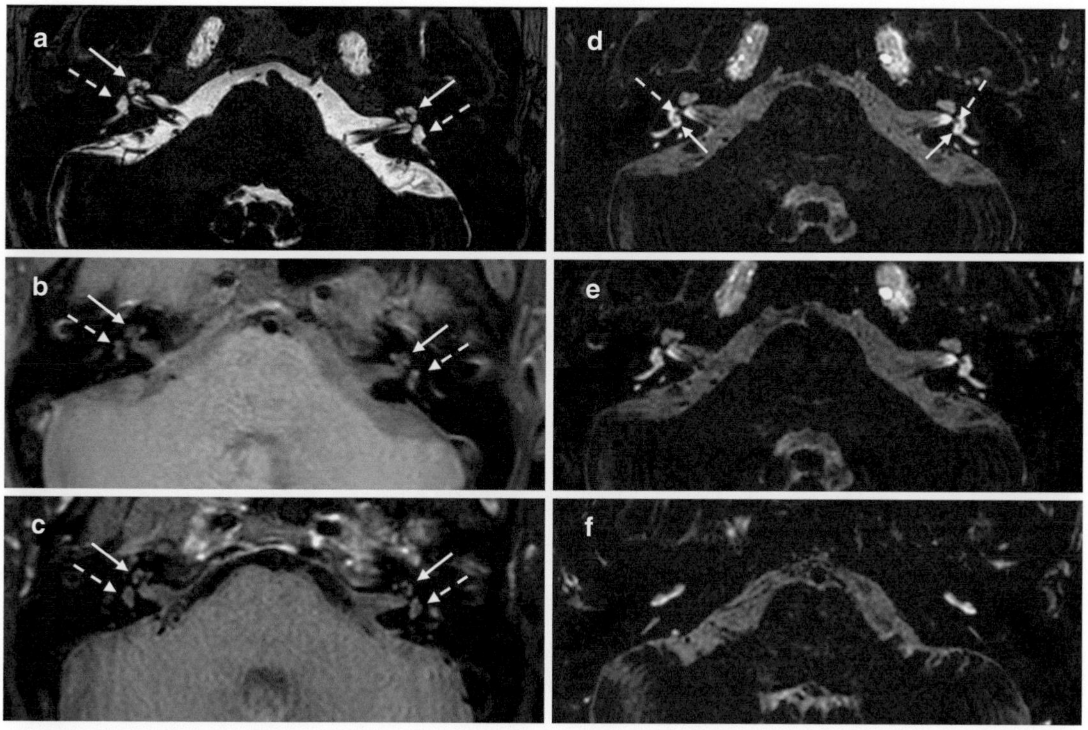

Fig. 9.28 **Constitutional cochlear fragility in a patient with suspected bilateral Menière disease.** (**a**) Axial 3D TSE-T2W, (**b**) axial FSE-T1W, and (**c**) axial contrast-enhanced 3D TSE-T1W BB show normal signal intensity of the bilateral inner ear structures: cochlea (arrows) and vestibule (dashed arrows). (**d–f**) Axial 4-h delayed contrast-enhanced 3D-FLAIR sequences demonstrate no visualization of the utricle bilaterally (arrows in **d**), consistent with atelectasis of the utricle. The saccule appears normal bilaterally (dashed arrows in **d**). Given the bilaterality, a hypothesis of constitutional fragility is considered. *Abbreviations*: TSE = turbo spin echo; FSE = fast spin echo; BB = black blood; FLAIR = fluid-attenuated inversion recovery

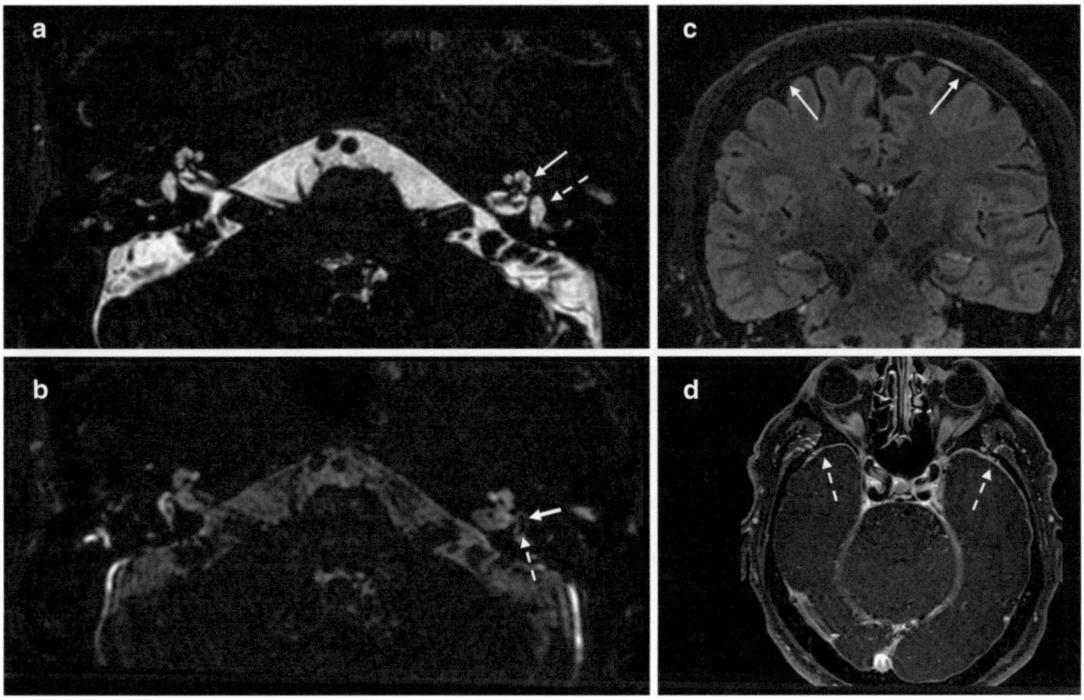

Fig. 9.29 **Left cochleo-vestibular hydrops in a patient with spontaneous intracranial hypotension**. (**a**) Axial 3D TSE-T2W sequence shows normal T2 signal intensity of the left inner ear structures, including the cochlea (arrow) and the vestibule (dashed arrow). (**b**) Axial 4-h delayed contrast-enhanced 3D-FLAIR sequence demonstrates grade 2 left cochleo-vestibular hydrops, with an enlarged saccule (small arrow), which is confluent with the utricle (dashed arrow). (**c**) Coronal 3D-FLAIR reveals bilateral thin subdural effusions (arrows), more prominent on the left. (**d**) Axial contrast-enhanced 3D FFE-T1W with fat suppression sequence shows mild dural thickening with linear enhancement (dashed arrows). Findings in **c** and **d** are suggestive of spontaneous intracranial hypotension. *Abbreviations*: TSE = turbo spin echo; FLAIR = fluid-attenuated inversion recovery; FFE = fast field echo

Fig. 9.30 **Left cochleo-vestibular hydrops in a patient with spontaneous intracranial hypotension (continuous from Fig.** 9.29). (**a**) Axial 3D TSE-T2W sequence shows normal T2 signal intensity of the left inner ear structures: cochlea (arrow) and vestibule (dashed arrow). (**b**) Axial 4-h delayed contrast-enhanced 3D-FLAIR sequence demonstrates resolution of the left cochleo-vestibular hydrops following treatment of intracranial hypotension. The left vestibule shows a normal saccule (small arrow) and utricle (dashed arrow). *Abbreviations*: TSE = turbo spin echo; FLAIR = fluid-attenuated inversion recovery

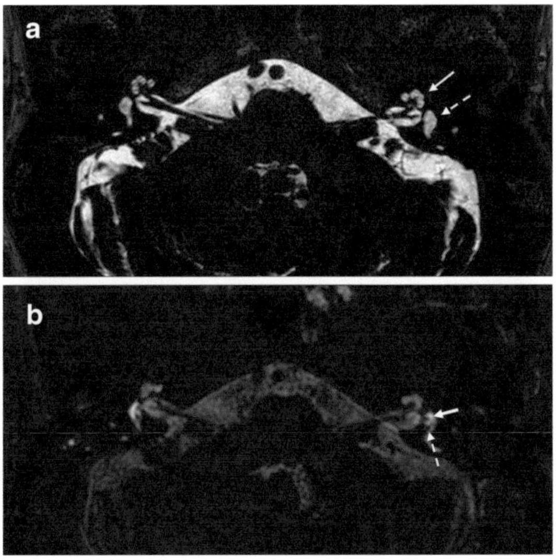

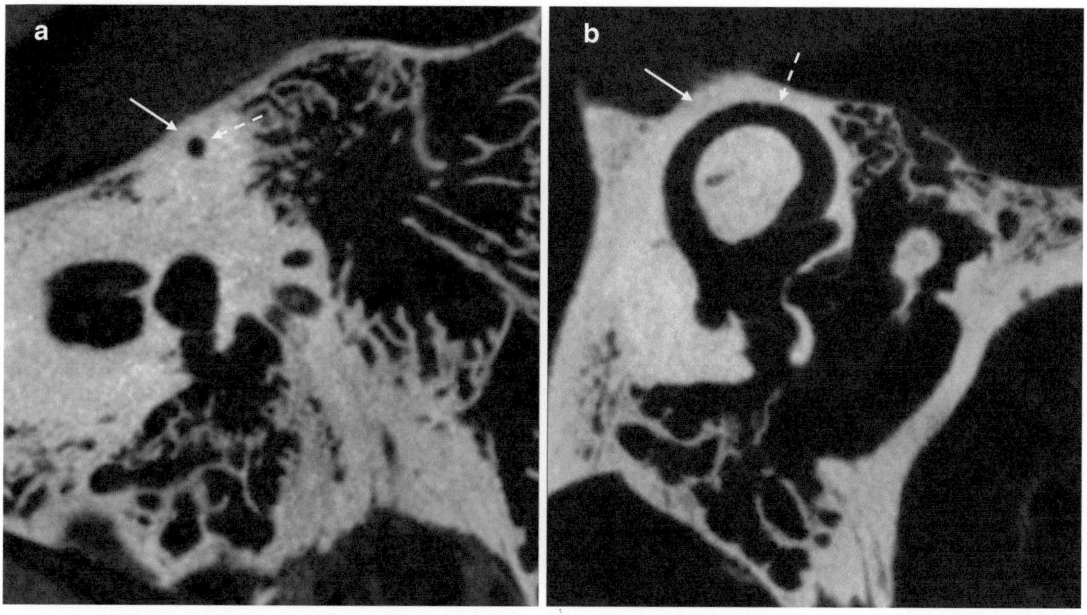

Fig. 9.31 Normal bony roof of the superior semicircular canal. These post-mortem CBCT images demonstrate a normal bony roof of the SSC, highlighting anatomical variability among different subjects. High-resolution imaging is essential for accurate evaluation of the bony roof of the superior semicircular canal, with CBCT offering significant advantages over MDCT. The isotropic voxels and sub-millimetric resolution of CBCT allow for more precise visualization, significantly reducing the risk of overdiagnosis of SSC dehiscence. (**a**) Oblique-coronal reformatted post-mortem CBCT, (**b**) Oblique-sagittal reformatted post-mortem CBCT images show a bony roof (arrow) of the superior semicircular canal (dashed arrow), measuring approximately 1.1 mm. *Abbreviations*: CBCT = cone-beam computed tomography; SSC = superior semicircular canal; MDCT = multi-detector computed tomography

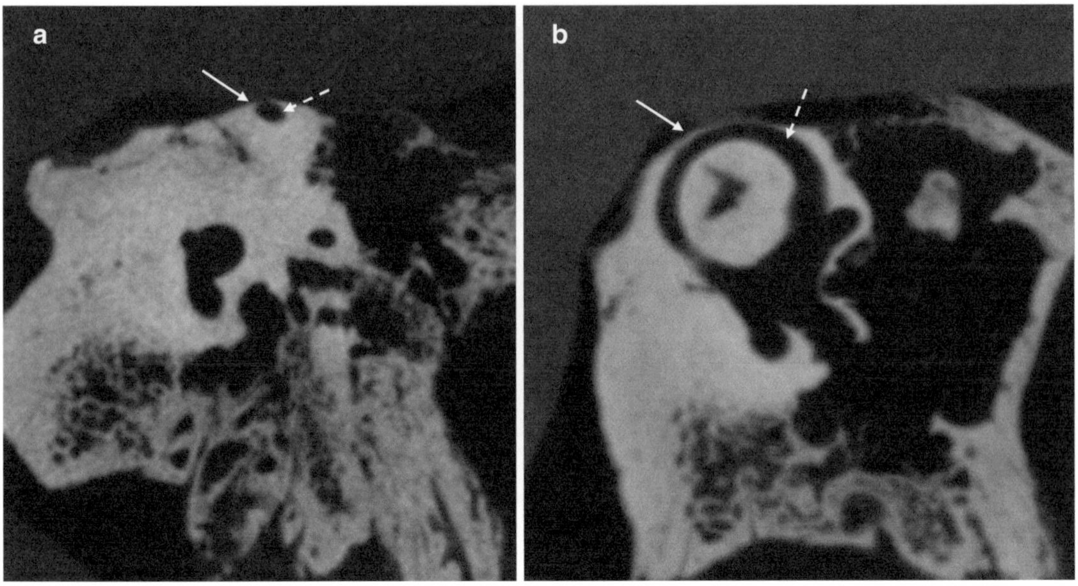

Fig. 9.32 Normal bony roof of the superior semicircular canal (continues from Fig. 9.31). (**c**) Oblique-coronal reformatted post-mortem CBCT, (**d**) Oblique-sagittal reformatted post-mortem CBCT show a bony roof (arrow) of the SSC (dashed arrow), measuring approximately 0.18 mm. In case of a very thin bony roof of SSC the sub-millimetric resolution of CTCB allows for the proper diagnosis of normal finding without dehiscence. *Abbreviations*: CBCT = cone-beam computed tomography; SSC = superior semicircular canal

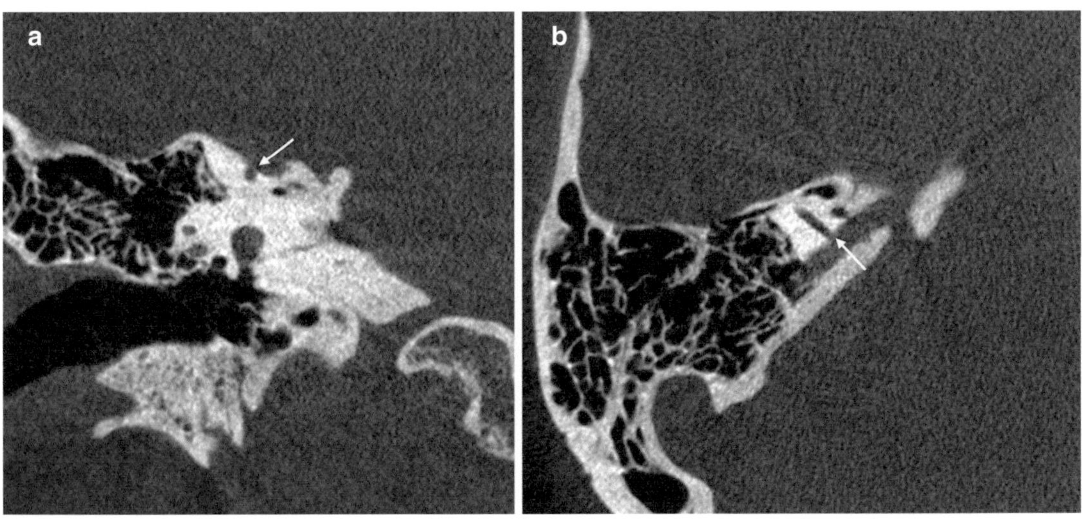

Fig. 9.33 Superior semicircular canal dehiscence causing Minor syndrome. (**a**) Oblique-coronal reformatted CBCT (**b**) axial reformatted CBCT show the dehiscence of the bony roof of the superior semicircular canal (arrow) at the level of the sulcus of the superior petrous sinus. *Abbreviation*: CBCT = cone-beam computed tomography

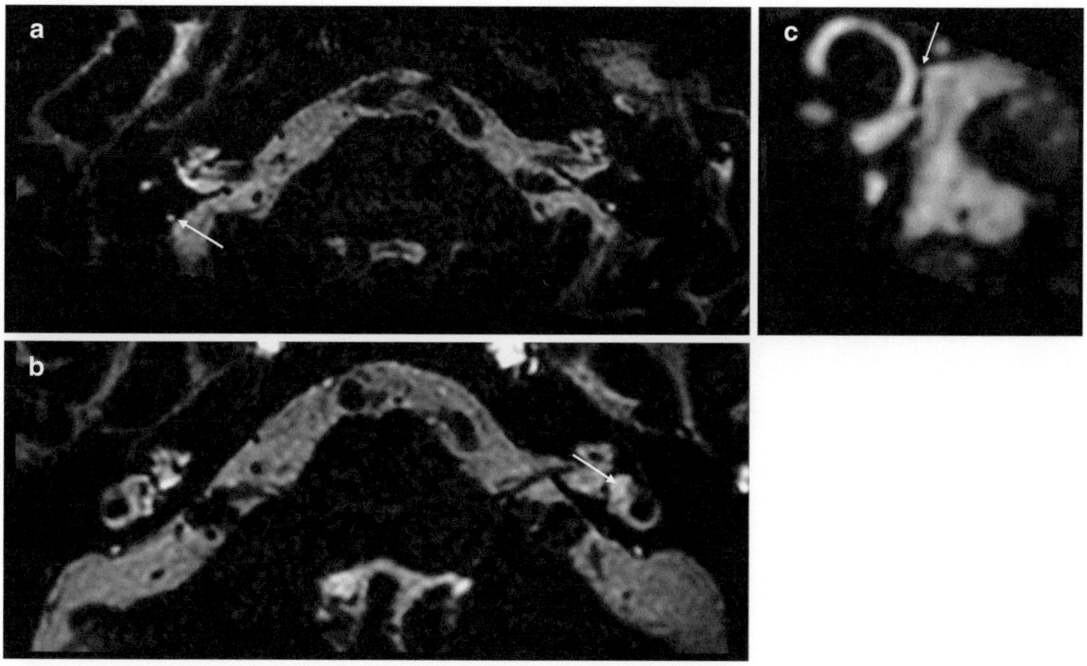

Fig. 9.34 **Right superior semicircular canal dehiscence and left saccule atelectasia in a patient with Minor syndrome**. (**a** and **b**) Axial 4-h delayed contrast-enhanced 3D-FLAIR shows right superior semicircular canal dehiscence (arrow in **a**) with posterior cranial fossa and left saccule atelectasis (arrow in **b**). (**c**) Oblique-sagittal reformatted 4-h delayed contrast-enhanced 3D-FLAIR better shows the dehiscence of the superior semicircular canal (arrow). *Abbreviation*: FLAIR = fluid-attenuated inversion recovery

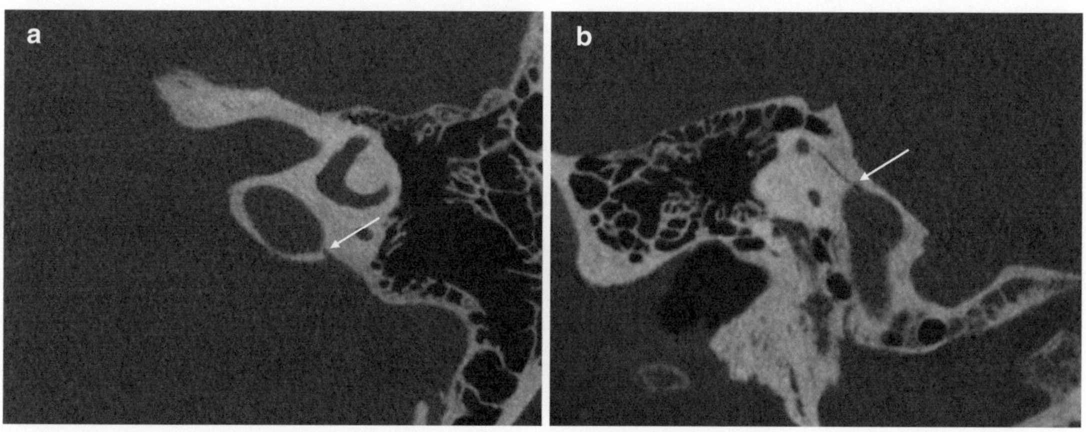

Fig. 9.35 **Left jugular bulb-vestibular aqueduct dehiscence**. Vestibular aqueduct dehiscence involving the jugular bulb is a condition commonly classified among inner ear dehiscence syndromes. It typically occurs when a high-riding jugular bulb extends abnormally superiorly and erodes into the vestibular aqueduct. This anatomical anomaly can cause a range of auditory symptoms, including pulsatile tinnitus, hearing loss, and autophony, as well as vestibular symptoms such as vertigo, dizziness, or imbalance. (**a**) Axial CBCT image demonstrates dehiscence of the left vestibular aqueduct into the jugular bulb (arrow). (**b**) Oblique coronal reformatted CBCT image confirms the dehiscence of the left vestibular aqueduct into the jugular bulb (arrow). *Abbreviation*: CBCT = cone-beam computed tomography

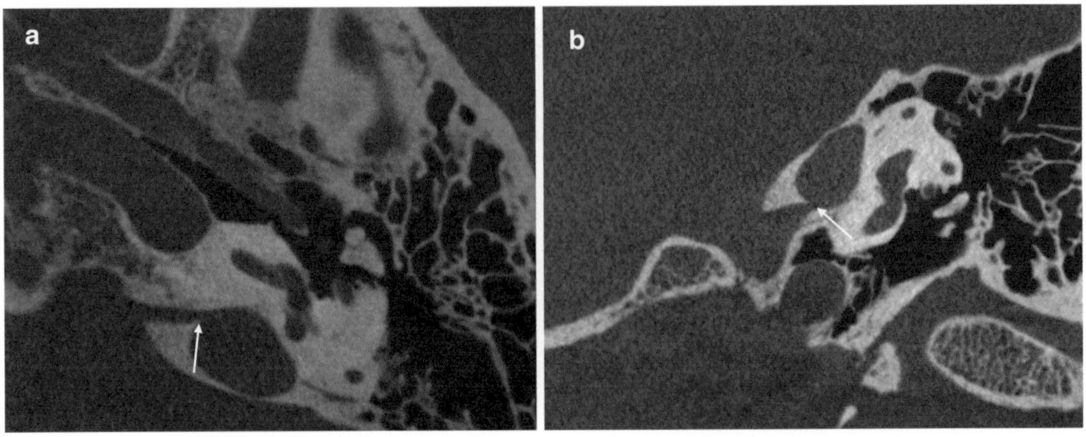

Fig. 9.36 Left jugular bulb-cochlear aqueduct dehiscence. Jugular Bulb–Cochlear Aqueduct Dehiscence is an uncommon pathological condition in which a high-riding or dehiscent jugular bulb erodes into or lies adjacent to the cochlear aqueduct. It is grouped under inner ear dehiscence syndromes. Usually it manifest with pulsatile tinnitus and hearing loss. (**a**) Axial CBCT, (**b**) Oblique-coronal reformatted CBCT show cochlear duct dehiscent in the jugular bulb (arrows). *Abbreviation*: CBCT = cone-beam computed tomography

Fig. 9.37 Dislocated stapedial prosthesis and perilymphatic fistula. (**a**) Axial 3D TSE-T2W sequence shows dark material in the right vestibule (arrow), representing a dislocated stapes prosthesis. (**b**) Axial 4-h delayed contrast-enhanced 3D-FLAIR sequence demonstrates enhancement in the right round window (arrow), consistent with a perilymphatic fistula where the contrast medium leaks from the perilymphatic space to middle ear via the round window.
Abbreviations: TSE = turbo spin echo; FLAIR = fluid-attenuated inversion recovery

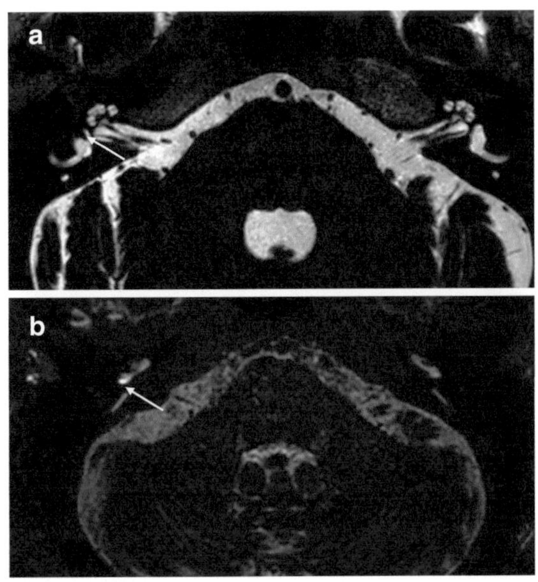

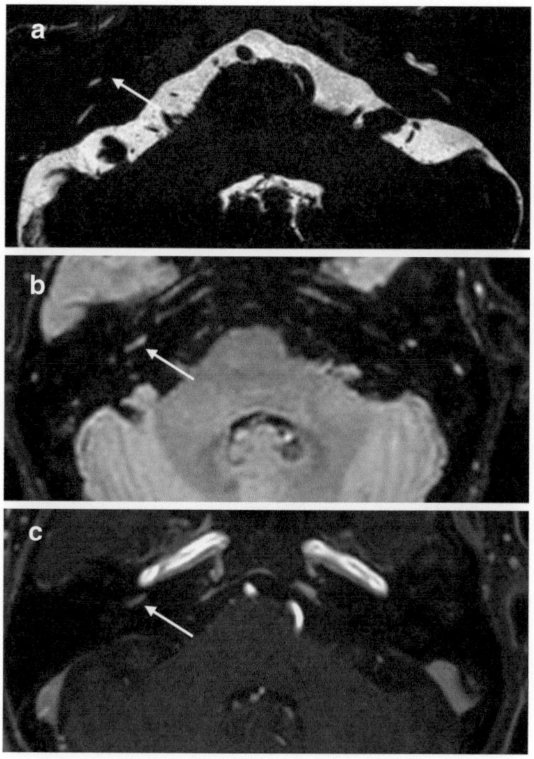

Fig. 9.38 Right cochlear schwannoma. (**a**) Axial 3D TSE-T2W shows partial absence of the T2 signal in the basal turn of the cochlea (arrow). (**b**) Axial 3D-FLAIR shows high signal in the right basal turn of the cochlea (arrow). (**c**) Axial contrast-enhanced 3D FFE-T1 with fat suppression shows enhancement in the right basal turn of the cochlea consistent with cochlear schwannoma (arrow). *Abbreviations*: TSE = turbo spin echo; FLAIR = fluid-attenuated inversion recovery; FFE = fast field echo

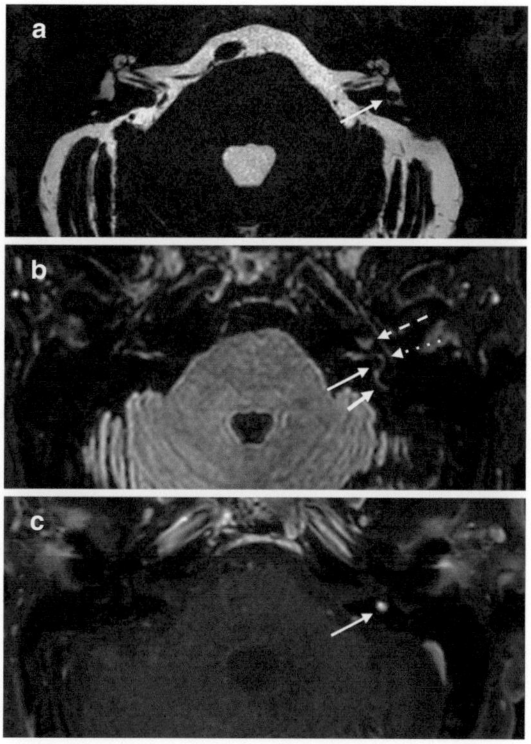

Fig. 9.39 Left vestibule schwannoma. (**a**) Axial 3D TSE-T2W sequence shows a millimetric round mass in the left vestibule (arrow). (**b**) Axial 3D-FLAIR sequence confirms the presence of a millimetric, round mass in the left vestibule (arrow). Additionally high signals are observed in the cochlea (dashed arrow), vestibule (dotted arrow), and lateral semicircular canal (small arrow), likely due to elevated protein content in the perilymph. This is caused by the presence of the labyrinthine schwannoma, which alters the normal dynamics of perilymphatic circulation. (**c**) Axial contrast-enhanced 3D FFE-T1W with fat suppression sequence demonstrates enhancement of the mass in the left vestibule (arrow), consistent with a vestibule schwannoma. *Abbreviations*: TSE = turbo spin echo; FLAIR = fluid-attenuated inversion recovery; FFE = fast field echo

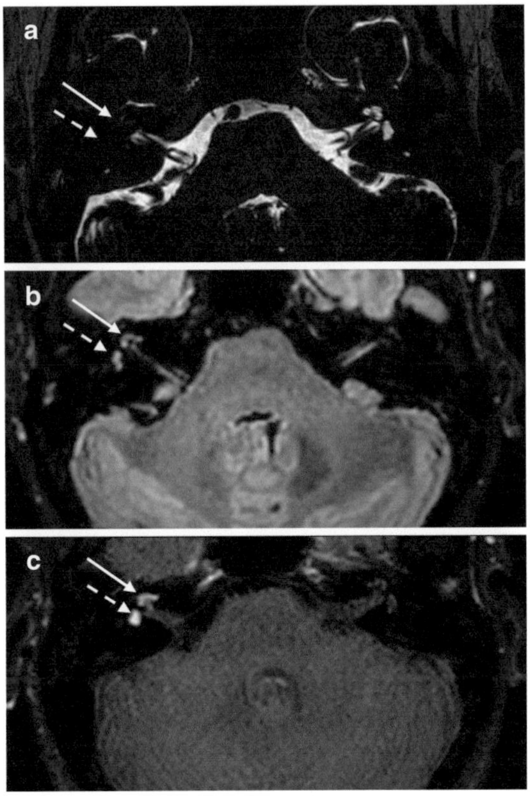

Fig. 9.40 Right cochleovestibular schwannoma. (**a**) Axial 3D TSE-T2W sequence shows the absence of the normal T2 signal in the right cochlea (arrow) and vestibule (dashed arrow). (**b**) Axial 3D-FLAIR sequence shows high signal intensity in the right cochlea (arrow) and vestibule (dashed arrow). (**c**) Axial contrast-enhanced 3D TSE-T1W BB sequence demonstrates enhancement of the right cochlea (arrow) and vestibule (dashed arrow). These imaging characteristics are consistent with a cochleovestibular schwannoma. *Abbreviations*: TSE turbo spin echo; FLAIR = fluid-attenuated inversion recovery; BB = black blood

References

1. Rauch SD. Idiopathic sudden sensorineural hearing loss. N Engl J Med. 2008;359(8):833–40.
2. Chandrasekhar SS, Tsai Do BS, Schwartz SR, Bontempo LJ, Faucett EA, Finestone SA, et al. Clinical practice guideline: sudden hearing loss (Update). Otolaryngol Head Neck Surg [Internet]. 2019 [cited 2025Jun30];161(S1). Available from: https://aao-hnsfjournals.onlinelibrary.wiley.com/doi/10.1177/0194599819859885
3. Ciorba A, Corazzi V, Bianchini C, Aimoni C, Skarzynski H, Skarzynski PH, et al. Sudden sensorineural hearing loss: is there a connection with inner ear electrolytic disorders? A literature review. Int J Immunopathol Pharmacol. 2016;29(4):595–602.
4. Li G, You D, Ma J, Li W, Li H, Sun S. The role of autoimmunity in the pathogenesis of sudden sensorineural hearing loss. Neural Plast. 2018;2018:1–9.
5. Chau JK, Lin JRJ, Atashband S, Irvine RA, Westerberg BD. Systematic review of the evidence for the etiology of adult sudden sensorineural hearing loss. Laryngoscope. 2010;120(5):1011–21.
6. Kuhn M, Heman-Ackah SE, Shaikh JA, Roehm PC. Sudden sensorineural hearing loss: a review of diagnosis, treatment, and prognosis. Trends Amplif. 2011;15(3):91–105.
7. Conte G, Di Berardino F, Zanetti D, Iofrida EF, Scola E, Sbaraini S, et al. Early magnetic resonance imaging for patients with idiopathic sudden sensorineural hearing loss in an emergency setting. Otol Neurotol. 2019;40(9):1139–47.
8. Buch K, Baylosis B, Fujita A, Qureshi MM, Takumi K, Weber PC, et al. Etiology-specific mineralization patterns in patients with Labyrinthitis Ossificans. AJNR Am J Neuroradiol. 2019;40:551.
9. Merchant SN, Adams JC, Nadol JB. Pathophysiology of Meniere's syndrome: are symptoms caused by endolymphatic hydrops? Otol Neurotol. 2005;26(1):74–81.
10. Loureiro RM, Sumi DV, Tames HLDVC, Soares CR, Salmito MC, Gomes RLE, et al. Endolymphatic hydrops evaluation on MRI: practical considerations. Am J Otolaryngol. 2020;41(2):102361.
11. Bernaerts A, Vanspauwen R, Blaivie C, Van Dinther J, Zarowski A, Wuyts FL, et al. The value of four stage vestibular hydrops grading and asymmetric perilymphatic enhancement in the diagnosis of Menière's disease on MRI. Neuroradiology. 2019;61(4):421–9.

10 Pathology of the Internal Auditory Canal and Cerebellopontine Angle

Antonia Valentina Genovese, Guido Del Vecchio, Eleonora Piccin, Flavia Bino, Sabrina Avignone, Silvia Casale, Fabio Triulzi, Elisa Scola, and Giorgio Conte

10.1 Introduction

The cerebellopontine angle (CPA) is a cerebrospinal fluid space located in front of the cerebellar hemispheres, posterior to the pyramid and lateral to the pons. Cranially and inferiorly it is delimited by the inferior and superior cerebellopontine fissure. It extends into the petrous part of the temporal bone as the internal auditory canal (IAC), with the porus acusticus being the medial opening of IAC. The CPA cistern contains cranial nerves (CN) and vessels, specifically the facial nerve (VII CN), the vestibulocochlear nerve (VIII CN), the superior cerebellar and anterior inferior cerebellar arteries, the labyrinthine artery, draining veins, and the choroid plexus protruding from the foramen of Luschka. The glossopharyngeal (IX CN), the vagus (X CN), and the accessory (XI CN) cranial nerves run in the inferior part of the CPA. Lesions in the CPA are often clinically nonspecific, as the symptoms presented are related to the involvement of nearby nerves or brain structures rather than the intrinsic characteristics of the lesions themselves [1].

Patients may experience symptoms such as hearing loss, tinnitus, vertigo, or facial nerve dysfunction, due to the compression or irritation of the cranial nerves in this region. Larger tumors may also cause headache, cerebellar signs, and trigeminal neuropathy. Lesions in the CPA can arise from the CPA cistern and other CPA structures or from embryological remnants. Tumors may also invade the CPA by extending from the petrous bone or skull base. Additionally, CPA lesions can be secondary to exophytic brain stem or ventricular tumors. Understanding these diverse origins is essential for accurate diagnosis and treatment planning [2]. Computed tomography (CT) and conventional and advanced magnetic resonance (MR) imaging are helpful in establishing a preoperative diagnosis.

Vestibular schwannoma, previously known as acoustic neurinoma, is the most frequent tumor found in the CPA, making up 70–80% of all CPA masses [1, 3]. These tumors arise from the Schwann cells and frequently stem from the

A. V. Genovese (✉) · G. Del Vecchio · S. Avignone
S. Casale · E. Scola
Neuroradiology Unit, Fondazione IRCCS Ca' Granda Ospedale Maggiore Policlinico, Milan, Italy
e-mail: valentina.genovese@policlinico.mi.it; guido.delvecchio@policlinico.mi.it; sabrina.avignone@policlinico.mi.it; silvia.casale@policlinico.mi.it; elisa.scola@policlinico.mi.it

E. Piccin · F. Bino
School of Medicine and Surgery, University of Milano-Bicocca, Milan, Italy
e-mail: ele.pic18@gmail.com; binoflavia@gmail.com

F. Triulzi · G. Conte
Neuroradiology Unit, Fondazione IRCCS Ca' Granda Ospedale Maggiore Policlinico, Milan, Italy

Department of Pathophysiology and Transplantation, University of Milan, Milan, Italy
e-mail: fabio.triulzi@policlinico.mi.it; giorgio.conte@policlinico.mi.it

G. Conte et al. (eds.), *Atlas of Normal and Pathological Findings in Otoneuroradiology*,
https://doi.org/10.1007/978-3-032-08232-9_10

inferior vestibular nerve within the IAC. Depending on their growth pattern, vestibular schwannomas can be entirely confined within the IAC, being defined intracanalicular or can extend both within the IAC and into the CPA cistern, creating what is described as an "ice-cream cone" appearance. Intracanalicular schwannomas can also present with a dumbbell-like lateral extension into the cochlea or vestibule.

In rare cases, vestibular schwannomas are purely intracisternal; unlike their intracanalicular counterparts, purely intracisternal vestibular schwannomas have more space to grow within the CPA, often delaying the onset of symptoms [1]. At CT, schwannomas are usually isodense to brain parenchyma and enhance after contrast administration. On MRI, they show T1 isointensity and T2 high signal with three contrast enhancing patterns: homogeneous (50–60%), heterogeneous (30–40%), and cystic (5–15%) [1]. These patterns are related not also on size of the lesion but also on histological Antoni subtype: Antoni A are usually small and homogeneous contrast enhancing mass, while larger, heterogeneous and cystic vestibular schwannomas are usually Antoni B pattern or a mix of type A and B [4]. DWI shows the solid component of vestibular schwannomas to be usually isointense to the brain tissue with apparent diffusion coefficient (ADC) values ranging from 1.1 to $1.7 \times 10 - 3\ \text{mm}^2/\text{s}$. One of the main differential diagnoses in CPA schwannomas is meningiomas. Diffusion and perfusion values may help: ADC is higher in schwannomas than meningiomas, probably related to the presence of increased amounts of extracellular water in the tumor matrix [3]. On the other hand, the relative tumor blood volume (rCBV) mean ratio is lower in schwannomas (2.2–4.4) than in meningiomas (3–18). Magnetic resonance spectroscopy (MRS) is rarely performed for tumors of the CPA. However, it can be useful in distinguishing schwannomas, which show a myoinositol peak (3.55 ppm), from meningiomas, which show an alanine peak [1, 3]. The imaging report should include the size of the tumor, the distance between the lateral extremity of the intracanalicular portion of the tumor and the fundus, the position of facial nerve relative to vestibular schwannoma and the intralabyrinthine signal intensity. (Figs. 10.1, 10.2, 10.3)

Non-vestibular schwannomas are less common but present distinct diagnostic challenges and may derive from trigeminal (V CN) or facial (VII CN) nerves. Among non-vestibular schwan-

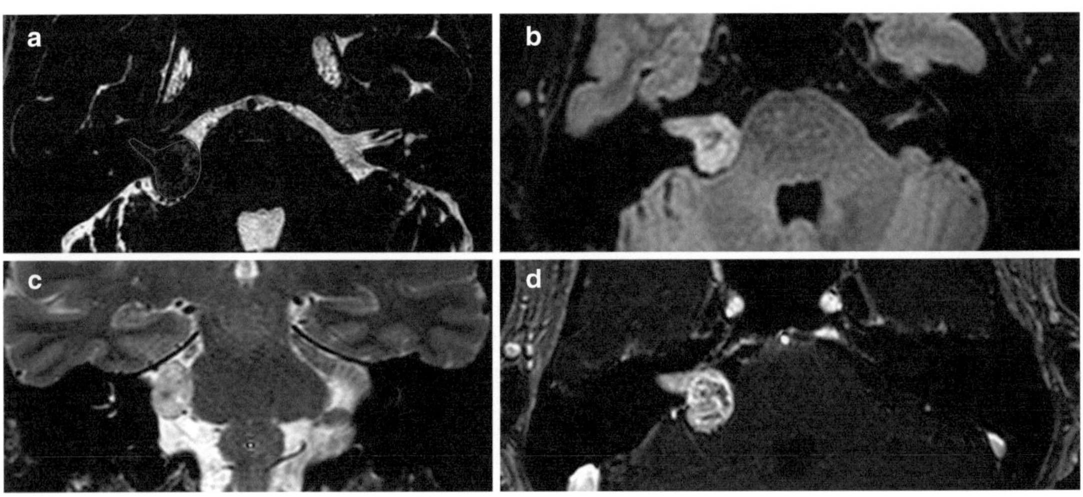

Fig. 10.1 Neurinoma of right VIII CN. An "ice cream cone-shaped" expansile lesion occupies the right IAC and extends into the CPA cistern (red shape in **a**). It shows slightly hyperintense signal on FLAIR and T2 sequences (**b** and **c**) and vivid and heterogeneous contrast enhancement after gadolinium injection (**d**), probably due to a cystic component. There is no mass effect on the brain stem. *Abbreviations:* CN = cranial nerve; IAC = internal auditory canal; CPA = cerebellopontine angle; FLAIR = fluid-attenuated inversion recovery

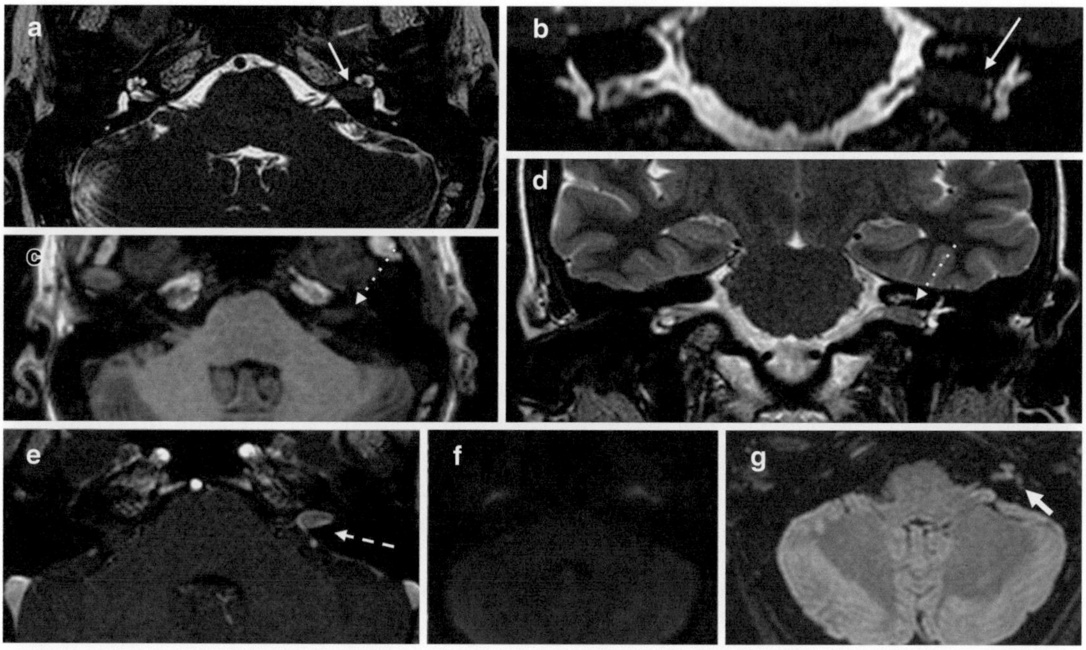

Fig. 10.2 Left intracanalicular neurinoma of VIII CN. The left IAC is occupied by a well-defined, oval intracanalicular mass along the course of the vestibulocochlear nerve with loss of the typical intracanalicular hyperintensity on 3D TSE T2W signal (**a** and **b**). The lesion shows hypointense signal on TSE T1W sequence and isointense signal on TSE T2W sequence (dotted arrows in **c** and **d**), along with intense enhancement (dashed arrow in **e**); DWI sequence does not show restriction (**f**). No evidence of extra canalicular extension (CPA component). In the FLAIR sequence, a hyperintensity of the cochlea and left vestibule can be appreciated, compatible with accumulation of proteinaceous material in the perilymph (short arrow in **g**). *Abbreviations:* CN = cranial nerve; IAC = internal auditory canal; TSE = turbo spin echo; DWI = diffusion-weighted imaging; CPA = cerebellopontine angle; FLAIR = fluid-attenuated inversion recovery

Fig. 10.3 Vestibular schwannoma or Scarpa's ganglion hypertrophy? 3D TSE T2W images show millimetric nodularity along the intracanalicular segment of the vestibular tract of the left VIII CN (arrows in **a** and **b**) is characterized by stippled mild contrast enhancement in TSE T1W images (dashed arrows on **c** and **d**). Given its location and morphological characteristics, the alteration is included in the differential diagnosis between vestibular schwannoma and hypertrophic cochlear ganglion (Scarpa's ganglion). The vestibular (Scarpa's) ganglion contains the bipolar cell bodies of the vestibular nerve and lies in the lateral internal auditory canal at the junction of its superior and inferior branches. *Abbreviations*: TSE = turbo spin echo; CN = cranial nerve.

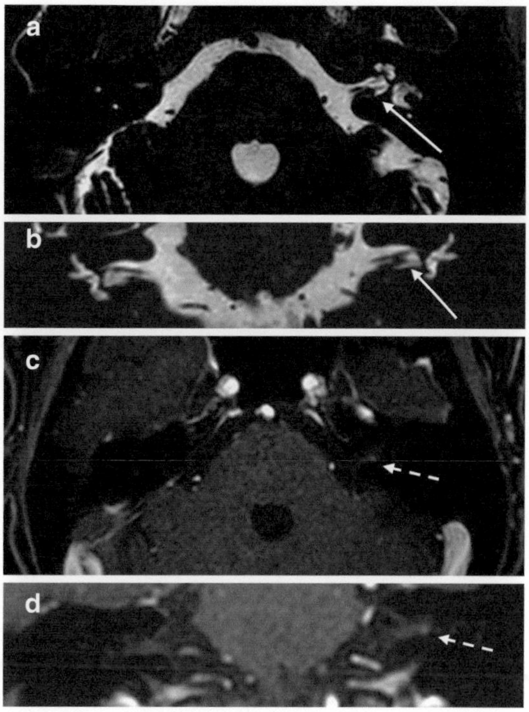

nomas, trigeminal schwannomas are the most frequent. These tumors extend in an anterior-posterior direction usually within the cranial portion of the CPA cistern and can grow into Meckel's cave and along the branches of the trigeminal nerve. Differential diagnosis between facial and vestibular schwannomas is challenging as they show similar appearance. Schwannomas of the glossopharyngeal (IX CN), vagus (X CN), and spinal accessory (XI CN) nerves, involving the jugular foramen, may extend upward with a significant component projecting into the CPA. These can mimic intracisternal vestibular schwannomas, but an enlarged jugular foramen is a key diagnostic feature [1].

Meningiomas are the second most common tumor found in the CPA, accounting for 10–15% of such tumors. These slow-growing masses originate from arachnoid meningo-epithelial cells and are more frequently seen in individuals over the age of 40. CPA meningiomas typically arise from the dura of the dorsal aspect of the petrous temporal bone. On CT scan, meningiomas often appear hyperdense in 70% of cases and calcified in about 20%, frequently accompanied by adjacent bone hyperostosis. MRI imaging reveals these tumors as isointense to the cerebral cortex on T1- and T2-weighted sequences, with strong post-contrast enhancement. A notable feature on MRI is the "dural tail sign," which indicates a thickened, nonneoplastic dura around the tumor and strongly suggests a meningioma diagnosis [1] (Fig. 10.4).

Epidermoid cyst is the third most common mass in CPA accounting for about 5%. These tumors originate during early embryogenesis from the inclusion of ectodermal epithelial tissue during neural tube closure. Their growth results from the desquamation and accumulation of keratin and cholesterol within cysts. On CT scan, epidermoid cysts typically appear hypoattenuating, almost iso-attenuating to cerebrospinal fluid (CSF), with irregular, lobulated margins. MRI scan shows these cysts with slightly higher signal intensity than CSF on T1- and T2-weighted images. They usually do not completely suppress the signal on FLAIR sequences and exhibit characteristic restricted diffusion on DWI due to their keratin content. DWI is also useful for confirming the presence of residual tumor postoperatively. The main differential diagnosis is an arachnoid cyst, which follows CSF signal intensity and does not

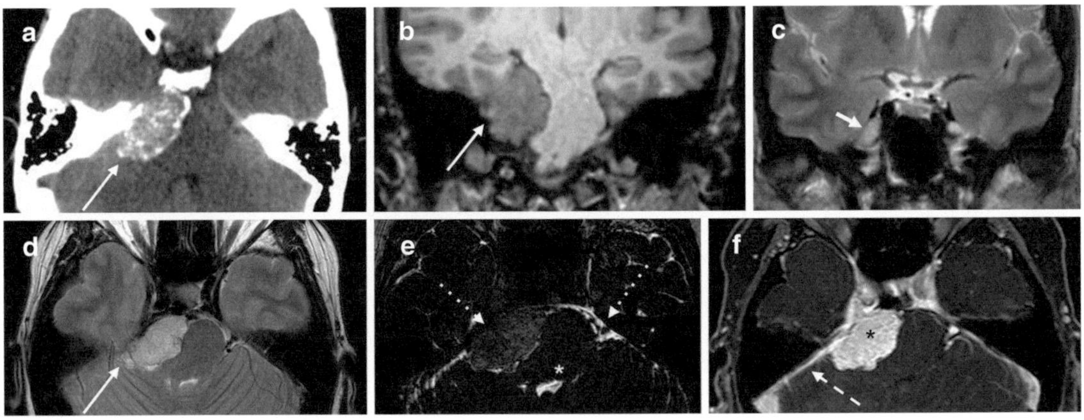

Fig. 10.4 Meningioma of right CPA. Right dural-based lesion at CPA has a hyperdense appearance on non-contrast MDCT image due to the calcific components (arrow in **a**). It shows iso-hypointense signal on T1 (**b**) and iso-hyperintense signal on T2 sequences (arrows in **c** and **d**) to the adjacent cerebellum. The mass occupies the right cerebellopontine angle and extends anteriorly into the right Meckel's cave (short arrow on **c**); it causes mass effect on the adjacent brainstem, displacing the pons and part of the midbrain; the fourth ventricle is minimally compressed (white asterisk on **e**). Due to compression, the ipsilateral acoustic facial and trigeminal nerves are not identifiable (dotted arrows on **e**). The lesion exhibits vivid and homogeneous contrast enhancement (black asterisk on **f**) along with thickening and enhancement of the dura (*dural tail sign*, dashed arrow on **f**). *Abbreviations*: CPA = cerebellopontine angle; MDCT = multidetector computed tomography

show restriction on diffusion images. Epidermoid tumors can occasionally present as "white epidermoids," which have reversed signal intensities with homogeneous high signal intensity on T1-weighted images and low signal intensity on T2-weighted images due to high proteinaceous content. Magnetic resonance spectroscopy (MRS) can assist in diagnosis, as epidermoids often show elevated lactate peaks [3]. While epidermoid tumors are typically benign, malignant transformation into squamous cell carcinoma can occur and should be suspected in cases of marked contrast enhancement [5] (Fig. 10.5).

Arachnoid cysts are congenital, benign, pouch-like lesions within the arachnoid membrane, filled with normal cerebrospinal fluid (CSF). They likely originate from a splitting of the embryonic meninges. Only 5–10% of arachnoid cysts are found in the posterior fossa [3]. Most arachnoid cysts are asymptomatic and are often discovered incidentally. However, in some cases, they may exert mass effect on lower cranial nerves, leading to clinical symptoms. On imaging, arachnoid cysts follow the CSF signal on both CT and MRI, showing no enhancement and increased apparent diffusion coefficient (ADC) values [3, 5]. They displace adjacent arteries and cranial nerves rather than encasing them, unlike epidermoid cysts. Arachnoid cysts have rounded edges, smoothly deforming adjacent brain tissue or scalloping the

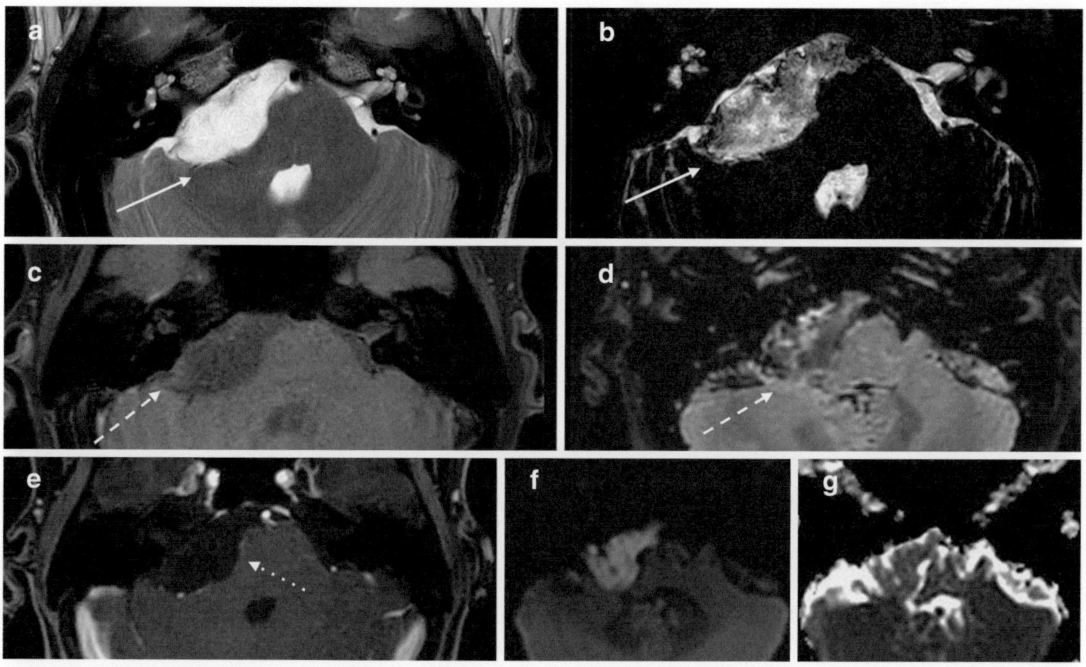

Fig. 10.5 Epidermoid cyst of right CPA. Epidermoid cyst originates during early embryogenesis from the inclusion of ectodermal epithelial tissue during neural tube closure. Their growth results from the desquamation and accumulation of keratin and cholesterol within cysts. Expansile mass in the cisterns of the right CPA with markedly hyperintense signal on TSE T2W and 3D T2W images (arrows in **a** and **b**), hypointense on T1, and heterogeneous signal on FLAIR (dashed arrows in **c** and **d**). The lesion does not show enhancement after contrast administration (dotted arrow in **e**) and is characterized by marked hyperintensity on DWI and low signal on ADC map (**f** and **g**). The right internal auditory canal is clear. The lesion exerts a mass effect on the brainstem, middle cerebellar peduncle, and cerebellar hemisphere, leading to a reduction in the size of the fourth ventricle, which is displaced to the left of the midline. No evidence of intraparenchymal edema is observed in the infratentorial region. The main differential diagnosis is an arachnoid cyst, which follows CSF signal intensity and does not show restriction on diffusion images. *Abbreviations:* CPA = cerebellopontine angle; TSE = turbo spin echo; FLAIR = fluid attenuated inversion recovery; DWI = diffusion-weighted imaging; ADC = apparent diffusion coefficient; CSF = cerebrospinal fluid

surrounding bony structures. Although rare, spontaneous or traumatic intracystic hemorrhage can occur, though this is seldom seen in the posterior fossa [2, 5] (Fig. 10.6).

Dermoid cysts originate from the inclusion of ectodermal elements during neural tube closure, possibly forming slightly earlier and containing elements from all skin layers. These cysts typically contain a mix of fat, hair, calcifications, and secretions from sebaceous glands along with desquamated keratinized epithelium. Dermoid cysts are usually midline lesions and rarely extend laterally into the CPA. On CT scans, dermoid cysts appear hypodense and may contain calcifications. MRI scans reveal these cysts with high signal intensity on T1-weighted images due to their fatty content, and they may exhibit a characteristic fat-fluid level [2] (Fig. 10.7).

Three other rare cystic lesions can be encountered in the CPA: *neurocysticercosis*, *neurenteric cysts*, and *neuroepithelial cysts* (Fig. 10.8). CPA structures can be involved by several pathological processess including vascular, inflammatory, granulomatous, infective or tumoral disorders as listed in Table 10.1 and shown in Figs. 10.9, 10.10, 10.11, 10.12, 10.14 and 10.15.

In Table 10.1 and in the flowchart the lesions of the CPA are listed according to anatomical localization and pattern of contrast enhancement.

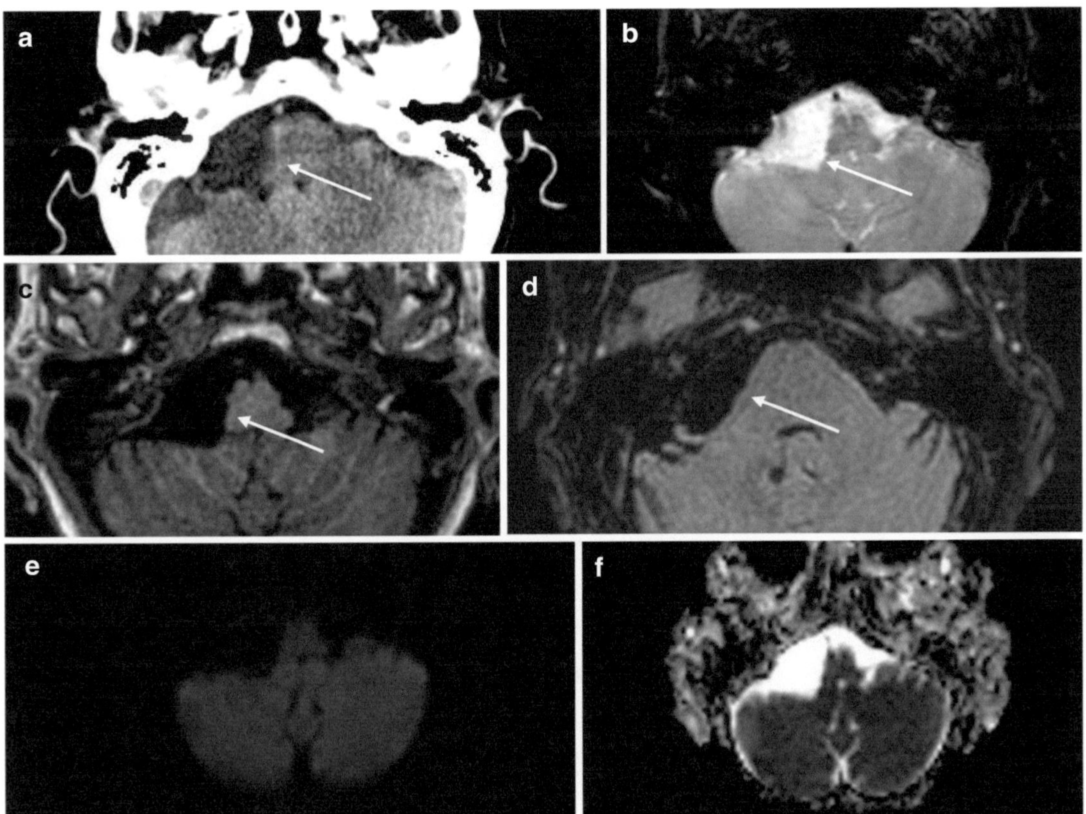

Fig. 10.6 Arachnoid cyst of right CPA. Arachnoid cysts are congenital, benign, pouch-like lesions within the arachnoid membrane, filled with normal CSF. They likely originate from a splitting of the embryonic meninges. Expansile cystic mass of the right CPA with CSF density on MDCT imaging (arrow in **a**) and CSF signal intensity on TSE T2W and TSE T1W sequences (arrows in **b** and **c**) with signal suppression in FLAIR (arrow in **d**); no diffusion restriction (**e** and **f**). Moderate mass effect on the medulla oblongata and the middle cerebellar peduncle along with mild displacement of the right cerebellar hemisphere. *Abbreviations:* CPA = cerebellopontine angle; CSF = cerebrospinal fluid; MDCT = multidetector computed tomography; TSE = turbo spin echo; FLAIR = fluid-attenuated inversion recovery

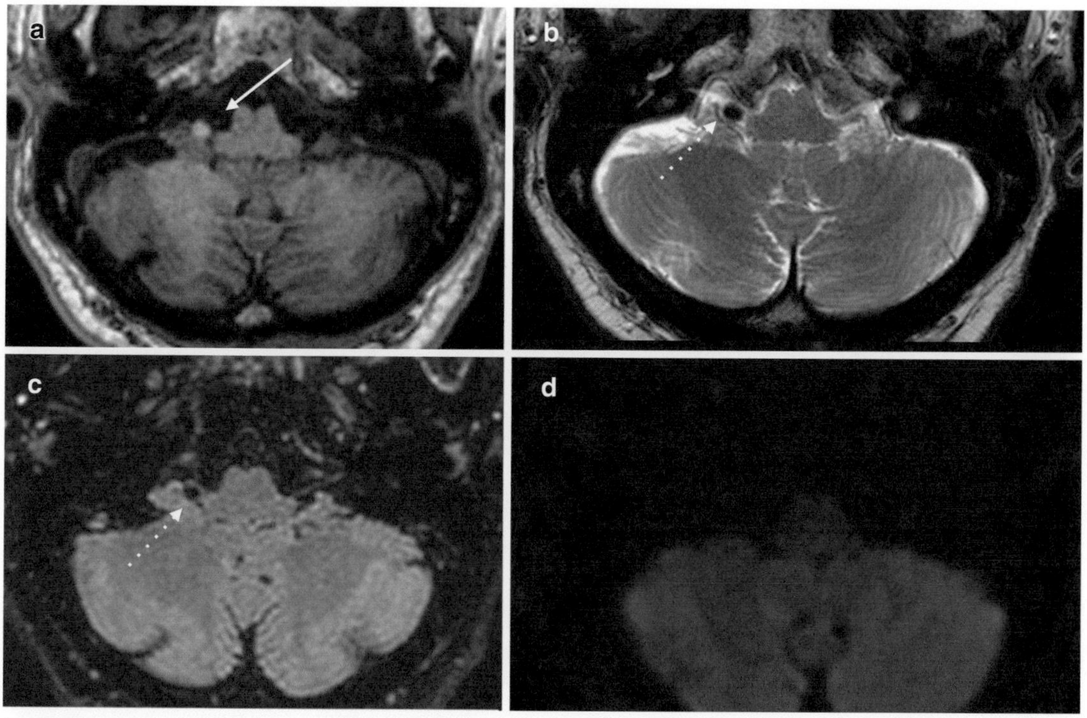

Fig. 10.7 **Dermoid cyst**. Dermoid cyst originates from the inclusion of ectodermal elements during neural tube closure, possibly forming slightly earlier and containing elements from all skin layers. These cysts typically contain a mix of fat, hair, calcifications, and secretions from sebaceous glands along with desquamated keratinized epithelium. Expansile round cystic mass localized anterior to the right cerebellar flocculus, in the subarachnoid spaces with hyperintense signal on TSE T1W (arrow in **a**) and hypointense on TSE T2W and FLAIR images (dotted arrow in **b** and **c**), suggesting a high protein content. The cyst does not have a diffusion restriction on DWI images (**d**). *Abbreviations:* TSE = turbo spin echo; FLAIR = fluid-attenuated inversion recovery; DWI = diffusion-weighted imaging

Neurovascular conflict In the CPA, vascular and neural structures are closely positioned. Neurovascular conflict is caused by direct contact between a blood vessel and the sensitive cisternal portion (the transition zone) of a cranial nerve, causing mechanical irritation that leads to neurovascular compression syndrome. The most common syndromes are trigeminal neuralgia (V CN) and hemifacial spasm (VII CN), vestibular paroxysmia (VIII CN), and glossopharyngeal neuralgia (IX CN).

The transition zone (TZ) has a central role in neurovascular conflict as an anatomical area with high mechanical vulnerability, where central myelin gradually changes into peripheral myelin, with oligodendrocytes being replaced by Schwann cells. The TZ varies in length and distance from the root entry/exit zone (REZ) for each cranial nerve. TZ is close to the REZ (1 mm or less) in CN V, VII, and IX, and it is longer and more distal from REZ in CN VIII [6].

Imaging identification of contact between CN and vessels is a frequent finding even in asymptomatic patients. Neurovascular contact is more likely responsible for neurovascular conflict when the REZ and TZ are involved, when there is a nerve root displacement, or, in more severe cases, when there is nerve root atrophy. Therefore, in clinically suspected cases, accurate anatomical identification of the TZ in relation to the REZ is helpful in understanding whether a neurovascular

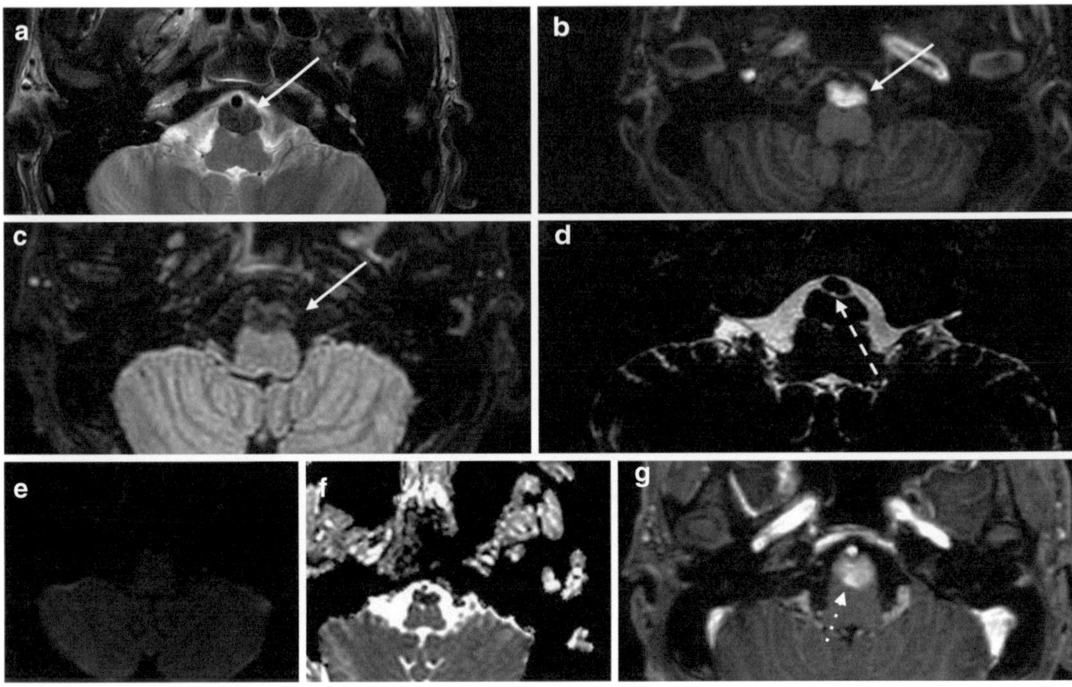

Fig. 10.8 Pre-pontobulbar neurenteric cyst. Neurenteric cysts likely originate from neurenteric canal dysgenesis. These cysts contain gastrointestinal or respiratory-like epithelium. Expansile oval mass with clear margins that show markedly hypointense signal on T2-weighted images (arrow in **a**) and hyperintense signal on T1-weighted images and FLAIR (arrow in **b** and **c**). It is located anterior to the medulla, exerting an impression on it, and posterior to the basilar artery, partially surrounding it (<180°) (dashed arrow in **d**). It does not show a clear restriction in the DWI and ADC map (**e** and **f**). After administration of the contrast medium, it shows minimal enhancement (dotted arrow in **g**). Neurenteric cysts, depending on the content of the cyst, could be isointense or slightly hyperintense to CSF; they typically show no calcification. *Abbreviations:* FLAIR = fluid-attenuated inversion recovery; DWI = diffusion-weighted imaging; ADC = apparent diffusion coefficient; CSF = cerebrospinal fluid

contact may be responsible for a symptomatic syndrome. Additionally, it should be noted that arteries are more likely responsible for neurovascular conflict.

High-resolution 3D T2-weighted imaging, combined with 3D time-of-flight (TOF) angiography and 3D T1-weighted gadolinium-enhanced sequences, represents the gold standard for precisely detecting the point of contact between vessels and cranial nerves. Moreover, imaging plays a crucial role in ruling out other potential causes of painful symptoms that may mimic neurovascular compression syndromes (Fig. 10.13).

Table 10.1 Lesions of the CPA are listed according to anatomical localization [1–3, 5, 7–9]

Extra-axial	
Vestibular schwannoma	Most frequent lesion of CPA; along VIII CN; ice-cream cone appearance
Meningioma	Second most common tumor of CPA; dural tail and hyperostosis; slow-growing mass
Epidermoid cyst	Third most common lesion of CPA; DWI +
Arachnoid cyst	CSF signal
Dermoid cyst	Fat or calcification
Neuroepithelial cyst	Rare; CSF signal; no calcification
Neurenteric cyst	Gastrointestinal or respiratory-like epithelium; isointense or slightly hyperintense to CSF, depending on the content of the cyst; no calcification
Non-vestibular schwannoma	Less common than the VIII CN schwannoma; along V, VI, IX, X, and XI CN
Lipoma	Homogeneous fat signal (high on T1) (Fig. 10.9)
Neurocysticercosis	Racemose lobulated cysts CSF signal, no bone erosion
Aneurysm	Strong enhancing, flow voids on T2-TSE (Fig. 10.10)
Metastasis	Heterogeneous, can be multiple
Meningeal inflammatory or infectious processes	
Tuberculosis	Leptomeningitis or tuberculoma; ring or thick/nodular enhancing (Fig. 10.11)
Sarcoidosis	Granulomatous inflammation of the meninges and hypothalamus, diffuse or plaque-like dural mass
Erdheim-Chester	Rare non-Langerhans histiocytosis, meningeal dural mass, infiltrative cerebellar lesions, osteosclerotic bone changes
Tumors extending from the petrous bone or skull base	
Cholesterol granulomas	Usually in the petrous bone apex; expansile lytic lesions; central T1 high signal intensity; hemosiderin peripheric rim; no DWI restriction
Paragangliomas (glomus tumors)	Benign but locally aggressive tumor, hypervascular soft-tissue masses with T2 flow void; moth-eaten bony erosion
Chondromatous tumors	Arise from cartilaginous remnants at the skull base, lytic heterogeneous mass
Chordomas	Arise from remnants of the notochord near the dorsum sellae, lobulated lytic heterogeneous mass, possible calcification
Endolymphatic sac tumors	Papillary adenomatous tumors, usually associated with Von Hippel Lindau syndrome. Lytic retrolabyrinthine petrous bone mass, intratumoral spiculated or reticulated bone can be seen, heterogeneous on MRI
Apex petrositis (petrous apicitis)	Enhancing mass at the petrous tip, with possible involvement of V and VI CN (i.e., Gradenigo syndrome)
Intra-axial extending to CPA	
Glioma	Enlarge brain stem, peripheral edema, heterogeneous enhancement (Fig. 10.14)
Lymphoma	Hypercellulated mass, DWI +
Metastasis	Heterogeneous, can be multiple (Fig. 10.12)
Hemangioblastoma	Hypervascular mass, solid or cystic with nodule, flow voids
Medulloblastoma	Heterogeneous enhancing mass, CSF dissemination, DWI +
Choroid plexus papilloma	Hypervascular mass, extending from choroid plexus near the Luschka foramen
Ependymoma	Heterogeneous, extending from the Luschka or Magendie foramen, "toothpaste tumor"

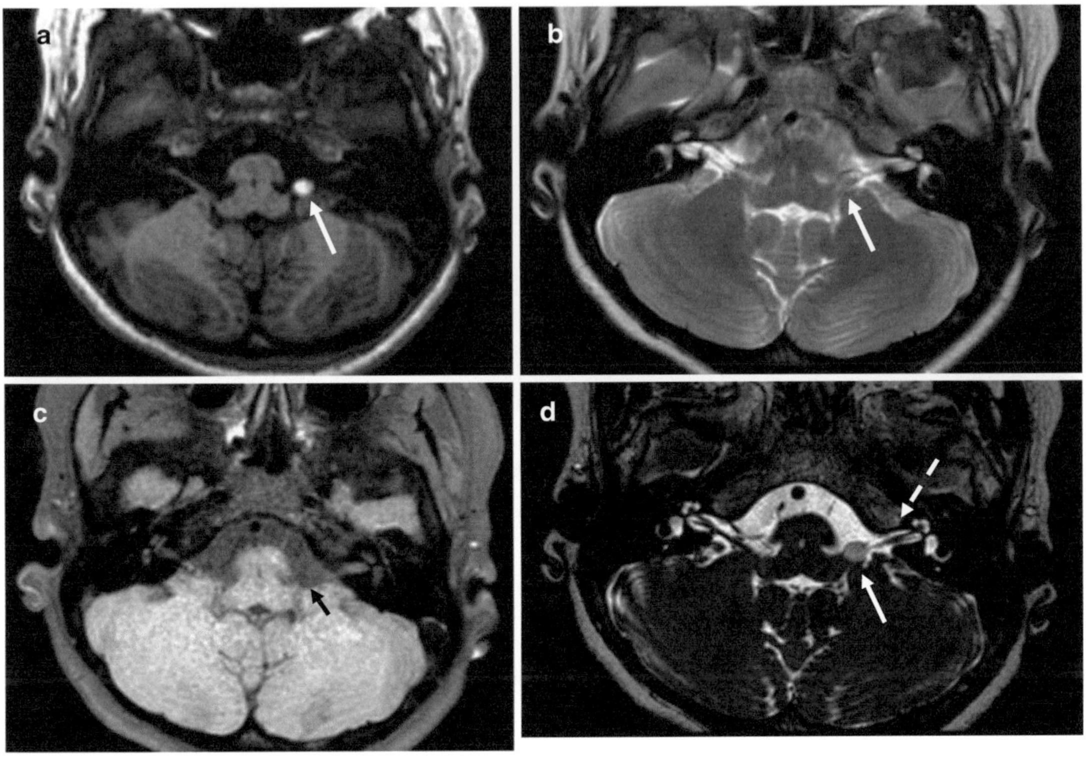

Fig. 10.9 Lipoma of the left cerebellar peduncle. Lipoma consists of mature adipose tissue resulting from an abnormal differentiation of the primitive meninx. Well-defined oval mass located near the left inferior cerebellar peduncle characterized by high signal on both in T1- and T2-weighted images (arrow in **a, b** and **d**). The signal follows that of adipose tissue and is suppressed on fat-suppressed sequences (short black arrow in **c**). Neurovascular structures can pass through the lipoma instead of being displaced (dashed arrow indicates VII and VIII CN in **d**). *Abbreviation:* CN = cranial nerves

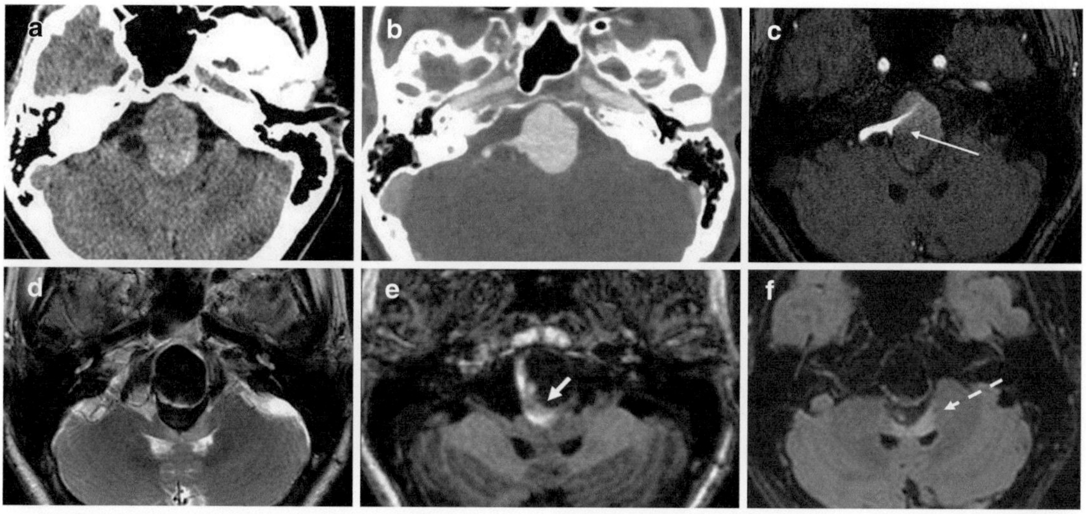

Fig. 10.10 Giant aneurysm of vertebrobasilar junction. Aneurysm, typically found in the vertebral and basilar arteries, can cause mass effects on the neural structures of the CPA. Non-contrast MDCT (**a**) and arterial phase of angio-CT (**b**) of a giant dissecting aneurysm in the region of the vertebrobasilar junction. It appears hyperintense in the angio-RM TOF sequence (arrow in **c**) and as flow voids on T2, T1, and FLAIR sequences (respectively, **d**, **e**, **f**). Thrombosed aneurysms may show variable high signal intensity (short arrow in **e**). It has a compressive effect on the structures of the trunk, mainly on the bulbo-pontine/pons junction, which are compressed and displaced posteriorly; furthermore, they show high signal in FLAIR (dashed arrow in **f**) as signs of tissue distress/edematous reaction. *Abbreviations:* CPA = cerebellopontine angle; MDCT = multidetector computed tomography; TOF = time of flight; FLAIR = fluid-attenuated inversion recovery

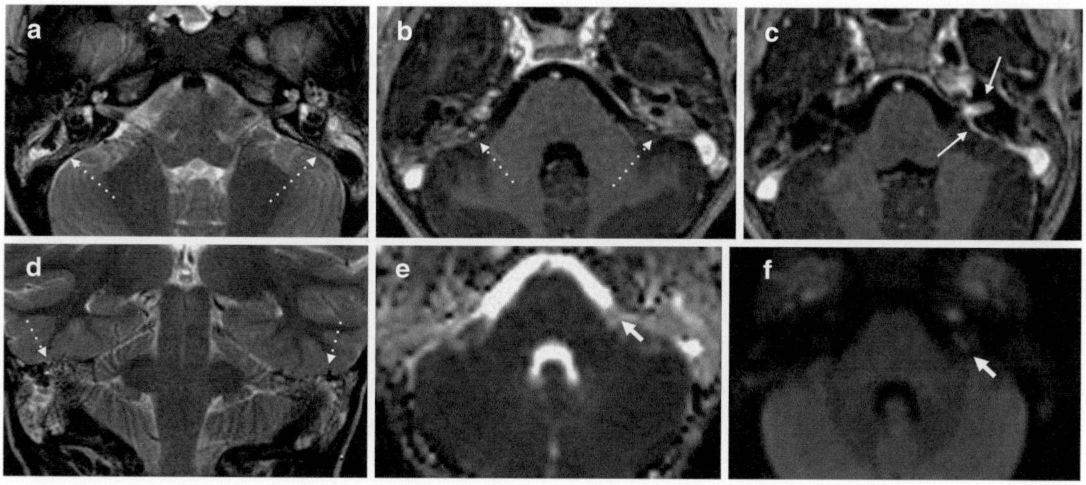

Fig. 10.11 Meningitis of the left posterior cranial fossa. Meningeal inflammatory or infectious processes, affecting the dura or leptomeninges, can involve the CPA cistern. Patient with bilateral acute otitis media: TSE-T2W images confirm the presence of hyperintense inflammatory tissue involving mastoids and tympanic cavities bilaterally (dotted arrows in **a** and **d**), with enhancement after contrast media administration (dotted arrow in **b**). Thickening and enhancement of the dura, consistent with meningitis, are observed in the left posterior cranial fossa, adjacent to the petrous apex, extending into the internal auditory canal (arrows in **c**). A mild diffusion restriction is noted in the CSF of the CPA, particularly near the left IAC (arrows in **e** and **f**). Differentiating these from metastatic disease (leptomeningeal carcinomatosis) through imaging alone is difficult, necessitating a thorough clinical history and often CSF analysis. *Abbreviations:* CPA = cerebellopontine angle; TSE = turbo spin echo; CSF = cerebrospinal fluid; IAC = internal auditory canal

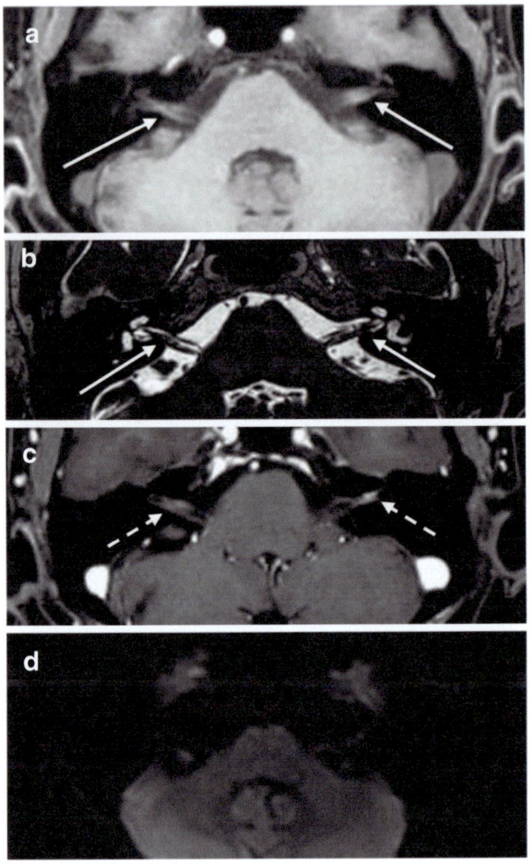

Fig. 10.12 Metastatic dissemination from breast cancer. MRI of a patient with breast carcinoma. Metastases are rare in the CPA and may mimic other CPA masses or present with leptomeningeal carcinomatosis. Bilateral intracanalicular VII–VIII CN appear slightly swollen (arrows in **a** and **b**), with pseudonodular thickening and mild contrast enhancement (dashed arrows in **c**). No abnormal high signal is observed on DWI (**d**). Common primary tumors include lung, breast, melanoma, and lymphoma. Specific imaging characteristics, like restricted diffusivity in adenocarcinoma metastases or T1 hyperintensity in melanocytic metastases, aid in diagnosis, but usually metastases have no specific feature. NF2 is a differential diagnosis due to multiple schwannomas. Clinical history plays a crucial role in the differential diagnosis. *Abbreviations:* CPA = cerebellopontine angle; CN = cranial nerves; DWI = diffusion-weighted imaging; NF2 = neurofibromatosis type 2

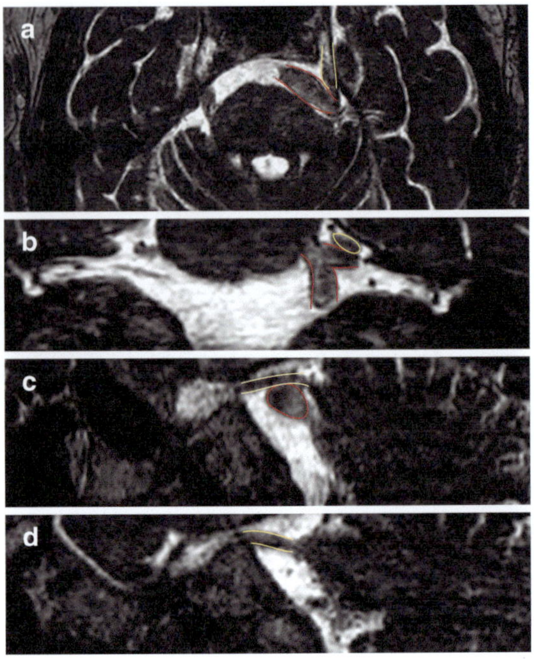

Fig. 10.13 Neurovascular conflict. Neurovascular conflict involves a vessel compressing a nerve at the root entry zone, most commonly affecting the trigeminal nerve, leading to trigeminal neuralgia. 3D TSE T2W axial (**a**), coronal (**b**), and sagittal (**c**) reconstructions show a dolichoectatic left vertebral artery and vertebrobasilar junction (red tracts) in close proximity to the cisternal segment of the left trigeminal nerve, causing compression and superior displacement of its course (yellow tracts). For comparison, (**d**) illustrates the normal contralateral cisternal course of the trigeminal nerve (yellow lines) without neurovascular conflict. *Abbreviation*: TSE = turbo spin echo

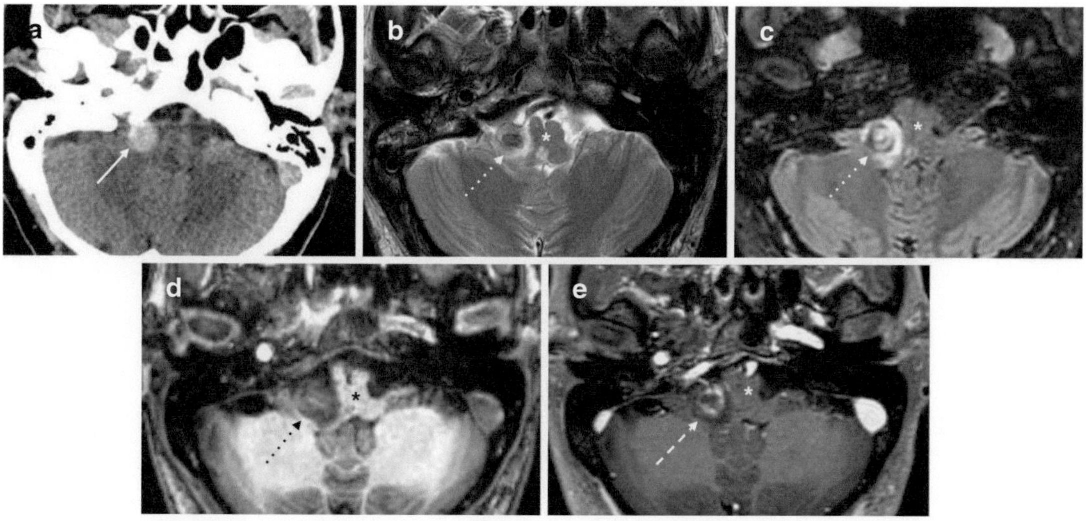

Fig. 10.14 Glioma of the right cerebellar peduncle. Intra-axial or intraventricular tumors such as gliomas, choroid plexus papillomas, lymphomas, hemangioblastomas, ependymomas, medulloblastomas, and dysembryoplastic neuroepithelial tumors can invade the CPA. Non-contrast MDCT shows a hyperdense glioma in the right cerebellar peduncle (arrow in **a**), likely due to hemorrhagic components. MRI reveals a heterogeneous signal consistent with a mixture of solid and hemorrhagic components, with probable blood-fluid levels, as seen on T2-weighted, FLAIR, and T1-weighted sequences (dotted arrows in **b**, **c**, and **d**, respectively). The lesion exhibits a ringlike enhancement pattern (dashed arrow in **e**). The mass displaces the fourth ventricle toward the left and exerts a mild mass effect with associated edema on the middle cerebellar peduncle and the pons on the right (asterisks in **b**, **c, d** and **e**). *Abbreviation:* CPA = cerebellopontine angle; MDCT = multidetector computed tomography; MRI = magnetic resonance imaging; FLAIR = fluid-attenuated inversion recovery

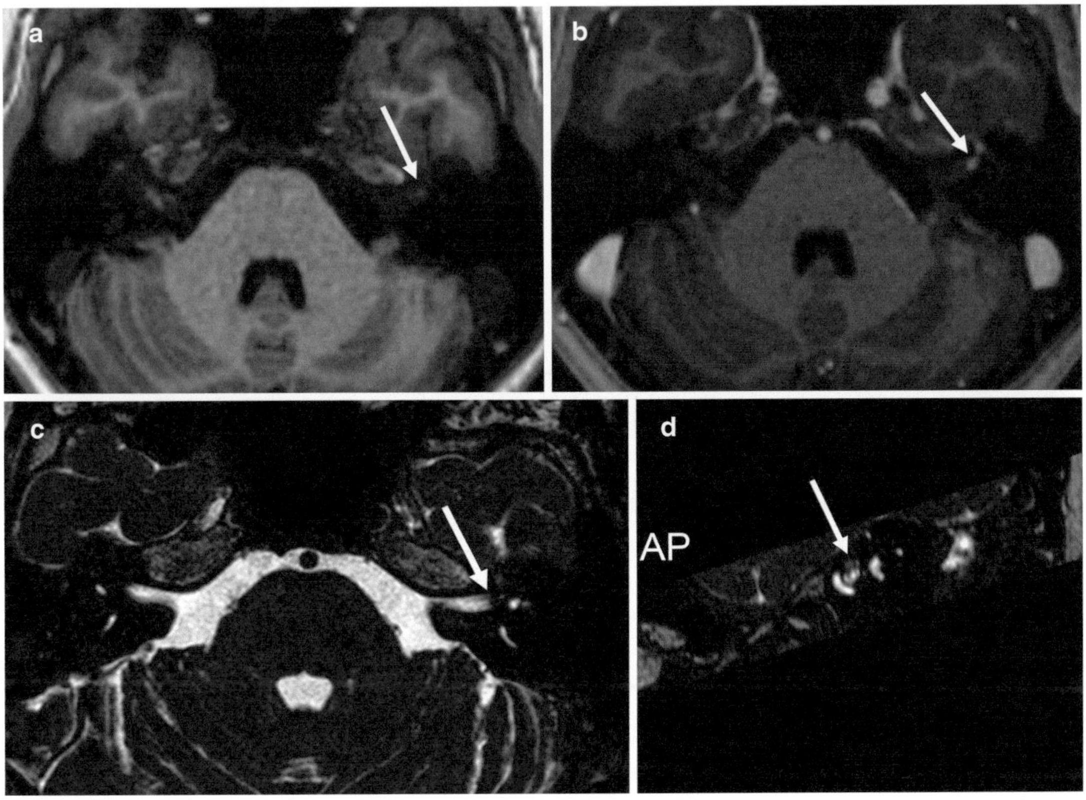

Fig. 10.15 **Left intracanalicular focal enhancement**. Patient with paralysis of left VII CN. The VII CN at the fundus of the left IAC and in the geniculate ganglion shows a focal gadolinium enhancement: the differential diagnosis is between an inflammatory process (Bell paralysis) and a small schwannoma of VII cranial nerve. In similar cases the clinical scenario can help in suggesting the diagnosis. Nevertheless the imaging follow-up is mandatory in order to evaluate the resolution in case of an inflammatory process or evolution of the finding in case of a neoplastic lesion. TSE T1W pre- and post-contrast images (**a** and **b**) show the focal enhancement (arrow); the 3D TSE T2W in axial and parasagittal planes (**c** and **d**) show the presence of a small focal thickening of the left VII CN (arrow). *Abbreviations:* CN = cranial nerve; IAC = internal auditory canal; TSE = turbo spin echo

Flowchart: Lesions of the CPA are listed according to anatomical localization and pattern of contrast enhancement. CPA= cerebellopontineangle

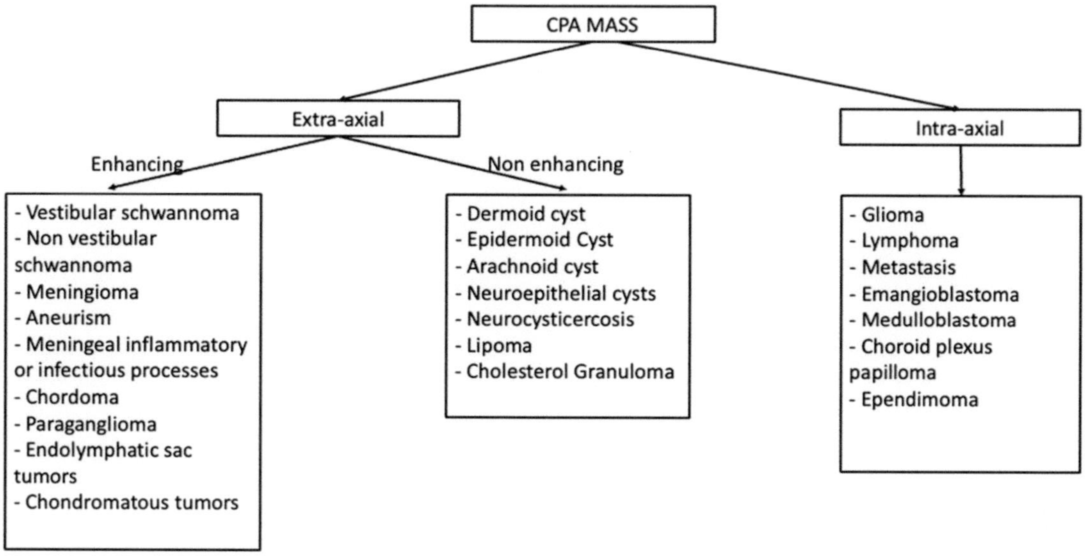

References

1. Bonneville F, Savatovsky J, Chiras J. Imaging of cerebellopontine angle lesions: an update. Part 1: enhancing extra-axial lesions. Eur Radiol. 2007;17(10):2472–82.
2. Bonneville F, Sarrazin JL, Marsot-Dupuch K, Iffenecker C, Cordoliani YS, Doyon D, et al. Unusual lesions of the cerebellopontine angle: a segmental approach. Radiographics. 2001;21(2):419–38.
3. Lakshmi M, Glastonbury CM. Imaging of the cerebellopontine angle. Neuroimaging Clin N Am. 2009;19(3):393–406.
4. Wippold FJ 2nd, Lubner M, Perrin RJ, Lämmle M, Perry A. Neuropathology for the neuroradiologist: Antoni A and Antoni B tissue patterns. AJNR Am J Neuroradiol. 2007;28(9):1633–8.
5. Bonneville F, Savatovsky J, Chiras J. Imaging of cerebellopontine angle lesions: an update. Part 2: intra-axial lesions, skull base lesions that may invade the CPA region, and non-enhancing extra-axial lesions. Eur Radiol. 2007;17(11):2908–20.
6. Haller S, Etienne L, Kövari E, Varoquaux AD, Urbach H, Becker M. Imaging of neurovascular compression syndromes: trigeminal neuralgia, hemifacial spasm, vestibular paroxysmia, and glossopharyngeal neuralgia. AJNR Am J Neuroradiol. 2016;37(8):1384–92.
7. Romano N, Federici M, Castaldi A. Imaging of cranial nerves: a pictorial overview. Insights Imaging. 2019;10(1):33.
8. Borges A, Casselman J. Imaging the cranial nerves: part I: methodology, infectious and inflammatory, traumatic and congenital lesions. Eur Radiol. 2007;17(8):2112–25.
9. Borges A, Casselman J. Imaging the cranial nerves: part II: primary and secondary neoplastic conditions and neurovascular conflicts. Eur Radiol. 2007;17(9):2332–44.

11 Pre and Post-surgical Imaging, Prosthesis and Cochlear Implant

Elisa Scola, Elisa Massullo, Silvia Casale, Francesco Maria Lo Russo, Fabio Triulzi, Giorgio Conte, Diego Zanetti, and Lorenzo Maria Gaini

11.1 Presurgical Evaluation

In preoperative radiological evaluation, anatomical conformation and variants should be acknowledged [1].

For the planning of mastoidectomy, the identification of the location of sigmoid sinus and jugular bulb as well as the temporal dura is really important. For cochlear implantation the presence of air cells around the facial recess (also called sentinel air cells) and the position of the facial nerve canal should be identified because they influence the accessibility of the round window and the subsequent feasibility of cochlear implant. The anatomical integrity of the whole acoustic route should be routinely assessed before cochlear implantation, evaluating all the structures of the external, middle, and inner ear as well as the cochlear nerve and nervous central acoustic pathway. For these purposes magnetic resonance imaging (MRI) and computed tomography (CT) scan are complementary [1].

The main anatomic structures and variants to be evaluated in presurgical imaging are reported hereinafter [2].

- *High jugular bulb* (Fig. 11.1): a CT-based classification of high jugular bulb is based on the position of the roof of the bulb on coronal planes: over the posterior semicircular canal, over the floor of the internal auditory meatus, or over the basal turn of the cochlea. Normally the upper border of the jugular bulb is under the hypotympanum. The position of the jugular bulb has clinical implications in microsurgical

E. Scola (✉) · S. Casale · F. M. Lo Russo
Neuroradiology Unit, Fondazione IRCCS Ca' Granda Ospedale Maggiore Policlinico, Milan, Italy
e-mail: elisa.scola@policlinico.mi.it; silvia.casale@policlinico.mi.it; francesco.lorusso@policlinico.mi.it

E. Massullo
Università degli Studi di Milano, Milan, MI, Italy
e-mail: elisa.massullo@unimi.it

F. Triulzi · G. Conte
Neuroradiology Unit, Fondazione IRCCS Ca' Granda Ospedale Maggiore Policlinico, Milan, Italy

Department of Pathophysiology and Transplantation, University of Milan, Milan, Italy
e-mail: fabio.triulzi@policlinico.mi.it; giorgio.conte@policlinico.mi.it

D. Zanetti
Audiology Unit, Department of Specialistic Surgical Sciences Fondazione IRCCS Ca' Granda, Ospedale Maggiore Policlinico Milan, Milan, Italy

Department of Clinical Sciences and Community Health University of Milan, Milan, Italy
e-mail: diego.zanetti@policlinico.mi.it

L. M. Gaini
Department of Otolaryngology and Head and Neck Surgery, Fondazione IRCCS Ca' Granda Ospedale Maggiore Policlinico, Milan, Italy
e-mail: lorenzo.gaini@policlinico.mi.it

G. Conte et al. (eds.), *Atlas of Normal and Pathological Findings in Otoneuroradiology*,
https://doi.org/10.1007/978-3-032-08232-9_11

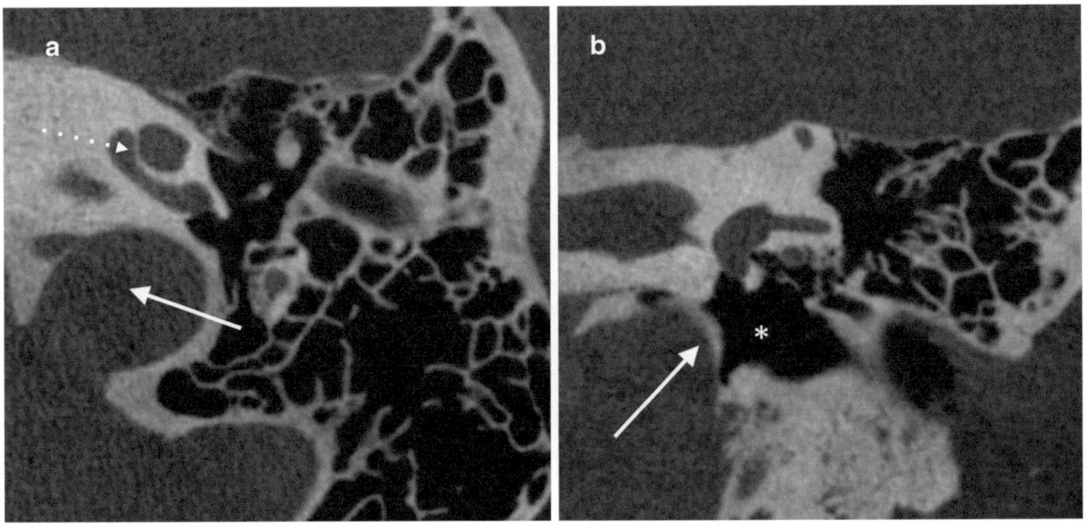

Fig. 11.1 Anatomical variants: high jugular bulb. Normally the upper border of the jugular bulb is under the hypotympanum. (**a**) Axial CBCT image shows the high prominent jugular bulb (arrow) on a plane passing through the basal cochlear turn (dotted arrow). (**b**) Coronal CBCT image passing through the vestibule shows the high prominent jugular bulb (arrow) located medially to the hypotympanum (asterisk). *CBCT* cone beam computed tomography

and endovascular interventions in otologic or neurosurgical conditions [3].

- *Dehiscent jugular bulb*: the sigmoid bony plate between a high riding jugular bulb and the tympanic cavity is absent; therefore, the bulb and the middle ear cavity are in direct contact. This may be a potential danger in surgery.
- *Jugular bulb diverticulum*: a protrusion of the jugular bulb; it can occur superiorly, medially, or posteriorly, with or without jugular bulb dehiscence.
- *Anteriorly located sigmoid sinus*: the position of sigmoid sinus is classified on axial plane according to its relation to three coronal lines: type 1, the sigmoid sinus is medial to the line parallel to the posterior semi-circular canal (line 1); type 2, the sigmoid sinus is located between line 1 and the line parallel to the tympanic segment of the facial nerve (line 2); type 3, the sigmoid sinus is located between line 2 and a plane parallel to the malleal-incudal axis (line 3); and type 4, the sigmoid sinus is located anteriorly to line 3. Types 3 and 4 are associated with difficult mastoidectomy [1].
- *Persistent petrosquamosal sinus*: it is an embryonic emissary vein that traverses the middle cranial fossa connecting intracranial dural sinuses with extracranial veins. It is located along the petrosquamosal fissure and usually involutes during fetal and early postnatal life. Its persistence may be a source of bleeding if encountered during surgery.
- *Mastoid emissary veins*: they are venous channels that connect the sigmoid sinus and the extracranial venous system, usually the posterior auricular or occipital vein, connecting the intracranial and extracranial venous systems. They can be multiple.
- *Persistent stapedial artery* (Fig. 11.2): the embryonic stapedial artery usually regresses in fetal life. When present it is seen as an abnormal small vessel that arises from the petrous portion of the internal carotid artery and crosses the middle ear as a linear soft-tissue density structure close to the cochlear promontory. Additionally, a small bony canal originating from the petrous segment of the internal carotid artery or a separate canal parallel to the facial nerve can be detected. The foramen spinosum can be aplastic or hypoplastic because of the absence or hypoplasia of the middle meningeal artery. The persistent stapedial artery can be associated with an aberrant internal carotid artery (Fig. 11.3).

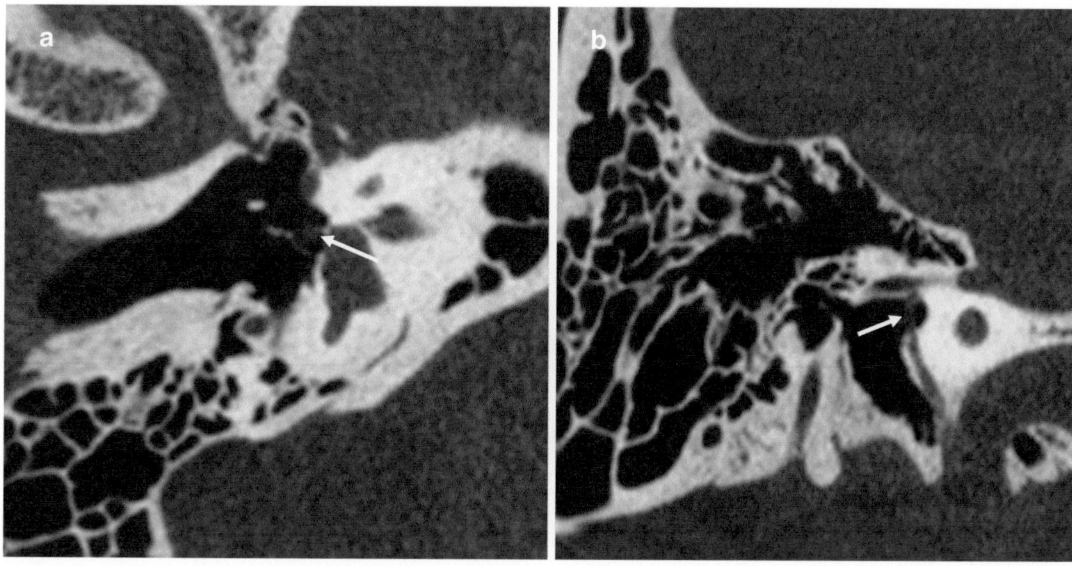

Fig. 11.2 Anatomical variants: persistent stapedial artery. The persistent stapedial artery is seen as an abnormal small vessel that arises from the petrous portion of the internal carotid artery and crosses the middle ear as a linear soft tissue density structure close to the cochlear promontory; it may pass through the stapedial crura. The foramen spinosum can be aplastic or hypoplastic because of the absence of hypoplasia of middle meningeal artery. The persistent stapedial artery can be associated with an aberrant internal carotid artery. (**a**) Axial CBCT image shows the persistent stapedial artery seen as a linear soft tissue density structure passing through the stapedial crura (arrow). (**b**) Coronal CBCT image shows the persistent stapedial artery seen as a linear soft-tissue density structure crosses the middle ear (arrow). *CBCT* cone beam computed tomography

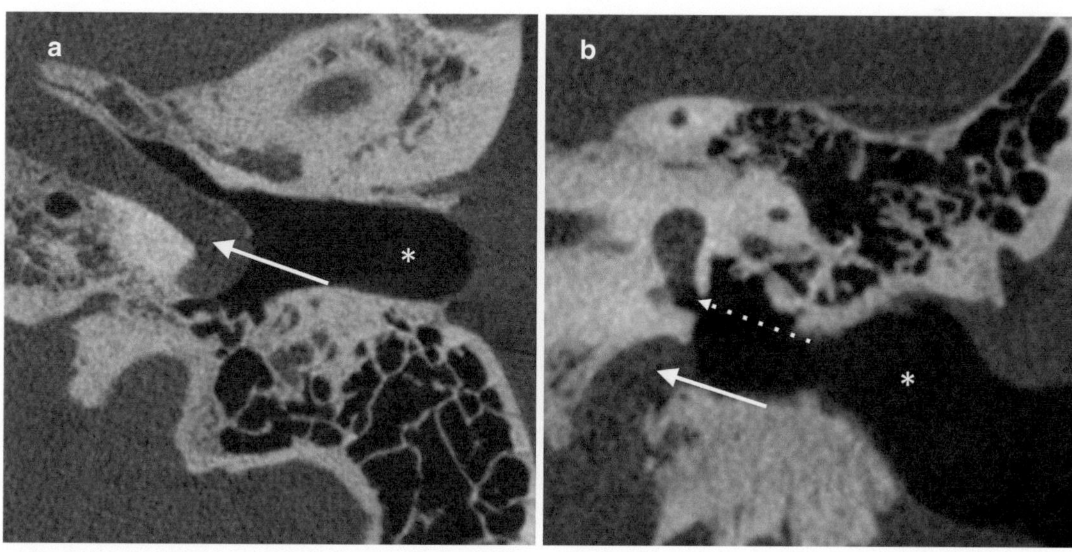

Fig. 11.3 Anatomical variants: aberrant internal carotid artery. The aberrant internal carotid artery can be associated with a persistent stapedial artery. (**a**) Axial CBCT image shows the aberrant internal carotid artery (arrow) as a retrotympanic mass at the level of mesotympanum and an absent carotid plate. The external auditory canal is indicated by the asterisk. (**b**) Coronal CBCT image shows the aberrant internal carotid artery (arrow) at the level of the posterior mesotympanum and inferiorly to the cochlear promontory and the round window (dotted arrow). The external auditory canal is indicated by the asterisk. *CBCT* cone beam computed tomography

Table 11.1 Presurgical checklist

Structures	What to check and tell the surgeon?
Mastoid and middle ear	Aerated vs sclerotic and/or signs of otomastoiditis When bone erosion (suspect of cholesteatoma)
Mastoid	Cellularity and aeration for planning of posterior tympanotomic access
Middle ear malformations and anatomical variants	Facial nerve canal position Presence of persistent stapedial artery High-riding jugular bulb
Ossicular chain (in particular stapes)	Morphology Position (dislocation) Fixation
Oval window accessibility	When narrow and/or obliterated
Round window accessibility	When narrow and/or obliterated and relationship with facial nerve canal
Inner ear malformations	Incomplete partition type III (high risk of gushing during surgery)
Superior semicircular canal condition	When dehiscent
Modiolar canal dimension	When wide
Internal auditory canal morphology and dimension	When narrow or globular
Vestibular aqueduct dimension	When dilated

- *Facial canal dehiscence*: Fallopian canal dehiscence and facial nerve exposure are diagnosed when there is a loss of integrity in the bone channel.
- *Deep sinus tympani*: when the depth of the recess is > or = 6 mm on an axial plane.
- *Meningocele*: the presence of prolapsing dura mater through a dehiscence of the tegmen antri or tegmen tympani should be acknowledged.
- *Hyrtl's fissure*: Hyrtl's fissure is a congenital cleft located posteriorly to the cochlear promontory on the axial plane. When open because of incomplete ossification, Hyrtl's fissure, also named tympano-meningeal fissure, connects the tympanic cavity and the posterior cranial fossa. A patent or a deep Hyrtl's fissure can be responsible for postoperative complications of cochlear implant surgery such as electrode misplacement or CSF fistulas.
- *Foramen of Huschke*: also known as foramen tympanicum, it is a bony defect that connects the external auditory canal to the temporomandibular joint. It is usually asymptomatic but can be occasionally responsible for recurrent otitis, temporomandibular joint septic arthritis, or masticatory tinnitus. The foramen tympanicum may close up to 5 years of age.

The presurgical checklist of anatomical structure is reported in Table 11.1.

For the explanation of congenital malformations of external, middle and inner ear, as well as cochlear nerve malformation, we refer to the correspondent Chap. 4.

Postsurgical imaging is often required after middle ear surgical intervention, such as cholesteatoma removal, or after positioning ossicular prosthesis and cochlear implant. Multi-detector computed tomography (MDCT) or cone beam computed tomography (CBCT) are the main techniques that are used in this context.

A recent classification of surgical procedures is proposed by the International Otology Outcome Group (IOOG) to categorize tympanomastoid operations according to the acronym SAMEO-ATO (stage of surgery, approach, mastoid bone extirpation, external bony wall repair, obliteration of the mastoid cavity, access to the middle ear, tympanic membrane reconstruction, and ossicular reconstruction) [4]. Nevertheless, middle ear surgery can be schematized as previously indicated by the American Academy of Otolaryngology—Head and Neck Surgery classification adapted in 1985 and displayed in Fig. 11.4.

Tympanoplasty without mastoidectomy includes myringoplasty and ossiculoplasty (com-

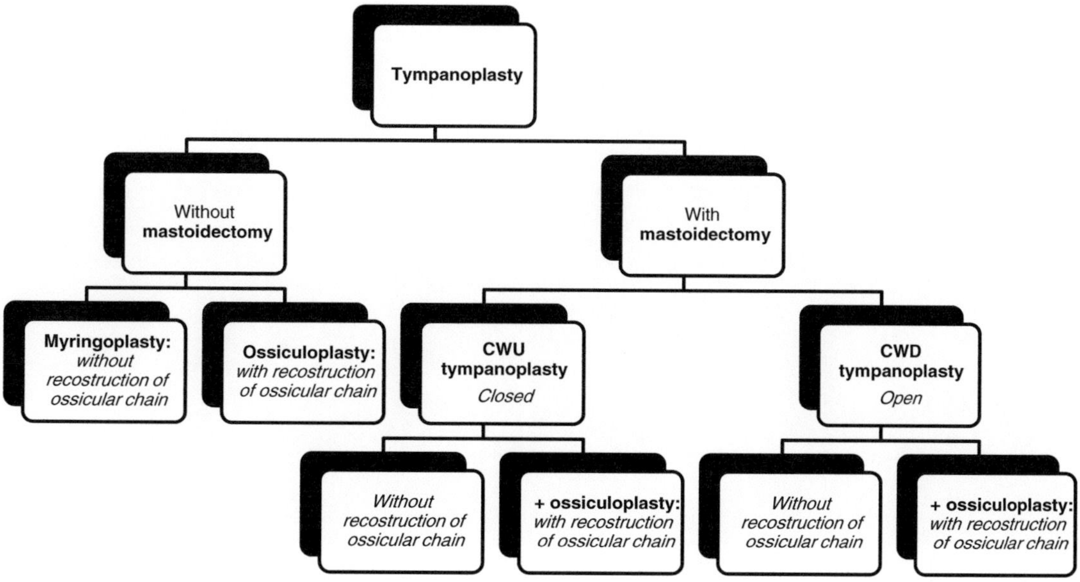

Fig. 11.4 **Middle ear surgery**. The middle ear surgery can be schematized as follows: tympanoplasty without mastoidectomy includes the myringoplasty and ossiculoplasty (comprehensive of stapedoplasty and prosthesis positioning). Tympanoplasty with mastoidectomy can be closed (CWU) or open (CWD). Both closed and open tympanoplasty with mastoidectomy can be associated or not with ossiculoplasty. CWU mastoidectomy consists in the removal of the mastoid cortex and the air cells and is aimed at preserving the posterosuperior wall of the EAC. CWD mastoidectomy involves the resection of the posterosuperior bony wall of the EAC and the scutum in addition to the removal of the mastoid cortex and the air cells. Ossiculoplasty or ossicular reconstruction surgery is used to reconnect the discontinued ossicular chain between the tympanic membrane and the oval window. The ossicular chain replacement prosthesis can be total or partial (TORP or PORP). *CWU* canal wall up, *CWD* canal wall down, *EAC* external auditory canal, *TORP* total ossicular chain replacement prosthesis, *PORP* partial ossicular chain replacement prosthesis

prehensive of stapedoplasty and prosthesis positioning). Tympanoplasty with mastoidectomy can be closed (canal wall up) Fig. 11.5 or open (canal wall down) Fig. 11.6. Both closed and open tympanoplasty with mastoidectomy can be associated or not with ossiculoplasty. Subtotal petrosectomy, also called petrous apicectomy, consists in a more demolitive surgery with the removal of all air cells of the temporal bone, including the middle ear and mastoid (Fig. 11.7). Complications of surgery include perilymphatic gusher, meningocele and meningoencephalocele.

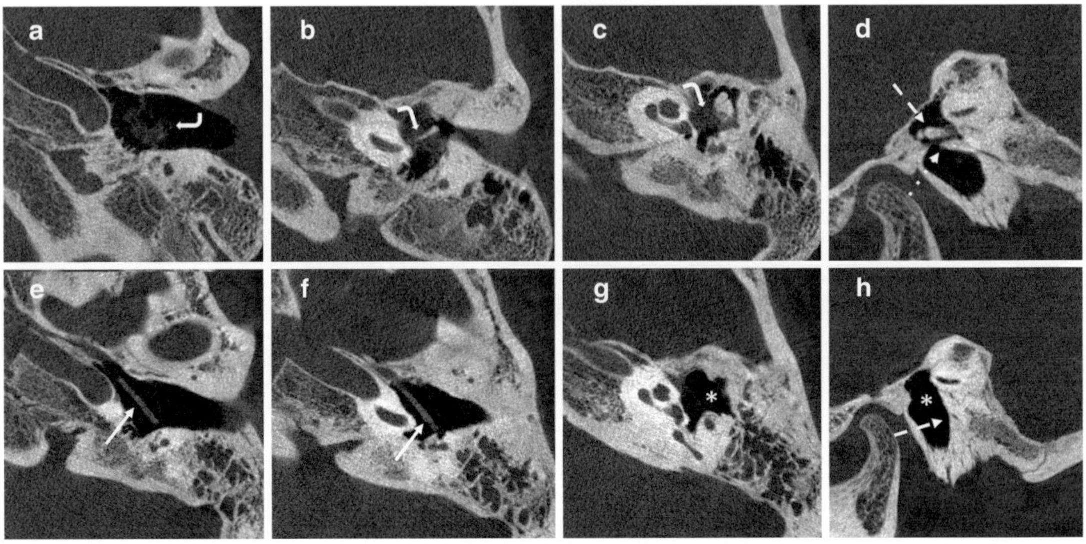

Fig. 11.5 **Canal wall up mastoidectomy**. CWU mastoidectomy is aimed at preserving the posterosuperior wall of the EAC. CBCT images of the left temporal bone before and after a CWU mastoidectomy for cholesteatoma are shown. CWU mastoidectomy involves the removal of the mastoid cortex and the air cells of epitympanum with the preservation of the posterosuperior bony wall of the EAC. The scutum is removed. This type of surgery is less invasive than CWD mastoidectomy but has a higher risk of cholesteatoma recurrence. The tympanic membrane was repaired using a tympanic patch. (**a–c**) Presurgical axial CBCT reformatted images passing below (**a**) and through the malleus handle (**b**) and the incus body (**c**) show cholesteatomatous tissue (curved arrow). (**d**) Presurgical sagittal CBCT reformatted image shows the ossicular chain (dashed arrow) and the scutum (dotted arrow) before surgery. (**e–g**) Postsurgical axial CBCT reformatted images show the result of demolition of the ossicular chain (asterisk) and the positioning of tympanic patch (arrow); after surgery the neo-tympanum is aerated. (**h**) Sagittal CBCT image shows the surgical cavity (asterisk) after the removal of ossicular chain and the scutum with the preservation of the posterior wall of EAC (dashed arrow). *CWU* canal wall up, *EAC* external auditory canal, *CBCT* cone beam computed tomography, *CWD* canal wall down

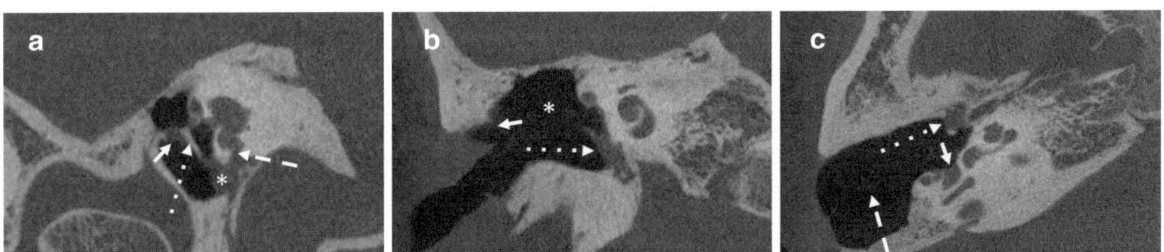

Fig. 11.6 **Canal wall down mastoidectomy**. CBCT images of the right temporal bone of a patient that underwent a CWD mastoidectomy for cholesteatoma. CWD mastoidectomy involves the removal of the mastoid cortex and the air cells and resection of the posterosuperior bony wall of the EAC and the scutum. This type of surgery is more invasive than CWU mastoidectomy, which is aimed at preserving the posterosuperior wall of the EAC, but ensures a lower risk of cholesteatoma recurrence. The tympanic membrane was repaired using tissue from temporalis fascia. (**a**) Coronal CBCT reformatted image of the right temporal bone passing through the malleus handle shows the results of partial surgical demolition of the eroded residual ossicular chain, with exclusive sparing of part of the malleus handle (dotted arrow) which is attached to the neomyrinx. After surgery the neo-tympanum is partially aerated, and residual soft-tissue density material is recognized adjacent to the manubrium of malleus (short arrow) and in the medial retrotympanum (asterisk) where it obliterates the niche of the round window (dashed arrow). (**b**) Coronal CBCT image of the right temporal bone passing through a more posterior plane shows that the soft-tissue density material also occupies part of the hypotympanum (dotted arrow). The large surgical cavity (asterisk) that remains after the removal of the mastoid cells and the scutum (short arrow) in association with the removal of the cholesteatomatous tissue is depicted. (**c**) Axial CBCT image of the right temporal bone depicts the results of removal of the posterior bony wall of the external auditory canal (dashed arrow). Soft-tissue density material is also recognizable anterior to the manubrium (dotted arrow) and in the sinus tympani (short arrow). *CBCT* cone beam computed tomography, *CWD* canal wall down, *CWU* canal wall up, *EAC* external auditory canal

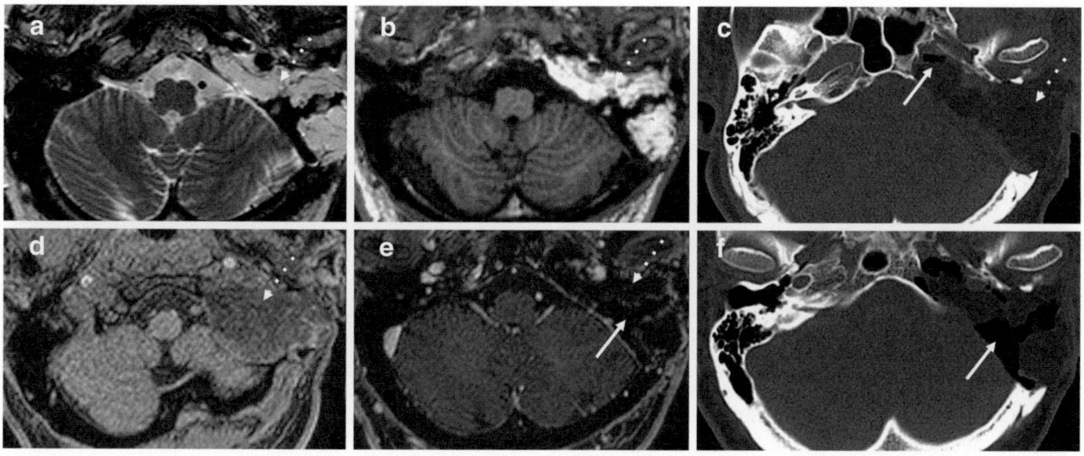

Fig. 11.7 **Subtotal petrosectomy**. Subtotal petrosectomy is also called petrous apicectomy and consists in the removal of all air cells of the temporal bone, including the middle ear and mastoid; only a few air cells in the petrous apex will remain. (**a**) TSE T2W axial image, (**b**) TSE T1W axial image, and (**d**) TSE T1W axial image with saturation of fat tissue show the subtotal petrosectomy; the cavity and the eustachian tube are filled with fat tissue (dotted arrow) and muscle. (**c**) MDCT axial image shows the subtotal petrosectomy and the surgical cavity that is filled with fat tissue and muscle. A small area of air infiltration is depicted in petrous apex (arrow). (**e**) Post-gadolinium TSE T1W axial image with saturation of fat tissue and (**f**) MDCT axial image follow-up after 1 year show the increase of air infiltration (arrow) within the surgical fat tissue that indicates fistulization. *TSE* turbo spin echo, *MDCT* multidetector computed tomograph

11.2 Myringoplasty

The repair of tympanic membrane defects can be done with underlay or overlay techniques according to the position of the graft over (laterally) or under (medially) the tympanic membrane edges. Compared to the underlay technique, the overlay technique has an increased risk of complications such lateralization of the graft and of blunting (fibrosis of the anterior edge of the tympanic membrane). Additionally the risk of cholesteatoma recurrence is higher in overlay technique because the native tympanic edges lay under the reconstructed eardrum: CT scan is therefore mandatory in the follow-up of patients undergoing this surgery.

11.3 Ossiculoplasty

Ossiculoplasty or ossicular reconstruction surgery (OCR) (shown in Figs. 11.8, 11.9, 11.10, 11.11, 11.12, 11.13, 11.14, 11.15, 11.16, 11.17, 11.18, 11.19, 11.20, 11.21, and 11.22) treats a conductive hearing loss: a prosthesis is used to reconnect the discontinued ossicular chain between the tympanic membrane and the oval window. Ossiculoplasty is the treatment for otosclerosis. Ossicular chain replacement prosthesis can be total or partial: total ossicular replacement prosthesis or partial ossicular replacement prosthesis (TORP or PORP). Ossicular chain prosthesis can be organic (the incus itself or the tragus cartilage) or synthetic. In ossiculoplasty the incus is disarticulated from the head of the malleus and rotated by 180° and then articulated again with the handle of the malleus with the long apophysis toward the oval window after demolition of the stapes.

Synthetic prosthesis includes bioinert materials (e.g., titanium) and bioactive materials (e.g., hydroxyapatite) or their combinations.

Multi-detector computed tomography (MDCT) or cone beam computed tomography (CBCT) assesses the position of stapes prosthesis. The type of the prosthesis should be known when assessing the penetration into the vestibule with CT as not all stapes prostheses are equally visualized on CT. Metallic prostheses are well visualized on CT scans, and their position is clearly depictable, even if their length may be overestimated on CT images. Conversely, the

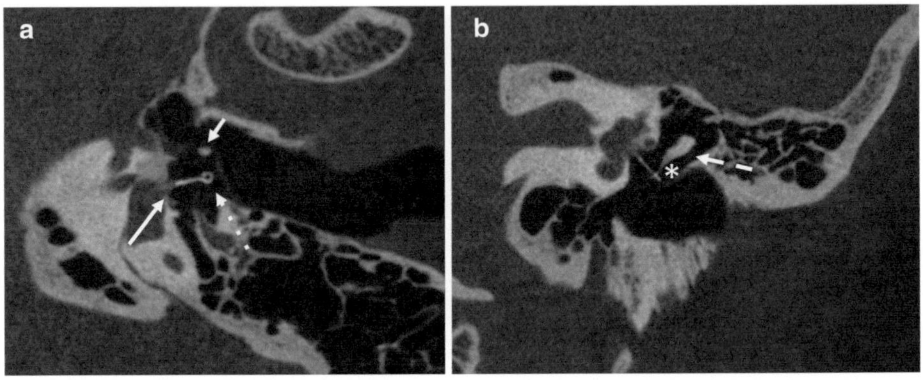

Fig. 11.8 Stapedotomy with platinum-fluoroplastic piston prosthesis replacement. The prosthesis was placed for fenestral otosclerosis. (**a**) Axial reformatted CBCT MPR images at the level of oval window show the stapedial prosthesis piston normally centered and articulated with the oval window (arrow). Also note the manubrium of malleus (short arrow) and the loop of the stapes prosthesis (dotted arrow). (**b**) Coronal reformatted CBCT MPR images at the level of oval window show the loop of the stapes prosthesis normally attached and articulated with the long process of the incus (asterisk). Also note the body of the incus (dashed arrow). *CBCT* cone beam computed tomography, *MPR* multiplanar recostruction

visualization of fluoroplastic pistons may be challenging. CBCT has shown advantages by reducing metal artifacts [5] with a lower dose of radiation [6] than multiplanar reconstruction (MPR) parallel to the stapes prosthesis is more accurate in the evaluation of prosthesis position.

Failures of OCR include extrusion, reabsorption (frequent in case of bioactive implants) and ankylosis, migration, and dislocation. Moreover, the necrosis of long process of incus is one of the most common causes of stapedectomy failure. It is probably caused by loss of blood supply or inflammation and bone erosion due to a poorly fit prosthesis [7]. Complications after stapes surgery are rare and include vertigo, hearing loss, dysgeusia, and tympanic membrane perforation. The malposition of the prosthesis with penetration into the vestibule may be responsible for hearing loss or vertigo [8]. CT scan is indicated in case of suspected ossicular chain dislocation.

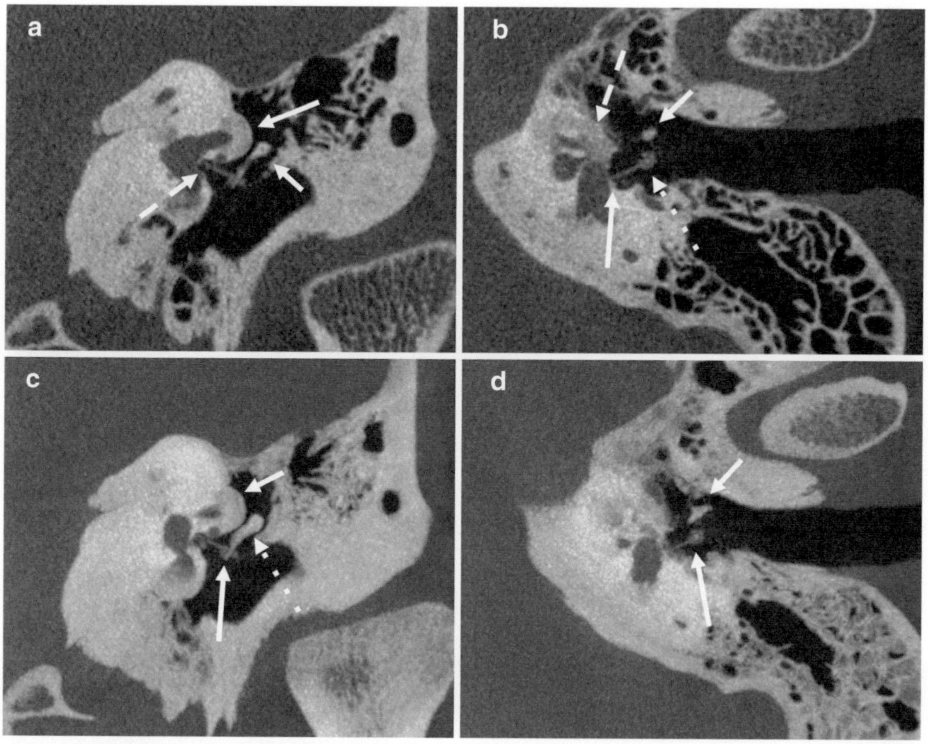

Fig. 11.9 Stapedotomy with insertion of a non-radiopaque stapes prosthesis (fluoroplastic loop). (**a**) Coronal reformatted CBCT MPR images show the distal prosthesis piston normally centered and articulated with the oval window (dashed arrow). Also note the body of the incus (short arrow) and the otospongiotic foci involving the otic capsule at the promontory (arrow). (**b**) Axial reformatted CBCT MPR images show the loop hooked into the long process of the incus (dotted arrow). Also note the medial end of the prosthesis normally centered and articulated with the oval window (arrow), the manubrium of malleus (short arrow), and the otospongiotic foci involving the otic capsule (dashed arrow) posterior to the vestibule and around the cochlear gyri. (**c**) Coronal reformatted CBCT MIP images show the loop of the stapes prosthesis normally attached and articulated with the long process of the incus (arrow). Also note the incus (dotted arrow) and the otospongiotic foci involving the otic capsule at the promontory (arrowhead). (**d**) Axial reformatted CBCT MIP images show normally located prosthesis (arrow). Also note the manubrium of malleus (short arrow). *CBCT* cone beam computed tomography, *MPR* multiplanar recostruction, *MIP* maximum intensity projection

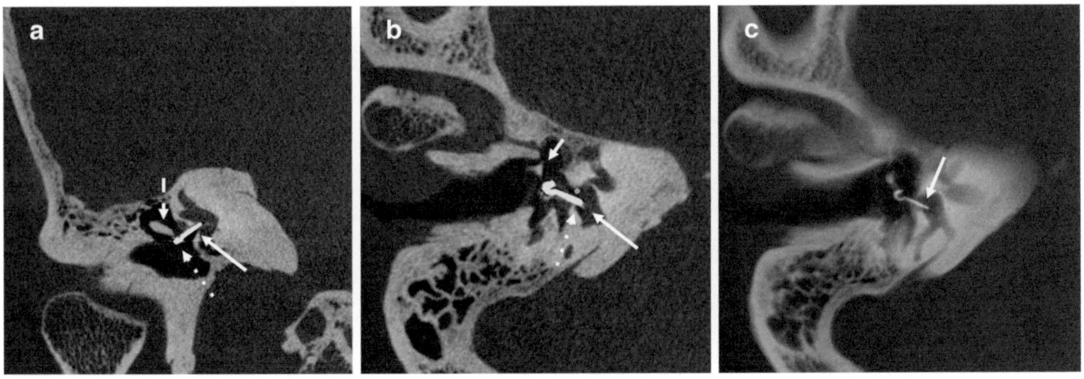

Fig. 11.10 Stapedotomy with insertion of radiopaque stapes titanium prosthesis. (**a**) Sagittal reformatted CBCT MPR images show the loop normally hooked into the long process of the incus (dotted arrow) and the medial end of the prosthesis centered at the oval window (arrow). Also note the body of the incus (dashed arrow). (**b**) Axial reformatted CBCT MPR images show the medial end normally centered at the base of the stapes (dashed arrow), but the apex of the prosthesis sinks into the vestibule for about 1.2 mm (arrow). Also note the manubrium of malleus (short arrow). (**c**) Axial reformatted CBCT MIP images better show the apex of the prosthesis sunk into the vestibule (arrow). This condition may be associated with the development of vertiginous symptomatology. *CBCT* cone beam computed tomography, *MPR* multiplanar recostruction, *MIP* maximum intensity projections

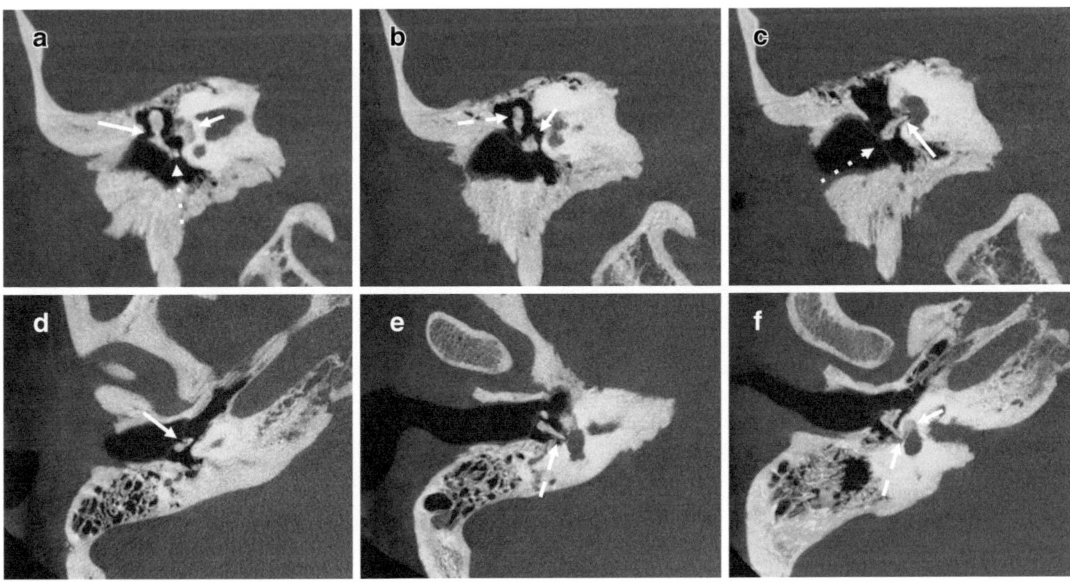

Fig. 11.11 Surgical outcomes of stapedotomy and ossiculoplasty. (**a–c**) Coronal reformatted CBCT MIP shows regular position and morphology of the malleus (arrow); the body of the incus (short arrow in **b**) is disarticulated from the head of the malleus and, after being rotated 180° and positioned more caudally, was rearticulated with the handle of the malleus (dashed arrow in **a**) by means of a small bony loggia excavated between the body and short process of the incus. The long apophysis then heads toward the oval window resting on the base of the stapes (arrow in **c**) after demolition of its overstructure. Also note the otospongiotic foci (short arrow in **a**) and the thickened tympanic membrane (dotted arrow in **c**). (**d–f**) Axial reformatted CBCT MIP better shows the small bony loggia excavated between the body and short process of the incus (arrow in **d**) and the long apophysis of the incus articulates with the plate of the stapes (dashed arrow in **e** and **f**). Also note the otospongiotic foci (short arrow in **f**). *CBCT* cone beam computed tomography, *MIP* maximum intensity projection

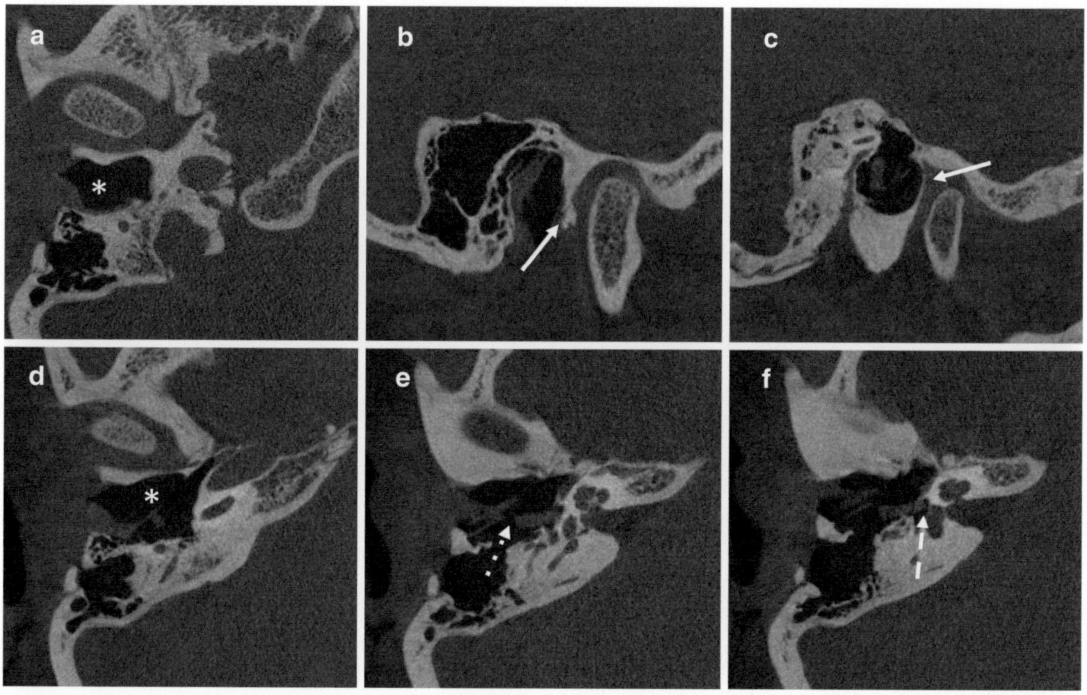

Fig. 11.12 Surgical outcomes of total ossicular replacement prosthesis. CWU mastoidectomy with TORP. Images show the removal of the ossicular chain and cartilaginous graft prosthesis. The prosthesis is dislocated: the lateral part does not articulate with the tympanic membrane, while the medial part properly articulates with the oval window. (**a–c**) CBCT axial images show the results of a CWU mastoidectomy with surgical cavity (asterisk in **a**) and the preservation of posterior wall of EAC (arrow in **b** and **c**). (**d–f**) CBCT axial images show surgical cavity (asterisk in **d**) and the cartilaginous prosthesis with the lateral part that does not articulate with the tympanic membrane (dotted arrow in **e**), while the medial part properly articulates with the oval window (dashed arrow in **f**). *TORP* total ossicular replacement prosthesis, *CBCT* cone beam computed tomography, *CWU* canal wall up, *EAC* external auditory canal

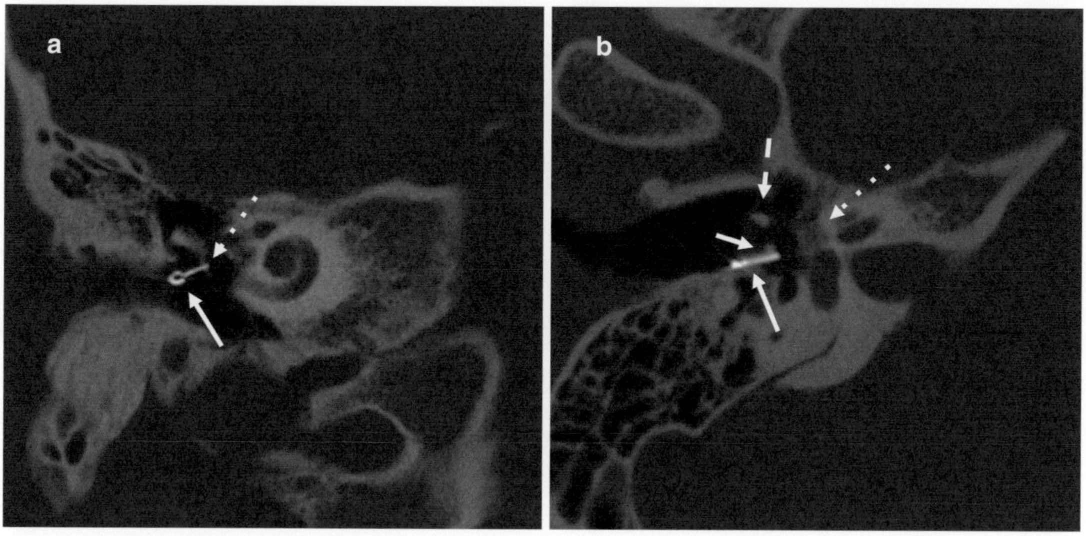

Fig. 11.13 Dislocated stapes prosthesis. (**a**) Coronal reformatted CBCT MPR images show a dislocated prosthesis with the lateral portion of the prosthesis placed near the tympanic membrane (arrow) and the medial portion of the prosthesis at the level of the long process of the incus (dotted arrow). (**b**) Axial reformatted CBCT MPR images better show the displaced prosthesis (arrow). Also note the long process of the incus (short arrow), the manubrium of malleus (dashed arrow), and the otospongiotic foci involving the otic capsule at the fissula ante fenestram (dotted arrow). *CBCT* cone beam tomography, *MPR* multiplanar recostruction

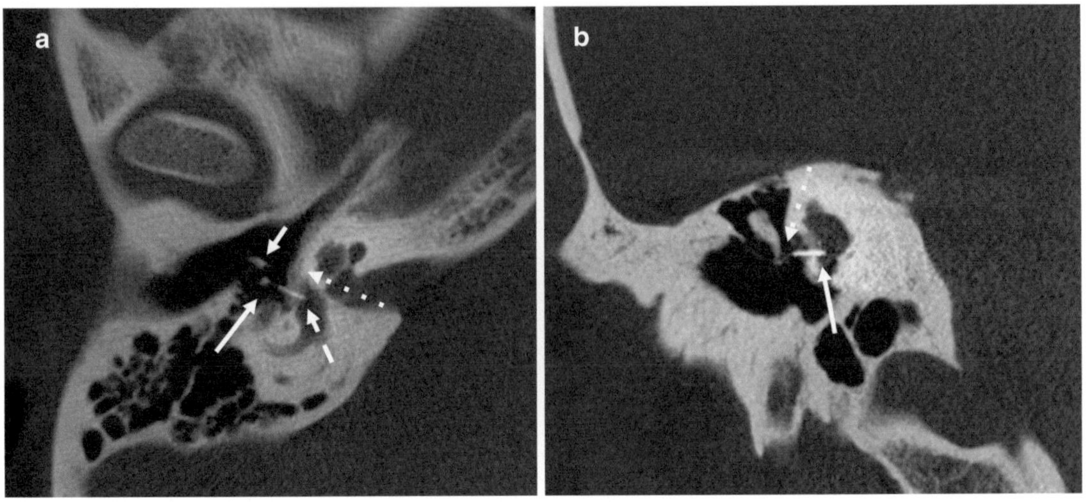

Fig. 11.14 Dislocated stapes prosthesis. (**a**) Axial reformatted CBCT MPR images shows the stapes prosthesis normally articulated with the lenticular process of the incus (arrow). The medial end of the stapes passes through the oval window with end point located within the vestibule (dashed arrow). Also note the manubrium of malleus (short arrow) and the otospongiotic foci involving the otic capsule at the fissula ante fenestram (dotted arrow). (**b**) Coronal reformatted CBCT MIP images better show the medial end of the prosthesis displaced within the vestibule (arrow). Also note the distal end of the prosthesis normally articulated with the long process of the incus (dotted arrow). *CBCT* cone beam computed tomography, *MPR* multiplanar recostruction, *MIP* maximum intensity projection

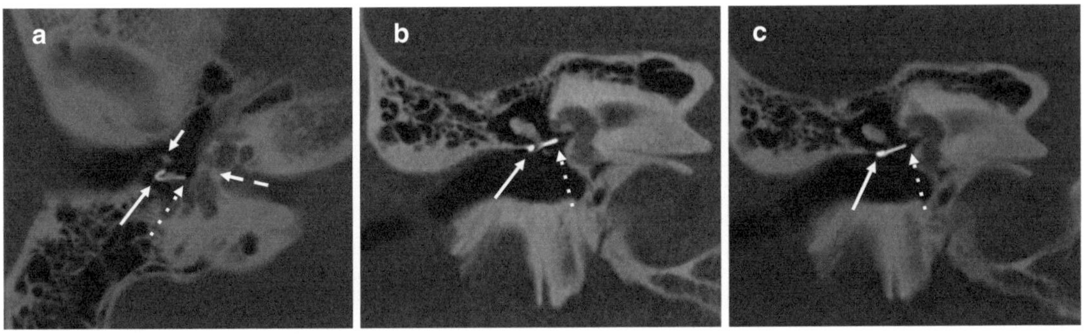

Fig. 11.15 Dislocated stapes prosthesis. (**a**) Axial reformatted CBCT MPR images show the prosthesis with lateralized positioning: the lateral end of the prosthesis is lateralized to the lenticular process of the incus (arrow); the medial end of the prosthesis also does not reach the oval window (dotted arrow). Also note the manubrium of malleus (short arrow) and the otospongiotic foci at the fissula ante fenestram that reaches the cochlear gyri (dashed arrow). (**b** and **c**) Coronal reformatted CBCT MPR images better show the laterally dislocated prosthesis: in particular, the distal portion is more lateral and higher than the long process of the incus (arrow). The medial end is not articulated with the oval window (dotted arrow). *CBCT* cone beam computed tomography, *MPR* multiplanar recostruction

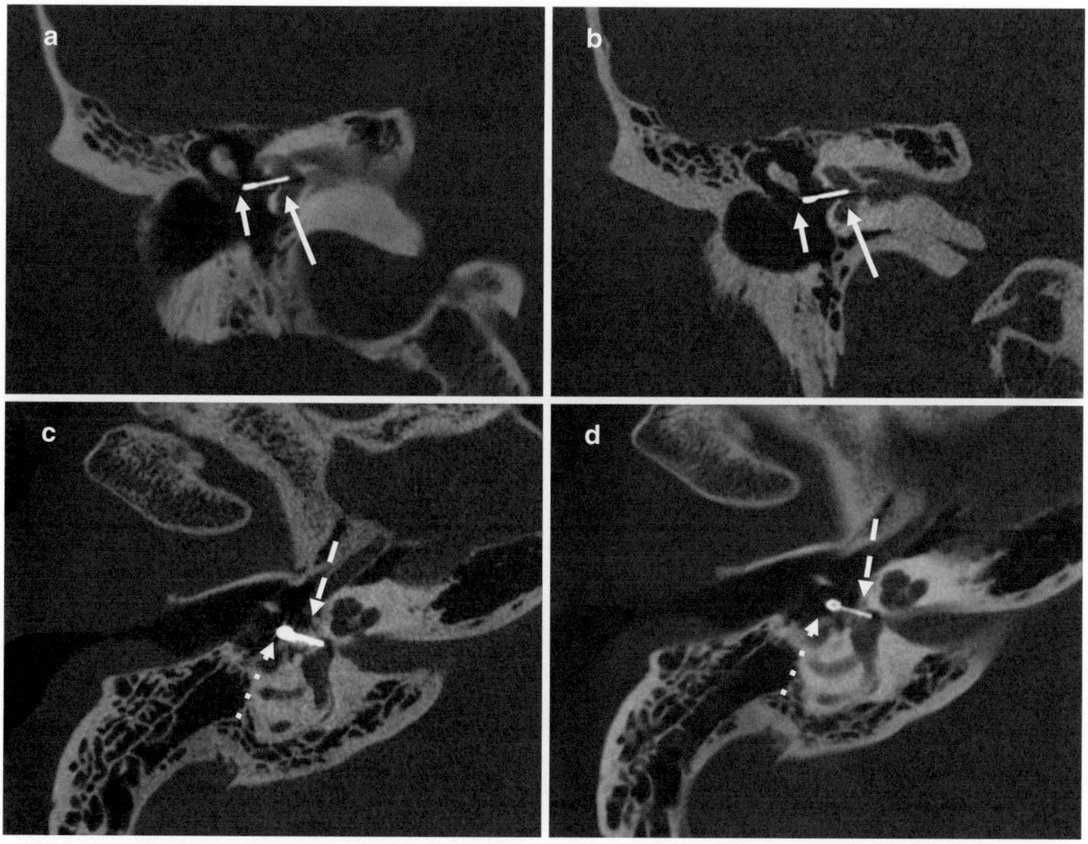

Fig. 11.16 Dislocated stapes prosthesis. (**a** and **b**) Coronal reformatted CBCT MPR images show the distal end of the stapes prosthesis protruded in the vestibule (arrow). Also note the medial end of stapes prosthesis disengaged from the long process of the incus (arrowhead). (**c** and **d**) Axial reformatted CBCT MPR images better show the stapes prosthesis disengaged from the long process of the incus (dotted arrow). The stapes axis is not perpendicular to the oval window, within which its distal end protrudes (dashed arrow). *CBCT* cone beam computed tomography, *MPR* multiplanar recostruction

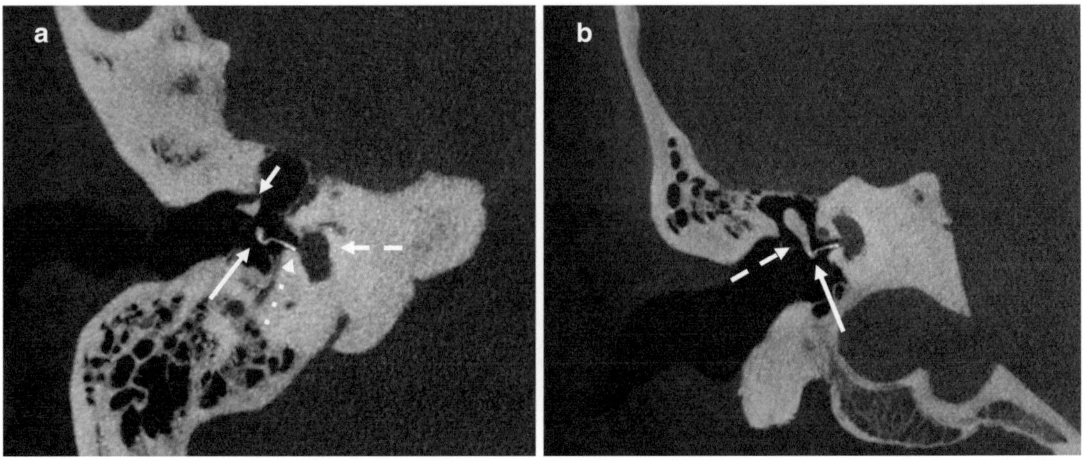

Fig. 11.17 Dislocated stapes prosthesis. (a) Axial reformatted CBCT MIP image shows the stapedial prosthesis normally attached to the long process of the incus (arrow). The distal end reaches and articulates with the oval window but in an off-center posterior position (dotted arrow). Also note the manubrium of malleus (short arrow) and the vestibule (dashed arrow). (**b**) Coronal reformatted CBCT MIP images better show the medial end of the prosthesis normally articulated with the long process of the incus (arrow). Also note the normal incus (dashed arrow). *CBCT* cone beam computed tomography, *MIP* maximum intensity projection

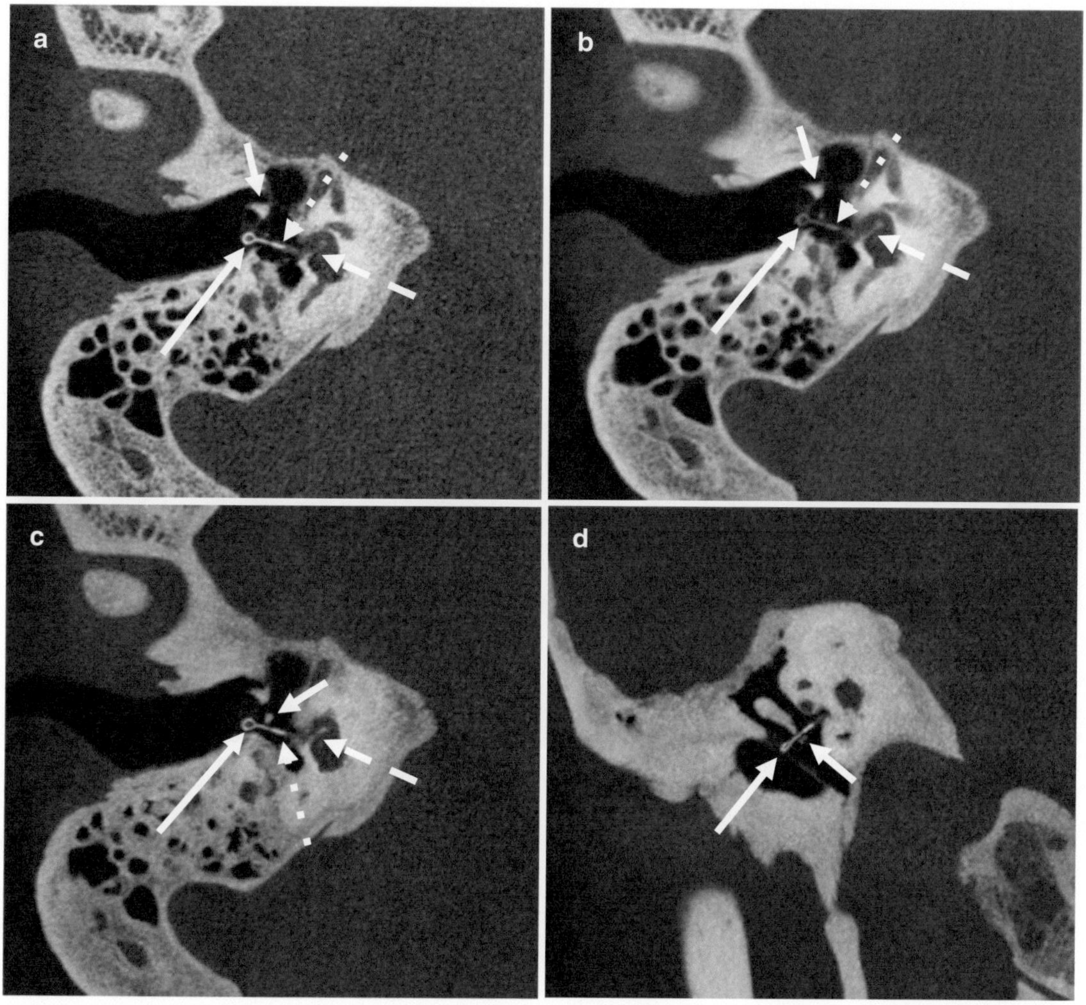

Fig. 11.18 Dislocated stapes prosthesis. (**a** and **b**) Axial reformatted CBCT MPR image shows the stapedial prosthesis detached from the long process of the incus and dislocated posteriorly and laterally in the tympanic cavity, with distal end near to the tympanic membrane (arrow). The medial end of the prosthesis (dotted arrow) does not reach the oval window. The stapes plate is sunk inside the vestibule (dashed arrow). Also note the manubrium of malleus (short arrow). (**c**) Axial reformatted CBCT MIP image better shows the lateral end of the prosthesis (arrow) dislocated from the lenticular process of the incus (short arrow). Note the stapes plate within the vestibule (dashed arrow) and the medial end of the prosthesis not articulated with the oval window (dotted arrow). (**d**) Coronal reformatted CBCT MIP image better shows the stapedial prosthesis detached from the long process of the incus with distal end near to the tympanic membrane (short arrow). Long process of incus (short arrow). *CBCT* cone beam computed tomography, *MPR* multiplanar reconstruction, *MIP* maximum intensity projection

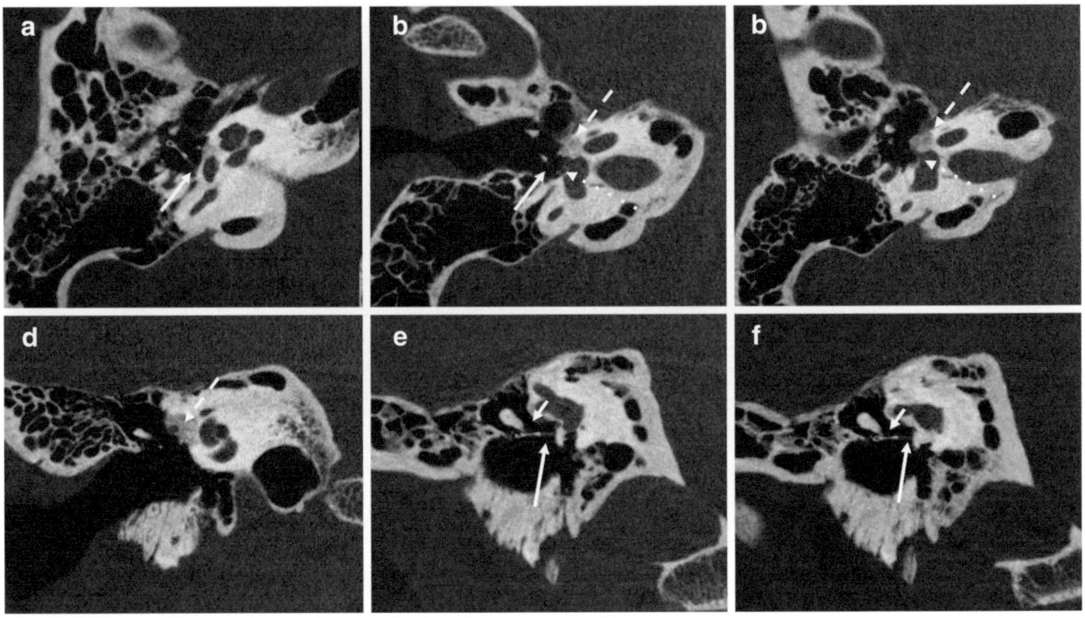

Fig. 11.19 Complication of stapedotomy and depositioning of stapes prosthesis: necrosis of long process of incus. CBCT images show the dislocation of stapes prosthesis due to erosion of the long process of incus. The necrosis and erosion of the long process of incus are the most frequent causes of stapedial prosthesis surgery failure. Note that in this case the medial part of the prosthesis is made of fluoroplastic material and it is not radiopaque. (**a–c**) Axial reformatted CBCT images show the dislocation of stapes prosthesis with the medial part (arrow) located inferiorly and posteriorly to the oval window (dotted arrow in **b** and **c**). An otospongiotic focus is present anteriorly to the oval window (dashed arrow in **b** and **c**). (**d–f**) Coronal reformatted CBCT images show the absence of the long apophysis of the incus (short arrow in **e** and **f**) and the dislocation of the stapes prosthesis (arrow) that ends inferiorly to the oval window. *CBCT* cone beam computed tomography

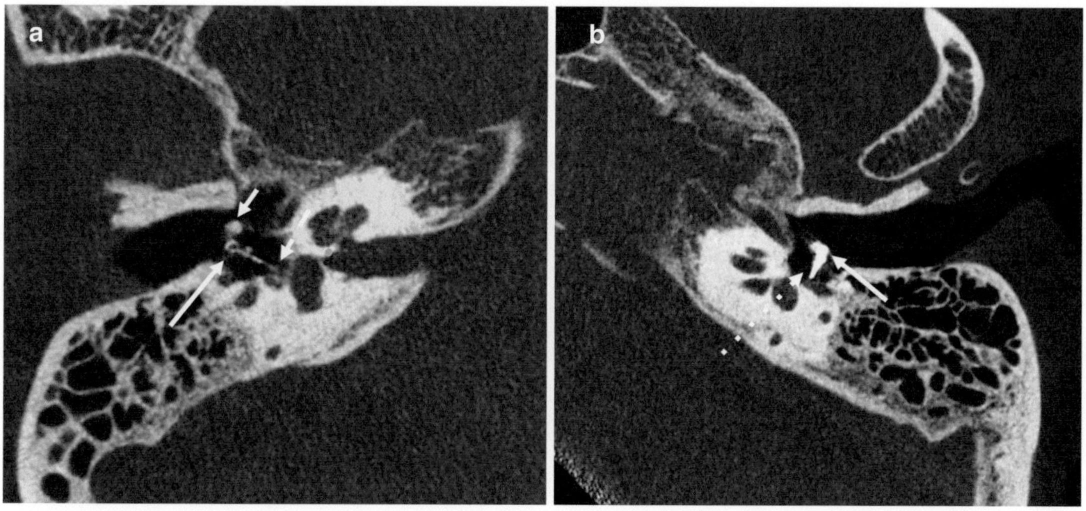

Fig. 11.20 Stapedotomy and bilateral prosthetic stapes replacement with different stapedial prostheses. Left and right prostheses are displaced. Note that the medial part of the prosthesis of the right side is made of fluoroplastic material and it is not radiopaque. (**a**) Axial reformatted CBCT shows the stapedial piston prosthesis disengaged from the long apophysis of the incus and lateralized almost close to the tympanic membrane (arrow). The medial end of the prosthesis is more difficult to depict as it is not radiopaque and it is located medially to the oval window (dashed arrow). Also note the manubrium of the malleus (short arrow). (**b**) Axial reformatted CBCT image shows the stapedial metallic piston prosthesis disengaged from the long apophysis of the incus, close to the tympanic membrane (arrow); the apex is dislocated posteriorly to the oval window toward the retrotympanum (dotted arrow). *CBCT* cone beam computed tomography

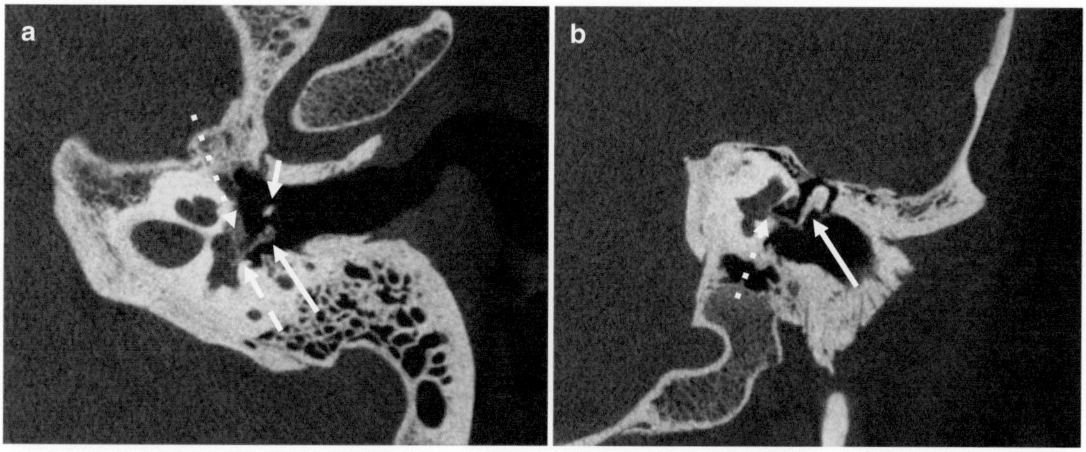

Fig. 11.21 Dislocated stapes prosthesis. (**a**) Axial reformatted CBCT MIP and (**b**) coronal reformatted CBCT MIP images show the stapedial prosthesis correctly attached to the long apophysis of the incus (arrow in **a**); the medial end of the prosthesis is not centered on the oval window but is displaced posteriorly close to the posterior crura remnant (dashed arrow in **a**) and plunged into the vestibule. The coronal reformatted image (**b**) better shows the medial end of the prosthesis posteriorly displaced in the oval window (dotted arrow in **b**). Also note the manubrium of malleus (short arrow in **a**) and the extensive otospongiotic foci at the fissula ante fenestram (dotted arrow in **a**). Note the long process of the incus (arrow in **b**). *CBCT* cone beam computed tomography, *MIP* maximum intensity projection

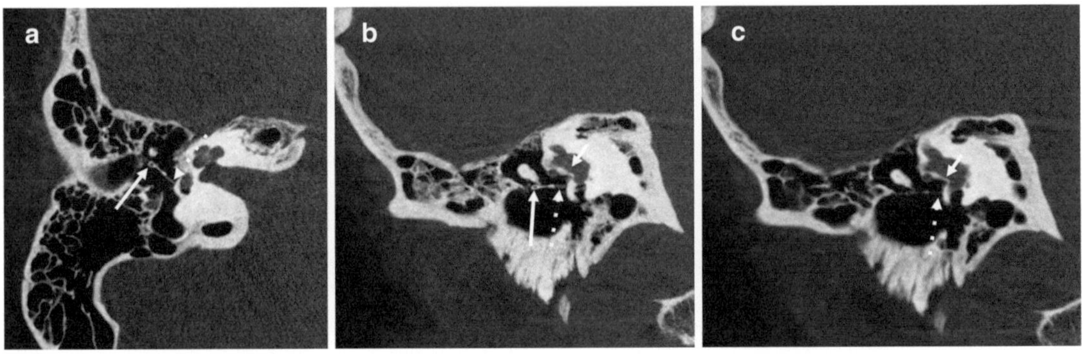

Fig. 11.22 **Dislocated stapes prosthesis**. (**a**) Axial reformatted CBCT MPR, (**b**) coronal reformatted CBCT MIP, and (**c**) coronal reformatted CBCT MIP show the stapedial prosthesis disengaged from the long apophysis of the incus (arrow in **a** and **b**), rotated clockwise in the axial plane. The medial part of the prosthesis is not centered on the base of the stapes but toward the posterior and inferior lips of the round window (dotted arrow in **a**–**c**). Note the position of the oval window (short arrow in **b** and **c**). *CBCT* cone beam computed tomography, *MIP* maximum intensity projection

11.4 Canal Wall Up Tympanoplasty with Mastoidectomy

Canal wall up (CWU) mastoidectomy (Fig. 11.5) consists in the removal of the mastoid cortex and the air cells and is aimed at preserving the posterosuperior wall of the external auditory canal (EAC). It is indicated in cases of cholesteatoma, chronic otitis media, and meningoceles. MR with non echo planar diffusion weighted imaging (non-EPI DWI) may replace the second-look surgery allowing the detection of cholesteatoma recurrences. The posterior wall or the EAC is the main site of recurrence due to the risk of interruption or defect after surgery. The risk of recurrence is higher in CWU than in canal wall down mastoidectomy (Fig. 11.6).

11.5 Atticotomy

During atticotomy the scutum is removed in order to access the epitympanum, usually for the removal of small cholesteatomas, and then the lateral attic wall and the tympanic membrane are reconstructed. The risk of cholesteatoma recurrence is high.

11.6 Canal Wall Down Tympanoplasty with Mastoidectomy

Canal wall down (CWD) mastoidectomy (Fig. 11.6) involves the resection of the posterosuperior bony wall of the EAC and the scutum in addition to the removal of the mastoid cortex and the air cells; the tympanic membrane is usually repaired using tissue from temporalis fascia. CWU and CWD mastoidectomies are the surgical approach to cholesteatoma removal. CWD is more invasive than CWU mastoidectomy but ensures a lower risk of cholesteatoma recurrence [9]. The indications for this surgery include the procidence in hypotympanum of the sigmoid sinus and of the jugular bulb and a poor visualization of the tympanic recesses at otomicroscopy, which can be resolved by the use of endoscopy.

11.7 Canal Wall Down Tympanoplasty with Other Mastoidectomies

CWD tympanoplasty may be modified into "radical" mastoidectomy (without the reconstruction of tympanic cavity and with obliteration of the

Eustachian tube) or to obliterative mastoidectomy. In the latter, obliteration of the surgical cavity with muscle, cartilage, or hydroxyapatite powder/granules is accomplished.

A Bondy mastoidectomy consists in CWD mastoidectomy with preservation of intact eardrum and ossicular chain.

11.8 Subtotal Petrosectomy

Subtotal petrosectomy (STP) (Fig. 11.7) is indicated in cases of recurrent and recalcitrant middle ear diseases after previous repeated surgeries or in case of intraoperative cerebrospinal fluid (CSF) leaks. It consists of the complete removal of all the air cells of the petrous bone including the antral, supralabyrinthine, infralabyrinthine, retrofacial, retrosigmoid, peritubal, and pericarotid air cells. The exenteration of cochlea and labyrinth is possible. Complication of middle ear surgery include perilymphatic gusher (Fig. 11.23), meningocele (Fig. 11.24) and meningoencephalocele (Fig. 11.25).

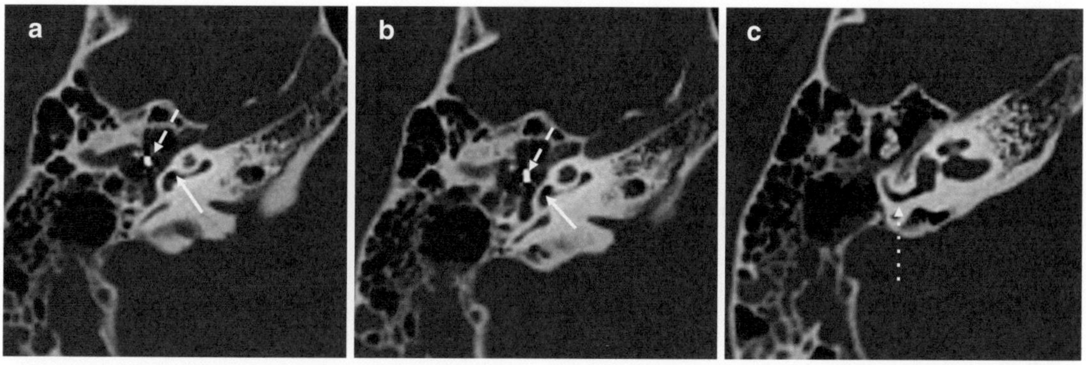

Fig. 11.23 Stapedectomy and stapedo prosthesis surgery complications: perilymphatic gusher. Gusher is a very rare phenomenon consistent of a perilymph flow after platinotomy. In adults it is associated to otosclerosis. (**a–c**) Postsurgical axial CBCT reformatted images passing through the basal turn (**a**), the basal and middle turns of the cochlea (**b**), and the modiolus (**c**) show air in the basal turn of the cochlea (arrow in **a** and **b**) and in the lateral semicircular canal (dotted arrow in **c**). The stapes prosthesis is depicted (dashed arrowin **b** and **c**)

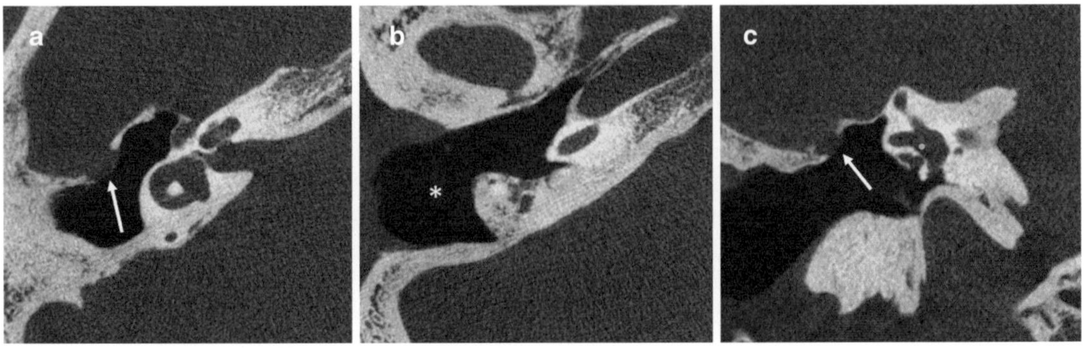

Fig. 11.24 **Canal wall down mastoidectomy complications: meningocele**. CBCT images of the right temporal bone of a patient that underwent a canal wall down mastoidectomy (CWD mastoidectomy) for cholesteatoma with removal of ossicular chain. CWD mastoidectomy involves the removal of the mastoid cortex and the air cells and resection of the posterosuperior bony wall of the EAC and the scutum. (**a**) Axial CBCT reformatted image of the right temporal bone shows the results of surgery and a bony defect of the tegmen tympani suggesting the presence of a meningocele (arrow). (**b**) Axial CBCT reformatted image of the right temporal bone shows the results of surgery: the large surgical cavity (asterisk) that remains after the removal of the mastoid cells, the scutum, and the posterior wall of EAC are depicted. (**c**) Coronal CBCT image of the right temporal bone shows the bony defect of the tegmen tympani suggesting the presence of a meningocele (arrow). *CBCT* cone beam computed tomography, *CWD* canal wall down mastoidectomy, *EAC* external auditory canal

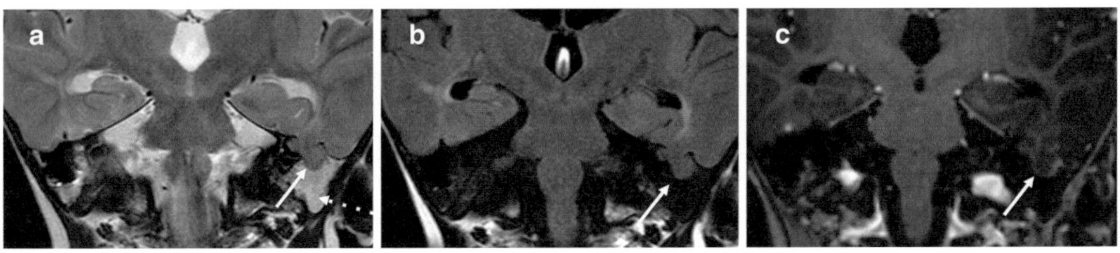

Fig. 11.25 **Postsurgical complications: meningoencephalocele**. MRI of a temporal postsurgical meningoencephalocele. (**a**) Coronal T2-weighted image, (**b**) coronal FLAIR image, and (**c**) coronal T1-weighted image after gadolinium injection show a bony defect of the tegmen tympani and a meningoencephalocele consisting of the herniation of meninges and fusiform gyrus through the defect of tegmen tympani (arrow). The mastoid is filled with fluid (dotted arrow in **a**). *MRI* magnetic resonance imaging, *FLAIR* fluid attenuated invertion recovery

11.9 Cochlear Implant

Cochlear implant (Figs. 11.26, 11.27, 11.28, 11.29, 11.30, 11.31, 11.32, 11.33, 11.34, 11.35, and 11.36) is composed of external and internal parts. The internal (implanted) components are the receiver/stimulator, the carrier cable, and the electrode array. The receiver/stimulator includes the radio frequency receiver, the coil antenna, the magnet, and the ground case contact (as a separate electrode in some models) [10, 11].

The surgical approach for cochlear implant insertion is a CWU mastoidectomy, with preservation of the posterior wall of the EAC, followed by posterior tympanotomy.

The drilling of the posterosuperior bony overhang of the round window niche allows a full exposure of the round window membrane. The electrode array of the cochlear implant is then inserted into the scala tympani. The scala tympani is located posteriorly to the scala vestibuli in axial planes. The electrode array lying close to the anterior wall of the cochlea indicates that the

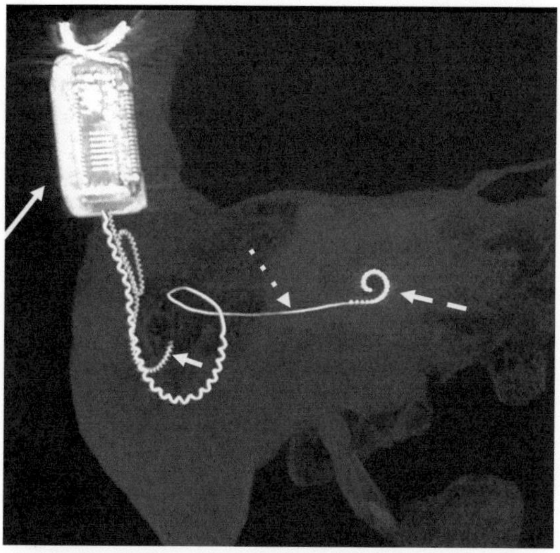

Fig. 11.26 Cochlear implant. The MIP CTCB image shows the cochlear implant inserted in the right temporal bone. Cochlear implant is composed of several parts: the receiver/stimulator (arrow), the electrode ground contact (dotted arrow), the implant electrode (dashed arrow), and the electrode array (short arrow). The receiver/stimulator includes the radio frequency receiver coil antenna, the magnet, and the ground case contact. *MIP* maximum intensity projection, *CBCT* cone beam computed tomography

array has inadvertently translocated into the scala vestibuli [12].

Complications of cochlear implant surgery are the malposition of the electrode array: it may migrate outside the cochlea in the tympanic cavity or be diverted into the vestibule and superior semicircular canal; in narrow or partially obstructed cochleas, an intracochlear fold over of its tip or the basal buckling of the electrode array can be observed. Additionally, malformation of the inner ear may predispose to complications. For example, the absence of the cribriform plate is the cause of the erroneous insertion and migration of the electrode array in the internal auditory canal and in the cerebellopontine angle. Other complications are the interruption of the tegmen tympani and facial nerve injury. Facial nerve injury is a rare occurrence in cochlear implantation and may present immediately or with delayed onset, hours, days, or weeks after surgery. The facial nerve may be injured directly by the drill bur or by the heat caused by prolonged drilling or by viral reactivation. In case of delayed injury, the mechanism is progressive nerve edema [13]. Additionally facial spasms may occur in case of facial nerve canal dehiscence or anatomical variant or when the facial nerve canal is close to the cochlear implant lead.CBCT provides images with higher spatial resolution than MDCT and minimizes metallic artifacts. It is suitable for the postsurgical evaluation of cochlear implant positioning. The factors that should be assessed and that are potentially related to cochlear implantation outcomes are the proper electrode position, the insertion depth, the scalar localization, the relationship to the facial nerve canal, and the surgical complications [14, 15].

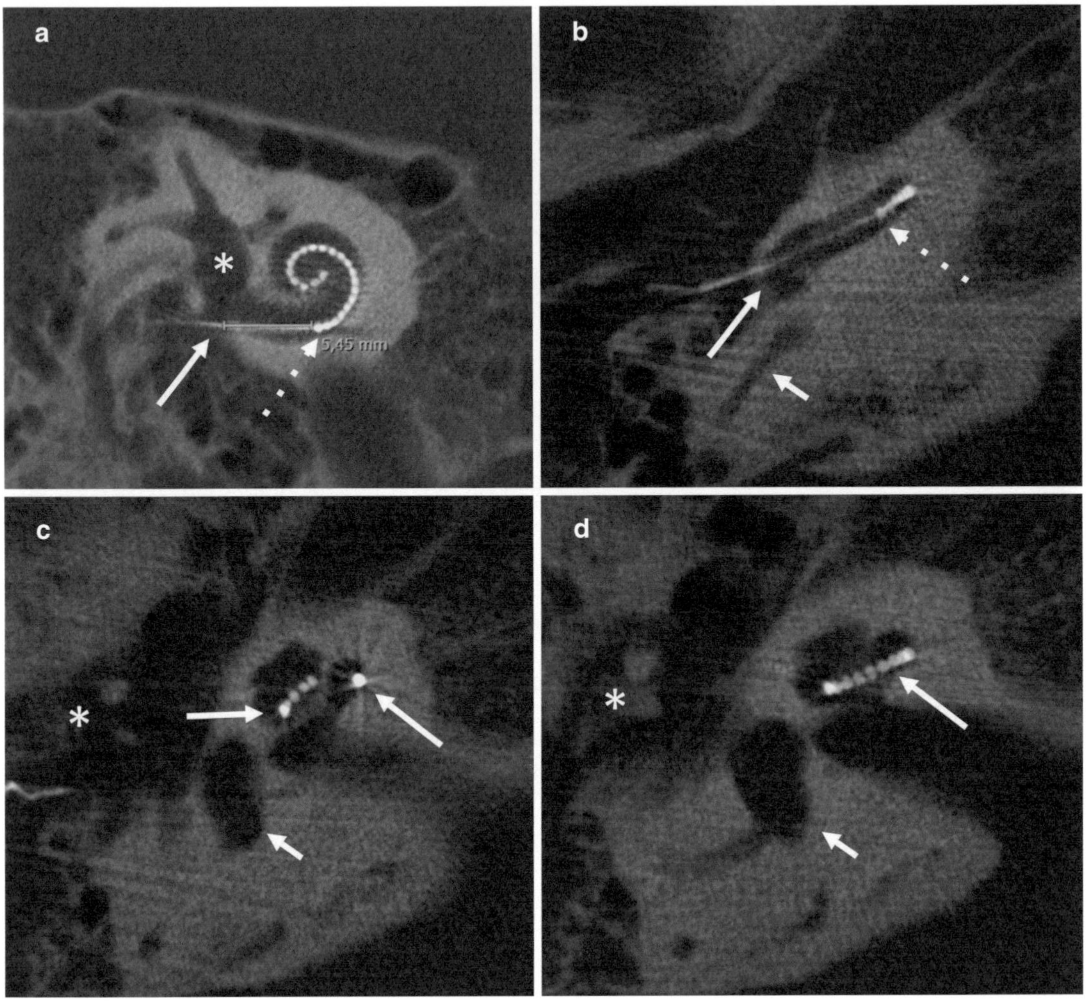

Fig. 11.27 Electrode position of cochlear implant. The surgical approach for cochlear implant insertion is a CWU mastoidectomy (with preservation of the posterior wall of the EAC) followed by posterior tympanotomy and the drilling of the posterosuperior bony overhang of the round window with a fully exposed round window membrane. (**a**) Coronal oblique reformatted MPVR CBCT at the level of the cochlea and vestibule (asterisk) shows the electrode array of cochlear implant correctly inserted into the cochlea. The most proximal electrode (dotted arrow) is within the cochlear basal turn at a 5.45 mm distance from the round window (arrow). (**b**) Axial reformatted MPVR CBCT at the level of the basal turn of the cochlea shows the electrode array of cochlear implant correctly inserted into the cochlea through the round window (arrow). The most proximal electrode (dotted arrow) is within the cochlear basal turn. Short arrow in **b** indicated the posterior semicircular canal. (**c**) Oblique reformatted MPVR CBCT on axial plane parallel to the modiolus and at the level of the medial and apical turn of the cochlea shows the electrode array of cochlear implant correctly inserted into the scala tympani of basal and medial turn (arrows). The scala tympani is located posteriorly to the scala vestibuli in axial planes. In the tympanic cavity (asterisk) the head of the malleus and the long process of the incus are depicted. The short arrow indicates the vestibule. (**d**) Oblique reformatted MPVR CBCT on axial plane parallel to the modiolus and at the level of the medial and apical turn of the cochlea shows the electrode array of cochlear implant correctly inserted into the scala tympani of medial turn (arrow). In the tympanic cavity the head of the malleus and the body of the incus are depicted (asterisk). The short arrow indicates the vestibule. *CWU* canal wall up, *EAC* external auditory canal, *CBCT* cone beam computed tomography, *MPVR* multiplanar volume reformatting

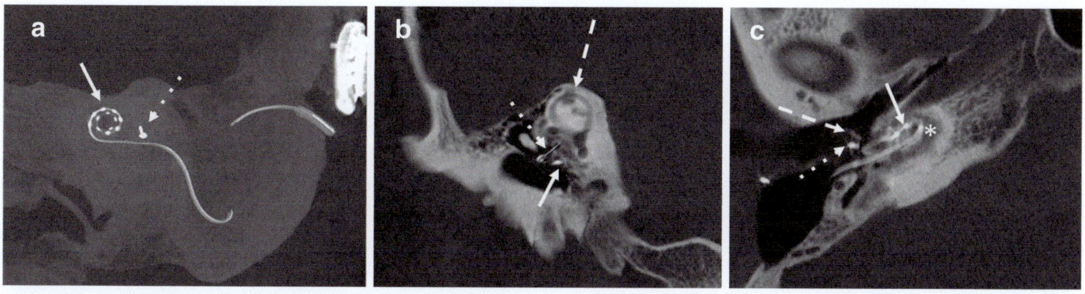

Fig. 11.28 Cochlear implant and stapedial prosthesis in a case of severe otospongiosis. (**a**) Coronal MIP image shows the cochlear implant (arrow) inserted in left temporal bone and the stapedial prosthesis (dotted arrow). (**b**) Oblique MPR image shows the stapedial prosthesis (dotted arrow) with the hook centered at the long process of the incus that is eroded and the medial extremity centered at the oval window. The electrode implant is depicted in the region of the round window (arrow). Superior semicircular canal is indicated by dashed arrow. (**c**) Axial MPR image shows the extensive areas of cochlear otospongiosis (asterisk) and the cochlear electrode array inserted (arrow). The stapedial prosthesis (dotted arrow) is depicted posteriorly to the handle of the malleus (dashed arrow). *MIP* maximum intensity projection, *MPR* multiplanar recostruction

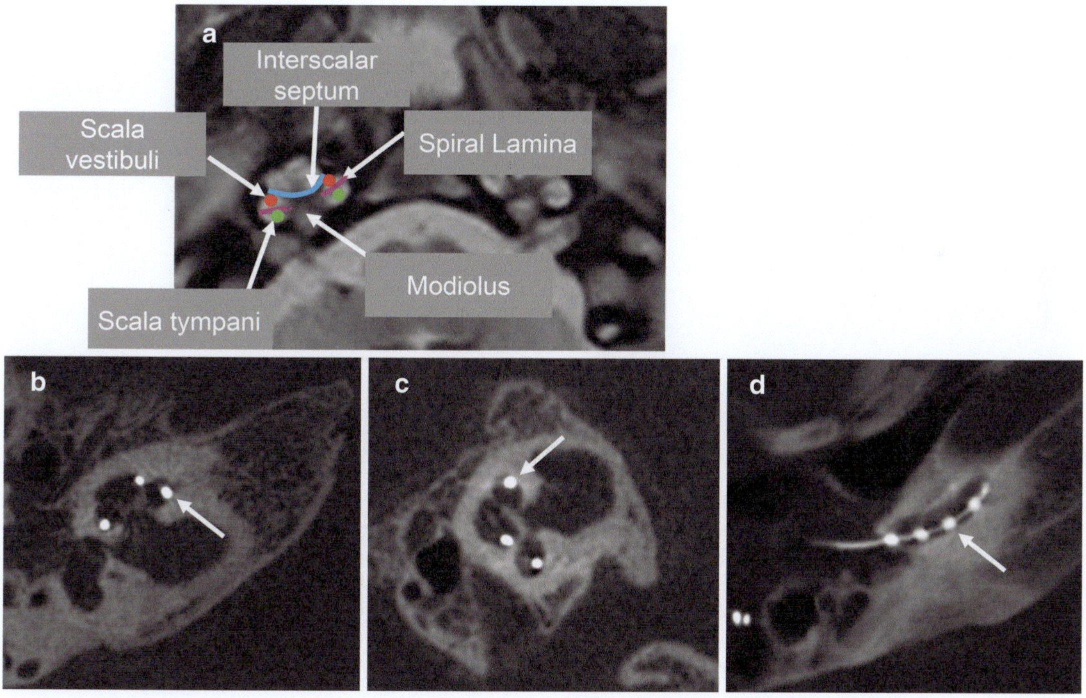

Fig. 11.29 Electrode array position of cochlear implant in the scala tympani. (**a**) Axial TSE T2W image shows the anatomy of the cochlea. Scala tympani is depicted by green dots and is posteriorly located to scala vestibuli that is indicated by red dots. (**b**) Axial reformatted MPR CBCT at the level of the middle and apical turns of the cochlea shows the electrode array of cochlear implant inserted into the cochlea and that is close to the posterior wall of the cochlea (arrow) indicating that the array is properly inserted in scala tympani. (**c**) Sagittal oblique reformatted MPR CBCT parallel to the modiolus shows the electrode array of cochlear implant properly inserted in scala tympani: the electrode array lays close to the posterior wall of the cochlea in basal turn (arrow) and middle turn of the cochlea. (**d**) Axial reformatted MPVR CBCT shows the electrode array of cochlear implant properly inserted in scala tympani: the electrode array lays close to the posterior wall of the cochlea in basal turn (arrow) of the cochlea. *TSE* turbo spin echo, *MPR* multiplanar reformatting, *CBCT* cone beam computed tomography, *MPVR* multiplanar volume reformatting

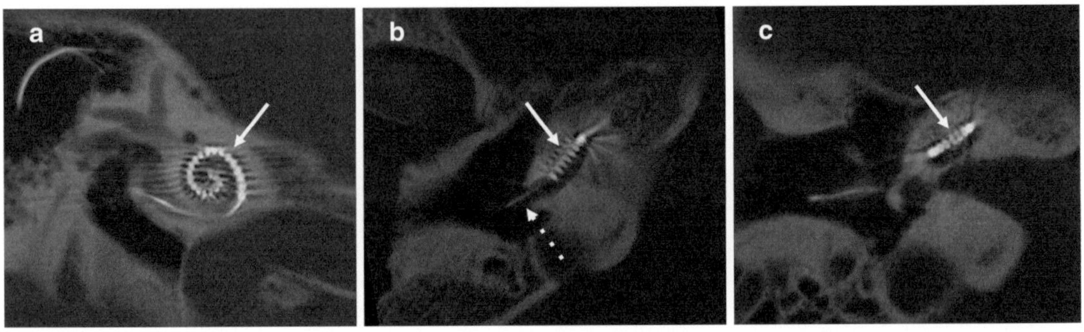

Fig. 11.30 Electrode array position of cochlear implant in scala vestibuli. (**a**) Coronal oblique reformatted MPVR CBCT at the level of the cochlea shows the electrode array of cochlear implant inserted into the cochlea (arrow). (**b**) Axial reformatted MPVR CBCT at the level of the basal turn of the cochlea shows the electrode array of cochlear implant inserted into the cochlea through the round window (dotted arrow). The electrode array lays close to the anterior wall of the cochlea (arrow) indicating that the array is erroneously inserted in scala vestibuli. In fact, the scala vestibuli is located anteriorly to the scala tympani in axial planes. (**c**) Axial reformatted MPVR CBCT on axial plane parallel to the modiolus and at the level of the medial turn of the cochlea shows the electrode array of cochlear implant erroneously inserted in scala vestibuli: the electrode array lays close to the anterior wall of the cochlea (arrow). *MPVR* multiplanar volume reformatting, *CBCT* cone beam computed tomography

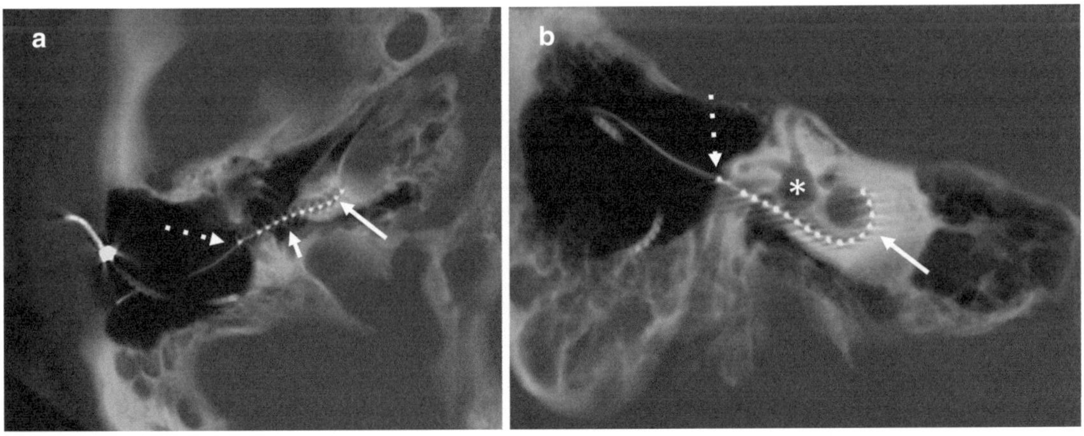

Fig. 11.31 CBCT after cochlear implantation: migration of cochlear array. MPR images show the electrode array (16 electrodes) inserted in the basal turn of the cochlea and migrated outside the cochlea in the tympanic cavity and in surgical cavity. (**a**) Axial CBCT MPVR image parallel to modiolus shows the electrode array partially inserted in the basal turn of the cochlea (arrow) and migrated in tympanic cavity (short arrow). The radiopaque mark can be identified at the deep border of mastoidectomy (dotted arrow). (**b**) Coronal CBCT image perpendicular to modiolus shows the electrode array partially inserted in the basal turn of the cochlea (arrow) and migrated in tympanic cavity with the radiopaque mark that is located at the deep border of mastoidectomy (dotted arrow). The electrodes from n. 1 to 11 are located in the cochlea, while the electrodes from n. 12 to 16 are outside the cochlea. The asterisk indicates the vestibule. *MPVR* multiplanar volume reformatting, *CBCT* cone beam computed tomography

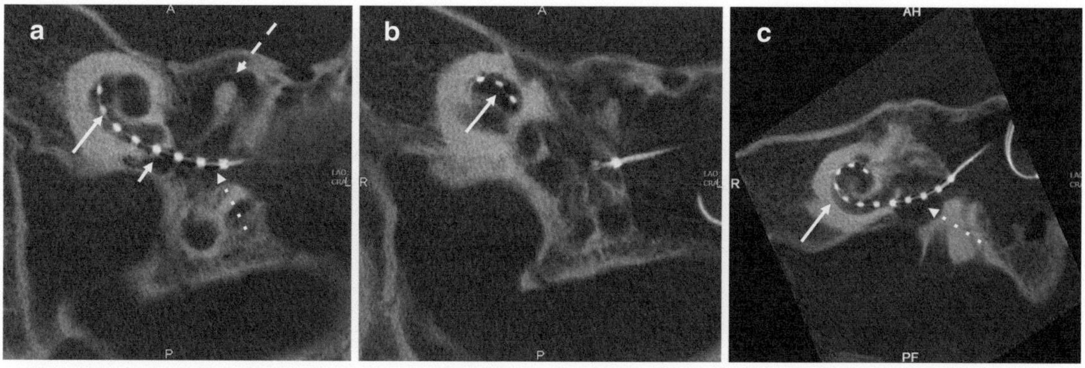

Fig. 11.32 **CBCT after cochlear implantation: migration of electrode array**. MPVR images show the electrode array in the basal and middle turn of the cochlea with the most proximal electrodes located outside the cochlea, in the tympanic cavity. (**a**) Oblique axial CBCT image parallel to modiolus shows the electrode array partially inserted in the basal turn of the cochlea (arrow) passing through the round window (short arrow) with the most proximal electrodes in the tympanic cavity (dotted arrow). The ossicular chain is indicated by dashed arrow. (**b**) Oblique axial CBCT image parallel to modiolus shows the electrode array inserted in the middle turn of the cochlea (arrow). (**c**) Coronal CBCT image perpendicular to modiolus shows the electrode array partially inserted in the cochlea (arrow) with the most proximal electrodes located laterally to the round window within the tympanic cavity (dotted arrow). *MPVR* multiplanar volume reformatting, *CBCT* cone beam computed tomography

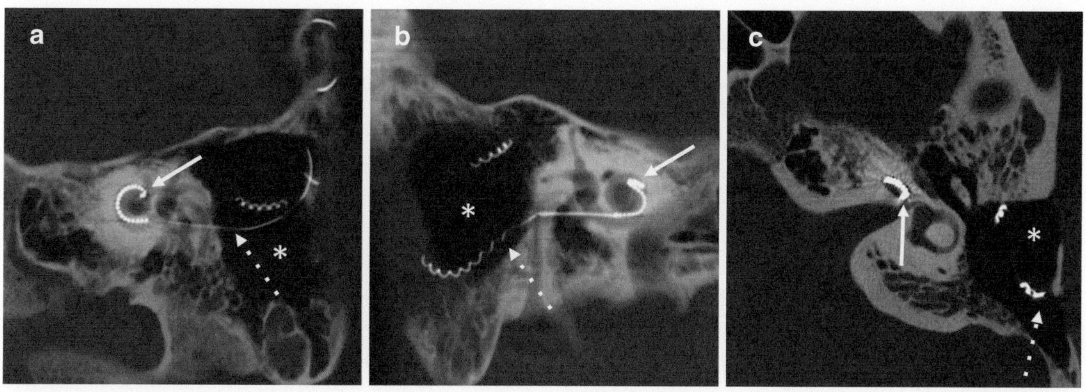

Fig. 11.33 **Fold over of electrode array of cochlear implant**. (**a**) Coronal MPVR CBCT shows the fold over of the tip of the electrode array in the middle turn of the cochlea (arrow). The wire of the cochlear implant (dotted arrow) is depicted in the mastoid surgical cavity (asterisk). (**b**) Oblique MPVR CBCT image shows the fold over of the tip of the electrode array in the middle turn of the cochlea (arrow): the apical electrodes seems to merge together because of the fold over (arrow). The wire of the cochlear implant (dotted arrow) is depicted in the mastoid surgical cavity (asterisk). (**c**) Axial CBCT image shows the fold over of the tip of the electrode array in the middle turn of the cochlea (arrow). The mastoidectomy cavity is indicated by asterisk, and the wire of the cochlear implant is visible (dotted arrow). *MPVR* multiplanar volume reformatting, *CBCT* cone beam computed tomography

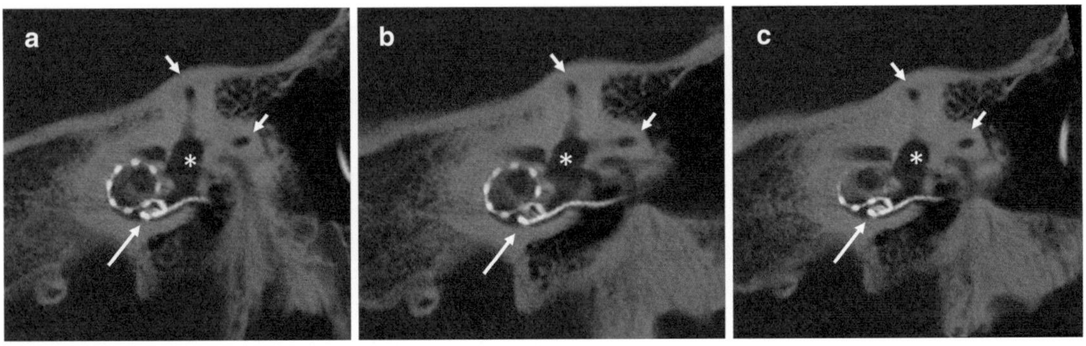

Fig. 11.34 Buckling of electrode array of cochlear implant. CBCT images show the buckling of a 12 electrodes array. (**a**–**c**) Coronal MPVR CBCT shows the buckling of the electrode array in the basal turn of the cochlea (arrow) with electrodes from 9 to 12 that are folded. The vestibule (asterisk) and the superior and lateral semicircular canal (short arrows) are visible. *MPVR* multiplanar volume reformatting, *CBCT* cone beam computed tomography

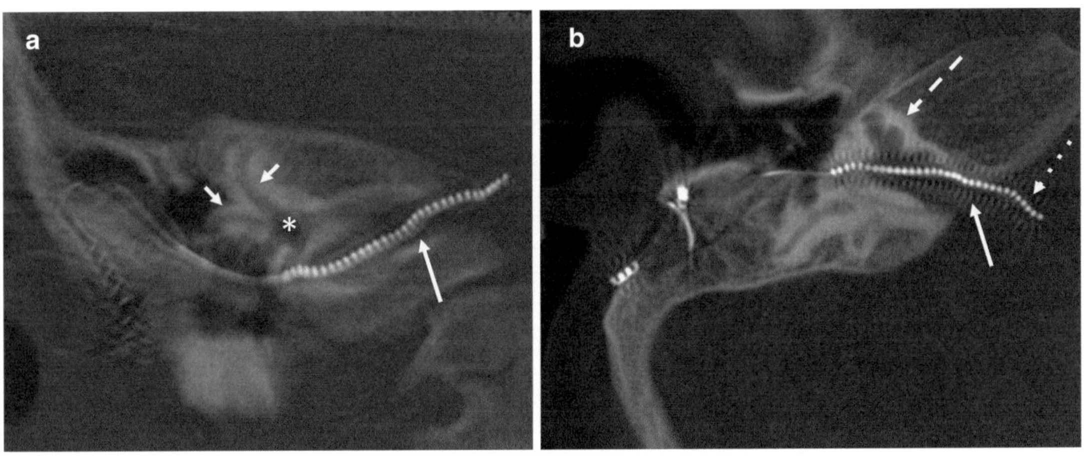

Fig. 11.35 CBCT of a complication after cochlear implantation. MPVR images show a case of cochlear implantation in a patient with cochlear incomplete partition type III (IP-III). IP-III is observed in X-linked deafness and is a non-syndromic genetic cochlear anomaly. It is a rare cause of mixed sensorineural and conductive hearing loss. The cochlea has a corkscrew appearance: the interscalar septa are present, but the modiolus is absent as well as the cribriform plate that normally separates basal turn of cochlea and IAC. The absence of the cribriform plate is the cause of the erroneous insertion and migration of the electrode array in the IAC and in the cerebellopontine angle. (**a**) Coronal CBCT MPVR image shows the electrode array partially inserted in the basal turn of the cochlea and migrated in the IAC (arrow). The asterisk indicates the vestibule and the short arrows the lateral and superior semicircular canals. (**b**) Axial CBCT MPVR image shows the electrode array partially inserted in the basal turn of the cochlea and migrated in the IAC (arrow) and in the cerebellopontine angle (dotted arrow). The cochlea has a corkscrew appearance consistent with cochlear IP-III (dashed arrow). *CBCT* cone beam computed tomography, *MPVR* multiplanar volume reformatting, *IP-III* cochlear incomplete partition type III, *IAC* internal auditory canal

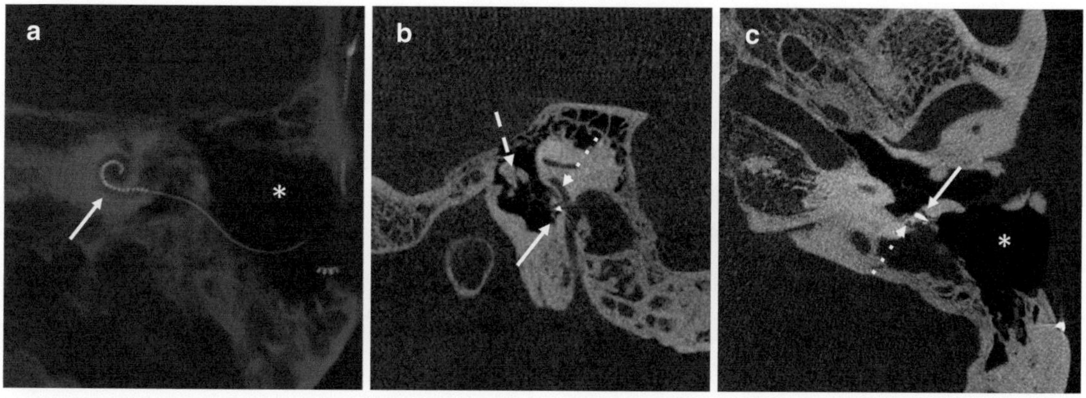

Fig. 11.36 Cochlear implantation and facial injury. The images show that a 22-electrode cochlear implant is correctly inserted in the cochlea in a patient suffering of facial nerve palsy. Facial nerve injury is a rare occurrence in cochlear implantation and may present immediately or with delayed onset, hours, days, or week after surgery. The facial nerve may be injured directly by the drill bur or by the heat caused by prolonged drill or by viral reactivation. In case of delayed injury, the mechanism is progressive neural edema. In the case presented the implant electrode is placed very close to the nerve facial canal. (**a**) Coronal CBCT MPVR shows cochlear electrode array (arrow) correctly inserted through the round window. The mastoidectomy cavity is clearly visible (asterisk). (**b**) Oblique CBCT image shows the implant electrode (arrow) placed very close to the mastoid segment of the facial nerve canal (dotted arrow). The ossicular chain is indicated with dashed arrow. (**c**) Axial CBCT image shows the implant electrode (arrow) placed very close to the mastoid segment of the facial nerve canal (dotted arrow). The mastoidectomy cavity is clearly visible (asterisk). *CBCT* cone beam computed tomography, *MPVR* multiplanar volume reformatting

References

1. Mandour M, Tomoum M, El Zayat S, Hamad H, Amer M. Surgeon oriented preoperative radiologic evaluation in ochlear implantation—our experience with a proposed checklist. Int Arch Otorhinolaryngol. 2019;23(2):137–41. https://doi.org/10.1055/s--0038-1648247. Epub 2018 May 9. PMID: 30956695; PMCID: PMC6449130.
2. Atalar MH, Başpınar N, Atalar DE. "Leave me alone": anatomical structures and variations seen on computed tomography of the temporal bone. Radiol Bras. 2023;56(1):27–35. https://doi.org/10.1590/0100-3984.2022.0030. PMID: 36926356; PMCID: PMC10013187.
3. Manjila S, Bazil T, Kay M, Udayasankar UK, Semaan M. Jugular bulb and skull base pathologies: proposal for a novel classification system for jugular bulb positions and microsurgical implications. Neurosurg Focus. 2018;45(1):E5. https://doi.org/10.3171/2018.5.FOCUS18106. PMID: 29961385.
4. Yung M, James A, Merkus P, Philips J, Black B, Tono T, Linder T, Dornhoffer J, İncesulu A. International otology outcome group and the international consensus on the categorization of tympanomastoid surgery. J Int Adv Otol. 2018;14(2):216–26. https://doi.org/10.5152/iao.2018.5553. PMID: 30100547; PMCID: PMC6354466.
5. Bremke M, Luers JC, Stenner M, Bovenschulte H, Dorn F, Unkel C, Hollering J, Beutner D. Radiologic examinations in human temporal bone specimens using digital volume tomography and high-resolution computed tomography after implantation of middle ear prosthesis and cochlear implant electrode array. Otol Neurotol. 2013;34:1321–8.
6. Aschendorff A, Kubalek R, Turowski B, Zanella F, Hochmuth A, Schumacher M, Klenzner T, Laszig R. Quality control after cochlear implant surgery by means of rotational tomography. Otol Neurotol. 2005;26:34–7.
7. Mohseni-Dargah M, Pastras C, Mukherjee P, Khajeh K, Asadnia M. Enhancing ossicular chain reconstruction through finite element analysis and advanced additive manufacturing: a review. Bioprinting. 2024;38:e00328.
8. Eisele DW. Complications in head and neck surgery. St. Louis, MO: Mosby; 1993.
9. Mor N, Finkel DA, Hanson MB, Rosenfeld RM. Middle ear cholesteatoma treated with a mastoidectomy: a systematic review of the measures used. Otolaryngol Head Neck Surg. 2014;151(6):923–9. https://doi.org/10.1177/0194599814549547. Epub 2014 Sep 5. PMID: 25193517.
10. Karkas A, Boureille P, Laroche N, Vico L, Bergandi F, Marotte H. Imaging of the human cochlea using micro-computed tomography before and after cochlear implantation: comparison with cone-beam

computed tomography. Eur Arch Otorrinolaringol. 2023;280(7):3131–40. https://doi.org/10.1007/s00405-022-07811-y. Epub 2023 Jan 6. PMID: 36604323.
11. Roland PS, Wright CG, Isaacson B. Cochlear implant electrode insertion: the round window revisited. Laryngoscope. 2007;117(8):1397–402.
12. Teymouri J, Hullar TE, Holden TA, Chole RA. Verification of computed tomographic estimates of cochlear implant array position: a micro-CT and histologic analysis. Otol Neurotol. 2011;32(6):980–6.
13. Carlson ML, Driscoll CL, Gifford RH, Service GJ, Tombers NM, Hughes-Borst BJ, Nef BA, Beatty CW. Implications of minimizing trauma during conventional cochlear implantation. Otol Neurotol. 2011;32(6):962–8.
14. Pearl MS, Roy A, Limb CJ. High-resolution secondary reconstructions with the use of flat panel CT in the clinical assessment of patients with cochlear implants. AJNR Am J Neuroradiol. 2014;35(6):1202–8. https://doi.org/10.3174/ajnr.A3814. Epub 2013 Dec 26. PMID: 24371026; PMCID: PMC7965126.
15. Postnov A, Zarowski A, De Clerck N, Vanpoucke F, Offeciers FE, Van Dyck D, Peeters S. High resolution micro-CT scanning as an innovative tool for evaluation of the surgical positioning of cochlear implant electrodes. Acta Otolaryngol. 2006;126(5):467–74.

Tinnitus 12

Luca Caschera, Elisa Massullo, Eleonora Piccin,
Andrea Fontana, Guido Del Vecchio,
Giulia Platania, Beatrice Modello, Elisa Scola,
Fabio Triulzi, and Giorgio Conte

12.1 Introduction

Tinnitus is the perception of a noise—typically buzzing, whistling, rustling, or hissing—heard in the ears or head without any external acoustic stimulus [1]. Subjective tinnitus is a "phantom" sound experienced only by the sufferer, making its underlying cause difficult to identify. It is especially common in people over 50 years of age [2]. Major contributing factors include excessive noise exposure, use of ototoxic medications, and inflammatory or degenerative inner ear conditions [3]. Objective tinnitus, unlike its subjective counterpart, can also be perceived by an external examiner. Its most frequently encountered etiologies include vascular abnormalities, temporomandibular joint disorders, bruxism, cervical spine dysfunction, and palatal or middle ear muscle myoclonus [4].

Tinnitus may be further classified into:

- Pulsatile tinnitus (PT)—characterized by rhythmic sounds synchronized with the patient's heartbeat
- Continuous tinnitus—marked by an uninterrupted, steady noise

PT is usually vascular in origin and subdivided into venous or arterial types:

- Venous PT stems from turbulence in veins or venous sinuses (e.g., transverse or sigmoid sinuses). This disturbance transmits through the temporal bone to the cochlea, resulting in perceived pulsations. The sound may be modulated by maneuvers that alter venous flow, such as jugular vein compression, head rotation/flexion, or the Valsalva maneuver [5, 6].
- Arterial PT remains unchanged by these maneuvers and typically arises from atherosclerosis, carotid aneurysms or dissections, or arteriovenous malformations/fistulas [6].

Tables 12.1 and 12.2 summarize the main causes of PT.

L. Caschera (✉) · E. Massullo · E. Piccin
G. Del Vecchio · G. Platania · B. Modello · E. Scola
Neuroradiology Unit, Fondazione IRCCS Ca' Granda Ospedale Maggiore Policlinico, Milan, Italy
e-mail: luca.caschera@policlinico.mi.it; massullo.elisa@policlinico.mi.it; guido.delvecchio@policlinico.mi.it; giulia.platania@pocliclinico.mi.it; beatrice.modello@policlinico.mi.it; elisa.scola@policlinico.mi.it

A. Fontana
Neuroradiology Unit, Fondazione IRCCS San Gerardo dei Tintori, Monza, Italy

F. Triulzi · G. Conte
Neuroradiology Unit, Fondazione IRCCS Ca' Granda Ospedale Maggiore Policlinico, Milan, Italy

Department of Pathophysiology and Transplantation, University of Milan, Milan, Italy
e-mail: fabio.triulzi@policlinico.mi.it; giorgio.conte@policlinico.mi.it

G. Conte et al. (eds.), *Atlas of Normal and Pathological Findings in Otoneuroradiology*,
https://doi.org/10.1007/978-3-032-08232-9_12

Table 12.1 Main causes of PT

Tumor related	Paraganglioma (glomus jugulare, glomus tympanicus)
Venous	Sigmoid plate dehiscence Sigmoid sinus diverticulum Transverse sinus stenosis High-riding jugular bulb Jugular bulb anomalies (e.g., dehiscence, diverticulum) Dilated emissary veins (mastoid, condylar, petrosquamosal vein) Extracranial jugular vein compression
Arterial	Aneurysms Arterial stenosis Carotid dissection Fibromuscular dysplasia Aberrant carotid artery Persistent stapedial artery Vascular loops Dural arteriovenous fistula Carotid cavernous fistula Arteriovenous malformations

12.2 Imaging Workup

The diagnostic imaging algorithm is outlined in Fig. 12.1 [6, 7].

For patients with continuous tinnitus, or tinnitus accompanied by vertigo, dizziness, or hearing loss, the first-line investigation should be a contrast-enhanced MRI (ceMRI) of the brain, inner ear, and internal auditory canal, including a delayed 3D-FLAIR sequence (~4 h post-contrast) targeting the ear in case of suspected hydropic ear disease. This protocol helps exclude both labyrinthine and intracranial pathologies.

In cases of PT, otoscopy is the initial step. If it reveals a potential intratympanic lesion, a cone beam CT (CBCT) of the temporal bone is useful to define lesion boundaries, assess tympanic cavity involvement, and identify relationships with structures like the internal carotid artery or a

Table 12.2 The conditions that are shown in the figures of the chapter are listed in the table with the corresponding figure number

Tinnitus		Figures
Jugulotympanic paraganglioma		Figs. 12.2, 12.3, 12.4,12.5,12.6,12.7,12.8, and 12.9
Dehiscent jugular bulb		Fig. 12.10
Sinus stenosis due to hypertrophic arachnoid granulation		Figs. 12.11 and 12.12
Sinus stenosis and sigmoid sinus diverticulum		Fig. 12.13
Enlarged mastoid emissary vein		Fig. 12.14
Aberrant anastomotic vein between the superior petrosal sinus and the jugular bulb		Fig. 12.15
Condylar vein		Fig. 12.16
High-riding jugular bulb		Figs. 12.17, 12.18, and 12.19
Bilateral dehiscent sigmoid sinus, left petrous venous anomaly		Fig. 12.20
Vestibular aqueduct	Enlarge vestibular aqueduct with internal jugular vein dehiscence and jugular bulb diverticula	Figs. 12.21 and 12.22
	Cochlear or vestibular aqueduct dehiscence into the high-riding jugular bulb	Fig. 12.23
Aberrant carotid artery		Fig. 12.24
Persistent stapedial artery		Figs. 12.25, 12.26, and 12.27
DAVF	Transverse-sigmoid sinus fistula	Figs. 12.28, 12.29, 12.30, and 12.31
	Condylar fistula	Figs. 12.32 and 12.33
	Cavernous sinus fistula	Figs. 12.34, 12.3, and 12.36
	Post-traumatic extracranial periauricular DAVF	Figs. 12.37, 12.38, and 12.39
AVM		Fig. 12.40

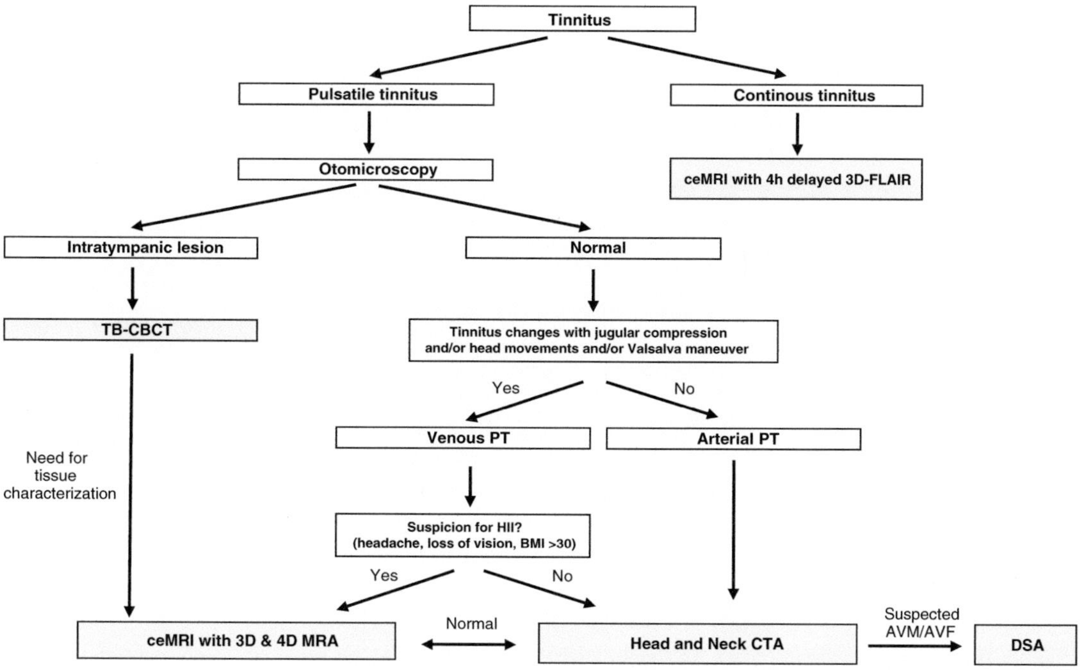

Fig. 12.1 Diagnostic imaging algorithm for patients with tinnitus. *Abbreviations:* AVM = arteriovenous malformation, AVF = arteriovenous fistula, CBCT = cone beam computed tomography, CTA = CT angiography, DSA = digital subtraction angiography, ceMRI = contrast-enhanced Magnetic Resonance Imaging, IIH = idiopathic intracranial hypertension, MRA = magnetic resonance angiography, PT = pulsatile tinnitus

dehiscent jugular bulb. However, ceMRI with eventually 3D and 4D magnetic resonance angiography (MRA) is often necessary to characterize the lesion more precisely.

If the otoscopic examination is normal, maneuvers such as jugular compression, head turning, or Valsalva should be tested. A change in tinnitus with these suggests a venous origin. At this point, it is important to assess for idiopathic intracranial hypertension (IIH)—especially in patients with headache, visual symptoms, or BMI >30. IIH is associated with pulsatile tinnitus in up to 40–60% of patients and is typically unilateral. If IIH is suspected, ceMRI should be performed eventually with 3D and 4D MRA. If ceMRI is negative, proceed to CT angiography (CTA) of the head and neck.

If tinnitus remains unchanged with maneuvers, suspect an arterial source and directly pursue head and neck CTA, which offers detailed assessment of vessel caliber, patency, stenosis, symmetry, dissections, aneurysms, and diverticula.

If CTA indicates a suspected arteriovenous malformation or fistula, digital subtraction angiography is recommended for detailed vascular characterization.

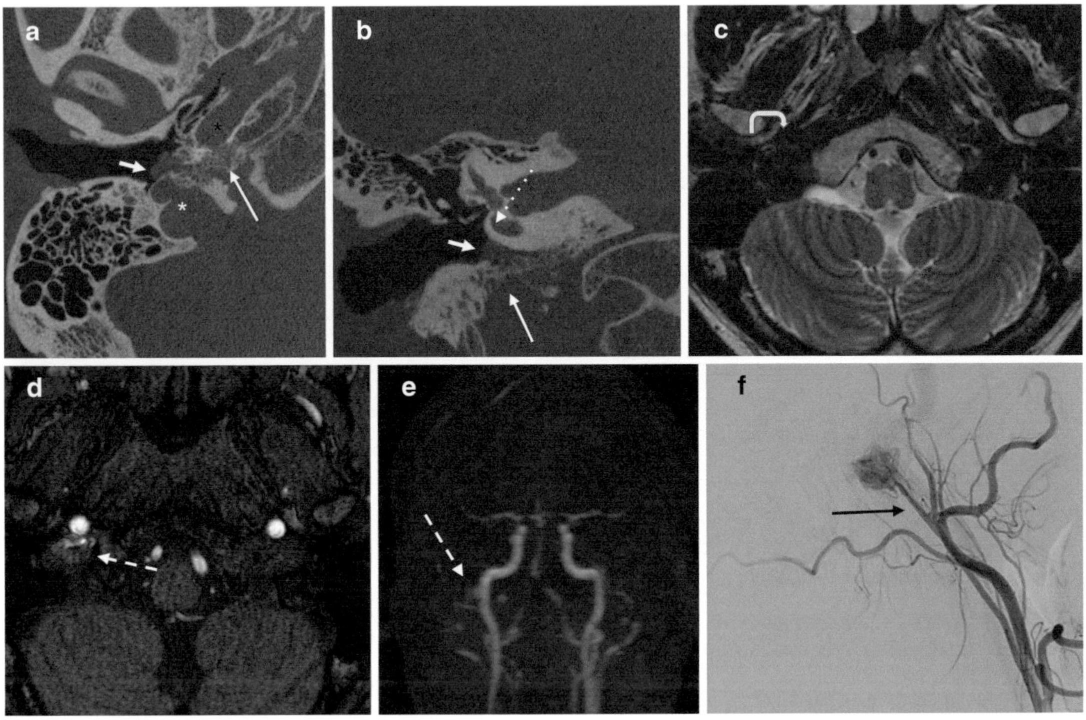

Fig. 12.2 Jugulotympanic paraganglioma. TP (also known as glomus tumor) is a highly vascular neoplasm and one of the most frequent causes of PT. It originates from paraganglionic tissue associated with the Jacobson's nerve (tympanic branch of the glossopharyngeal nerve). Depending on its extent, it may involve the jugular bulb (glomus jugulare), middle ear or mastoid (glomus tympanicum), or both (glomus jugulotympanicum). (**a** and **b**) Axial and coronal CBCT images show a right jugulotympanic paraganglioma occupying the hypotympanum (short arrow), located anterior to the jugular bulb (white asterisk), and extending along the cochlear promontory (dotted arrow). Irregular bone erosion (long arrow) is seen reaching the posterior margin of the carotid canal (black asterisk) and the anterior margin of the jugular foramen (white asterisk). (**c**) Axial TSE T2w MRI demonstrates the classic "salt-and-pepper" appearance of the lesion (curved arrow), reflecting flow voids from high vascularity. (**d**) 3D MRA reveals intralesional arterial signal. (**e**) 4D MRA shows lesion enhancement synchronous with arterial flow. (**f**) DSA highlights a prominent arterial blush supplied by the neuromeningeal trunk of the ascending pharyngeal artery (black arrow). *Abbreviations:* CBCT = cone-beam computed tomography; DSA = Digital subtraction angiography; MRA = magnetic resonance angiography; PT = pulsatile tinnitus; TP = Tympanic paraganglioma; TSE = turbo spin echo

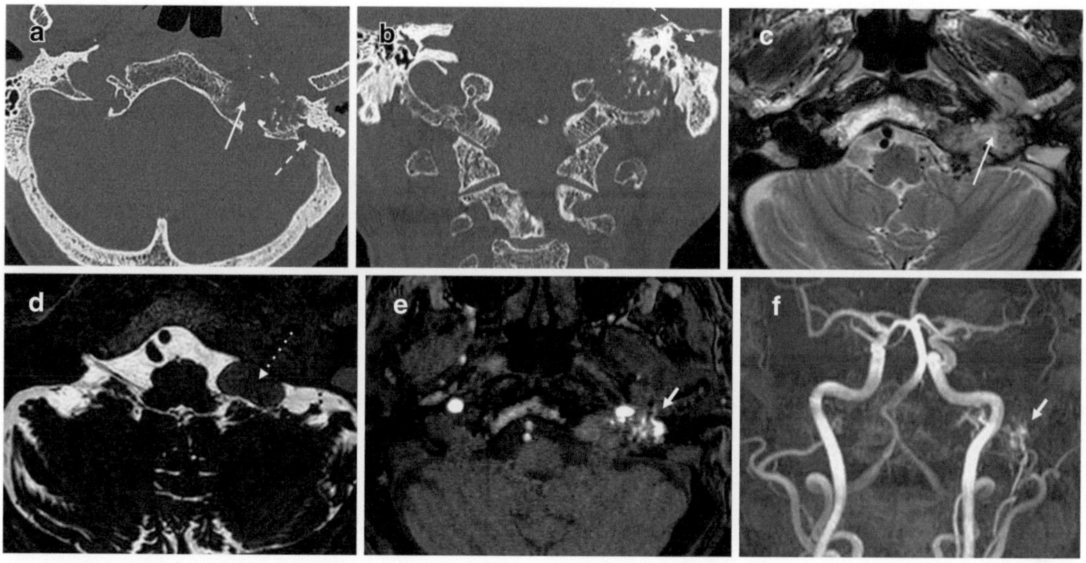

Fig. 12.3 Left tympano-jugular paraganglioma. (**a** and **b**) Axial and coronal CT images (bone algorithm) reveal a left tympano-jugular paraganglioma involving the petrous portion of the temporal bone and clivus, with erosion of the jugular foramen (arrow) and extension into the tympanic cavity (dashed arrow). (**c** and **d**) TSE T2w MRI shows a soft-tissue mass centered in the jugular foramen (arrow), with a prominent component extending into the left cerebellopontine angle cistern (dotted arrow). (**e**) 3D MRA and (**f**) corresponding MIP reconstruction demonstrate intralesional arterial signal (short arrow). *Abbreviations:* CT = computed tomography; MIP = maximum intensity projection; MRA = magnetic resonance angiography; TSE = turbo spin echo

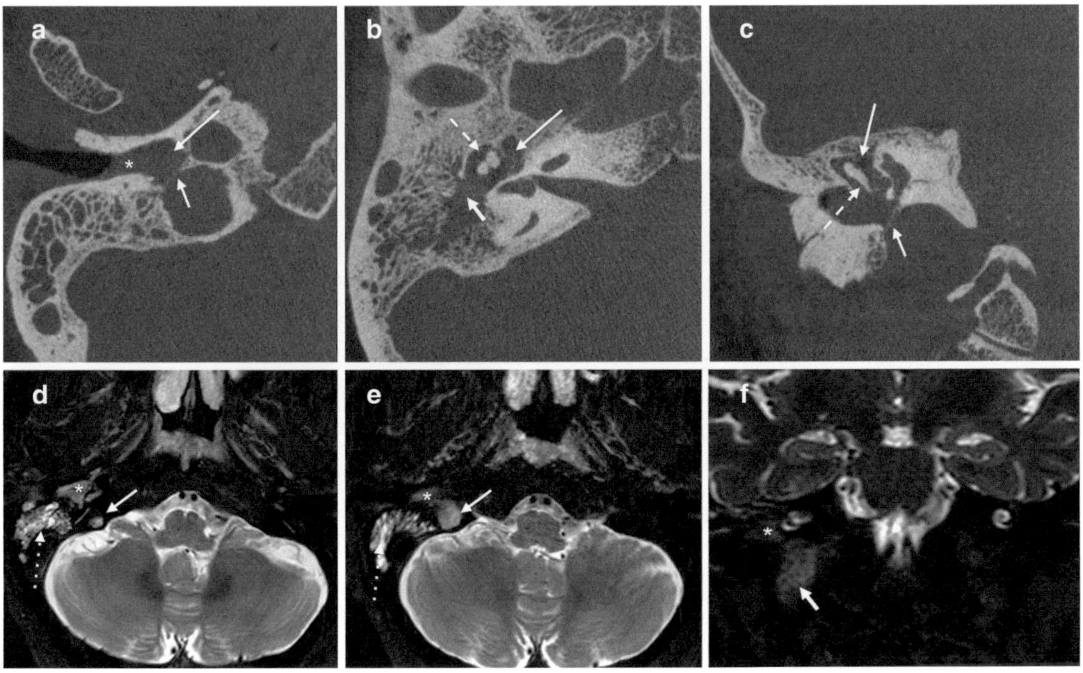

Fig. 12.4 Right tympano-jugular paraganglioma. (**a**–**b**) axial and (**c**) coronal CBCT images show a soft-tissue mass occupying the proximal segment of the EAC (asterisk), the tympanic cavity (long arrow), and the mastoid (arrowhead). The ossicular chain is preserved (dashed arrow), while thinning of the bony wall of the jugular bulb is observed (short arrow). (**d**–**e**) Axial and (**f**) coronal fat-suppressed TSE T2w MRI demonstrate a mildly hyperintense lesion centered at the jugular foramen (long arrow), with extension into the tympanic cavity (asterisk) and superior cervical vascular space (short arrow). Associated mastoid fluid effusion is noted (dotted arrow). *Abbreviations:* CBCT = cone-beam computed tomography; EAC = external auditory canal; MRI = magnetic resonance imaging; TSE = turbo spin echo

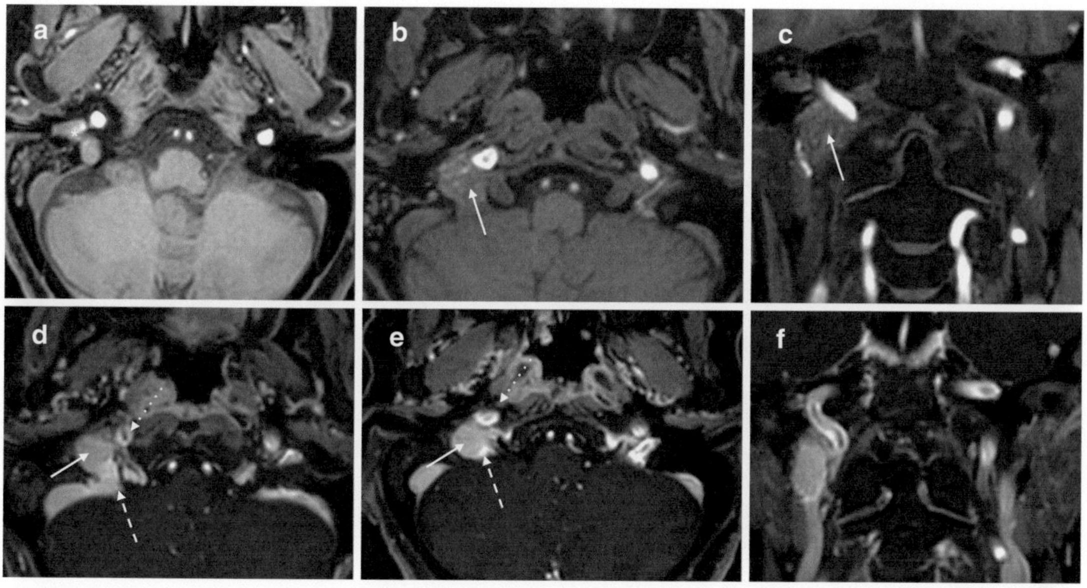

Fig. 12.5 Right tympano-jugular paraganglioma (continued from Fig. 12.4). (**a** and **b**) Non-contrast axial, and (**c**) coronal 3D FFE T1 with fat suppression images reveal a soft-tissue mass centered in the jugular foramen (arrow) with extension into the tympanic cavity (asterisks). Intralesional foci of high signal intensity are visible, consistent with flow-related signal from arterial vessels. (**d** and **e**) Contrast-enhanced axial, and (**f**) coronal post-contrast T1-weighted images demonstrate intense enhancement of the lesion (arrow), located adjacent to the petrous segment of the internal carotid artery (dotted arrow) and the jugular bulb (dashed arrow). *Abbreviation:* FFE = fast field echo

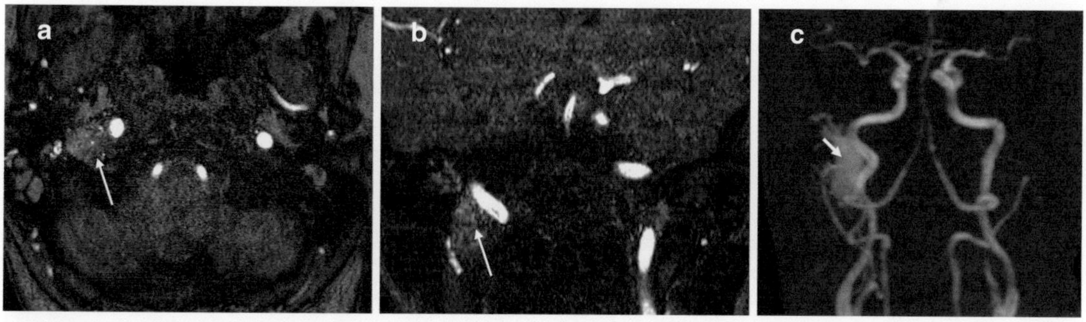

Fig. 12.6 Right tympano-jugular paraganglioma (continued from Figs. 12.4 and 12.5). (**a**) Axial and (**b**) coronal reformatted MRA images show multiple intralesional high-signal foci (arrow), corresponding to arterial vessels. (**c**) Time-resolved contrast-enhanced 4D MRA demonstrates early arterial-phase enhancement of the lesion (short arrow). *Abbreviation:* MRA = magnetic resonance angiography

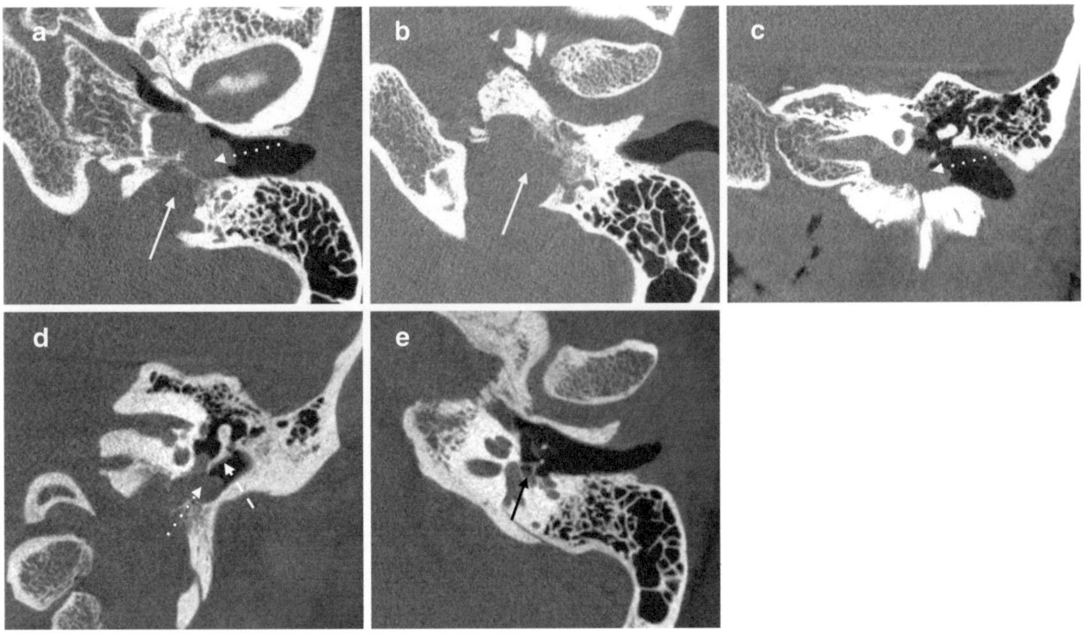

Fig. 12.7 Left tympano-jugular paraganglioma. (**a** and **b**) Axial and (**c**) coronal CBCT images show a soft-tissue mass centered at the level of the jugular foramen (arrow), extending into the hypotympanum of the tympanic cavity (dotted arrow). (**d**) Coronal and (**e**) axial CBCT images further demonstrate the lesion within the hypotympanum (dotted arrow), with partial encasement of the handle of the malleus (dashed arrow) and the posterior crus of the stapes (black arrow). *Abbreviation:* CBCT = cone-beam computed tomography

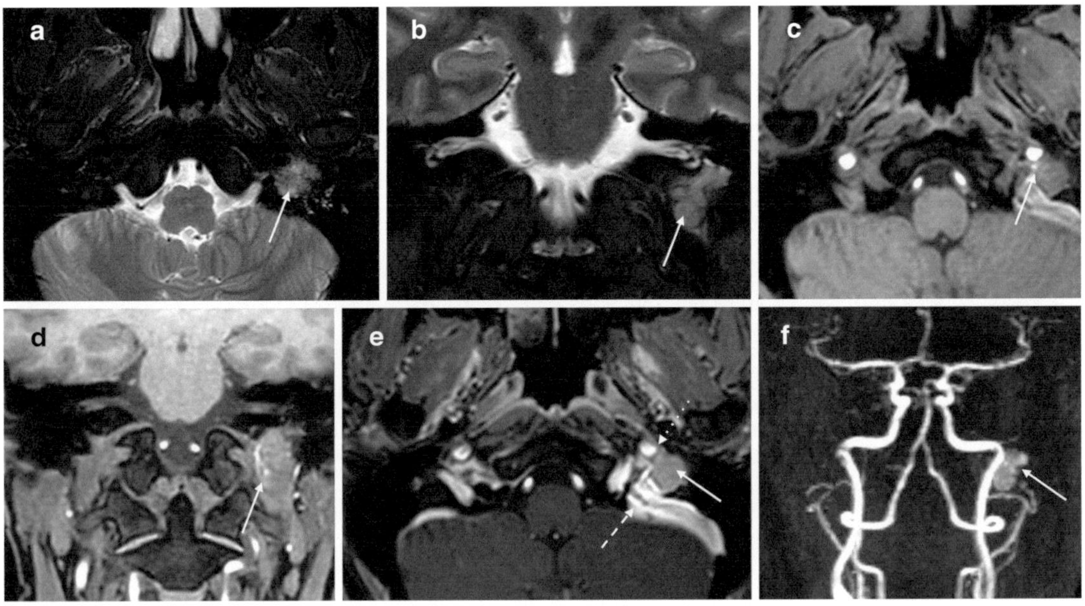

Fig. 12.8 Left tympano-jugular paraganglioma (continued from Fig. 12.7). (**a** and **b**) Axial and coronal 3D FFE T2 with fat suppression images show a hyperintense mass (arrow) centered in the jugular foramen with extension into the tympanic cavity. (**c** and **d**) Axial and coronal 3D FFE T1w with fat suppression images reveal an intermediate-signal lesion with intralesional foci of high signal intensity (arrow), corresponding to arterial vessels. (**e**) Axial contrast-enhanced 3D FFE T1w with fat suppression image demonstrates marked enhancement of the lesion (arrow), which is located adjacent to the petrous segment of the internal carotid artery (dotted arrow) and the jugular bulb (dashed arrow). (**f**) Time-resolved contrast-enhanced 4D MRA shows early arterial-phase enhancement of the lesion. *Abbreviations:* FFE = fast field echo; MRA = magnetic resonance angiography

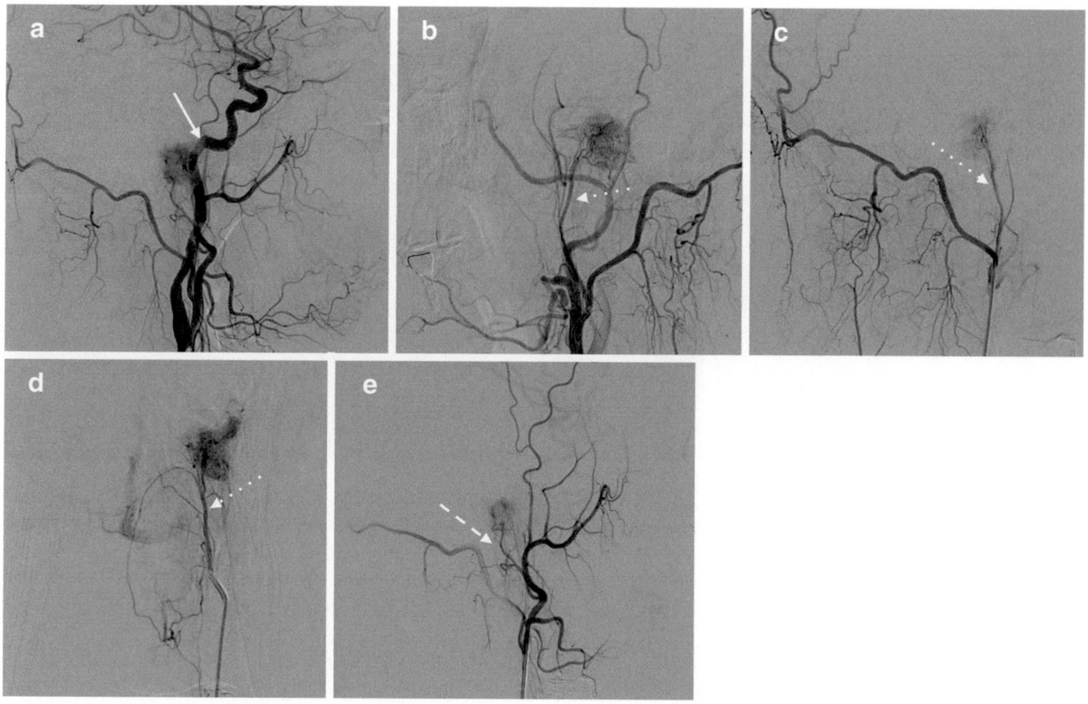

Fig. 12.9 Left tympano-jugular paraganglioma (continued from Figs. 12.7 and 12.8). Although DSA is not essential for diagnosis, it may be indicated when preoperative embolization is planned. (**a–e**) Selective DSA of the (a) common carotid artery, (**b**) external carotid artery, (**c**) occipital artery, (**d**) ascending pharyngeal artery, and (**e**) internal maxillary artery demonstrates the arterial supply to the paraganglioma. The lesion lies in close proximity to the distal cervical and foraminal segments of the ICA (arrow), and is primarily vascularized by the left neuromeningeal trunk (dotted arrow) and the left anterior tympanic artery (dashed arrow). *Abbreviations:* DSA = digital subtraction angiography; ICA = internal carotid artery

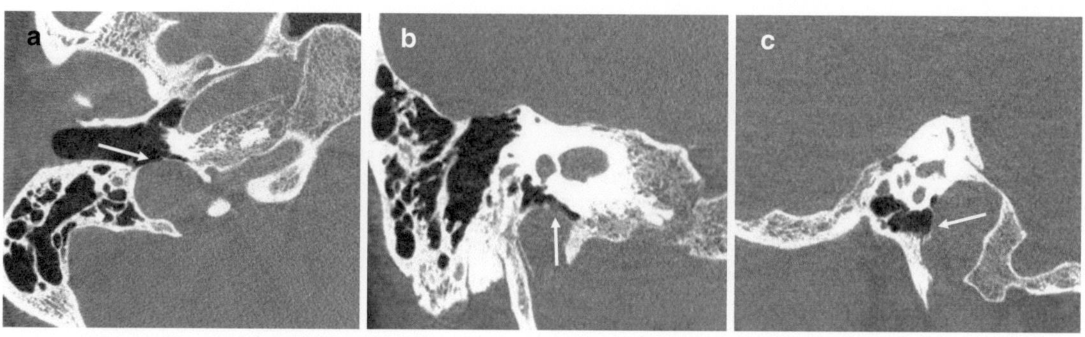

Fig. 12.10 Dehiscent jugular bulb. Jugular bulb dehiscence is characterized by thinning or a defect of the jugular plate, leading to turbulent venous flow transmitted to the cochlea through the skull base and mastoid air cells, resulting in venous PT. (**a–c**) Axial, coronal, and sagittal CBCT images demonstrate protrusion of the internal jugular bulb into the hypotympanum, with thinning of the bony jugular plate (arrow). *Abbreviations:* CBCT = cone-beam computed tomography; PT = pulsatile tinnitus

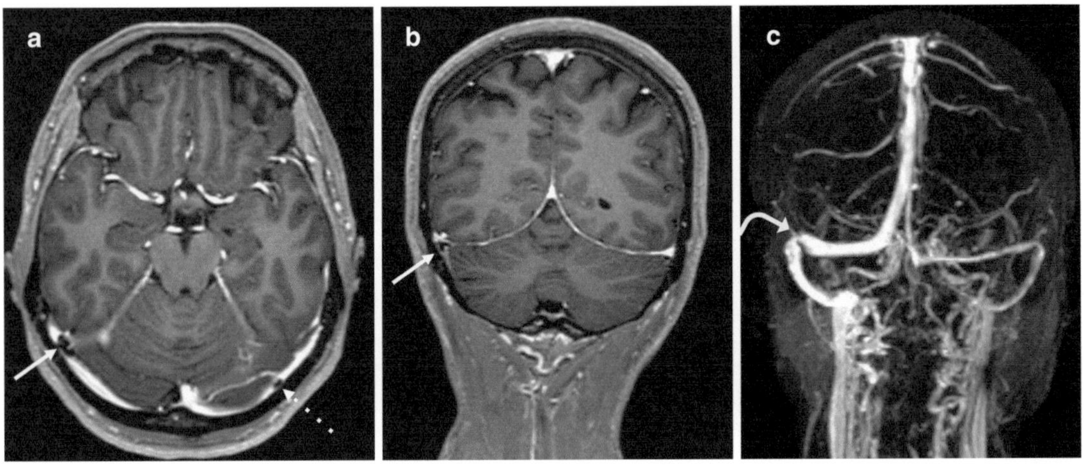

Fig. 12.11 Right transverse sinus stenosis due to hypertrophic arachnoid granulation. Dominant transverse sinus stenosis can increase blood flow velocity and turbulence near the inner ear and mastoid, potentially causing venous PT. Stenosis may arise from intrinsic or extrinsic causes. Intrinsic stenosis often results from intraluminal filling defects causing focal or segmental narrowing, such as hypertrophic arachnoid granulations. (**a** and **b**) Axial and coronal contrast-enhanced 3D FFE T1w without fat suppression show focal narrowing of the right dominant transverse sinus (arrow) due to an arachnoid granulation. A contralateral hypertrophic arachnoid granulation is also visible (dotted arrow). (**c**) Time-resolved contrast-enhanced 4D MRA demonstrates transverse sinus asymmetry with right-sided dominance and focal stenosis (curved arrow). *Abbreviations:* FFE = fast field echo; MR = magnetic resonance; PT = pulsatile tinnitus; MRA = magnetic resonance angiography

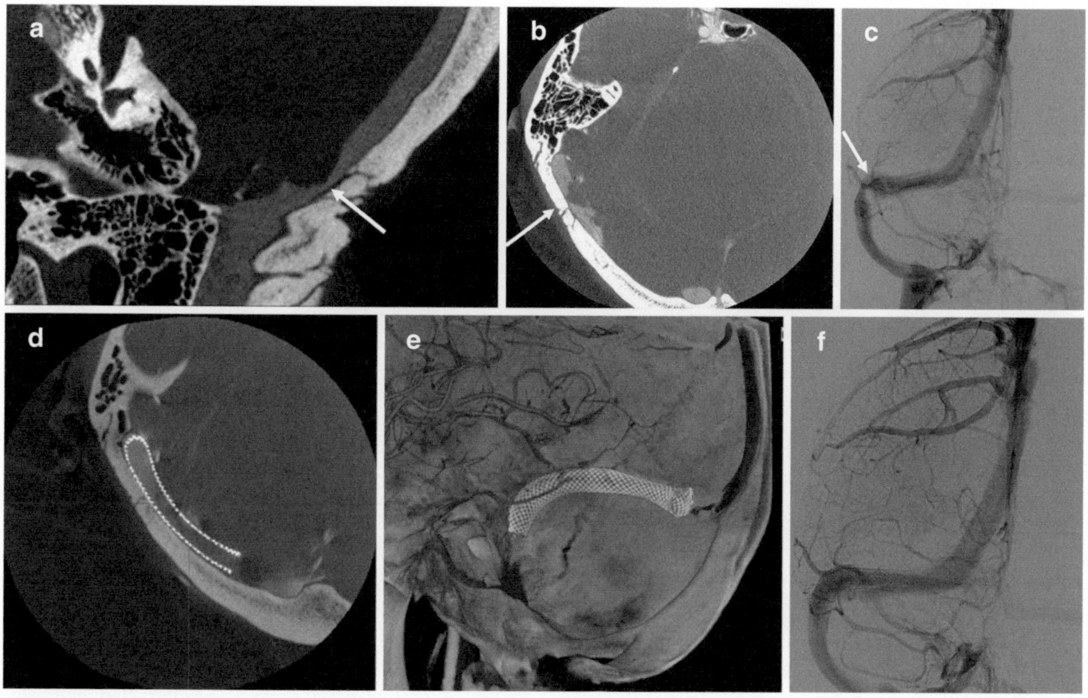

Fig. 12.12 Right transverse sinus stenosis due to hypertrophic arachnoid granulation (continued from Fig. 12.11). Stent placement may be considered in patients with debilitating PT caused by stenosis of the dominant transverse sinus when no other causes are identified. Preoperative imaging includes: (**a** and **b**) Sagittal and axial reformatted contrast-enhanced CBCT, and (**c**) DSA, which confirm focal stenosis of the lateral segment of the right transverse sinus (arrows). Post-intervention imaging demonstrates: (**d**) axial CBCT and (**e**) MIP reconstruction after endovascular stent placement, while (**f**) post-procedural DSA confirms restored patency of the transverse sinus. *Abbreviations:* CBCT = cone-beam computed tomography; DSA = digital subtraction angiography; MIP = maximum intensity projection; PT = pulsatile tinnitus

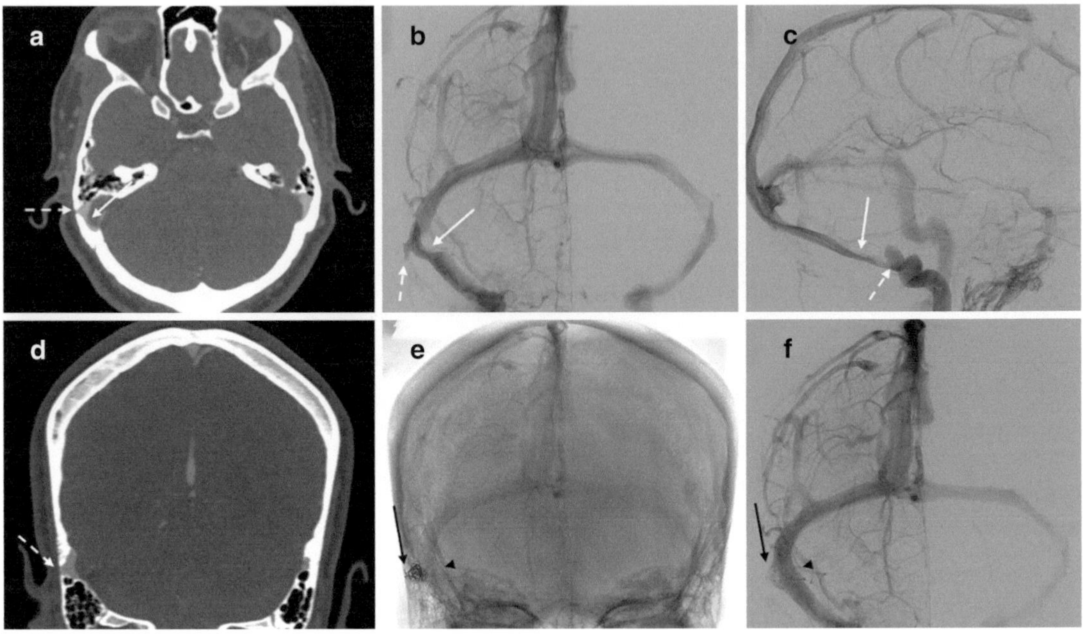

Fig. 12.13 Right transverse sinus stenosis and sigmoid sinus diverticulum in a patient with PT. (**a** and **d**) Axial and coronal CTA images demonstrate focal narrowing of the right dominant transverse sinus (arrow) and a sigmoid sinus diverticulum with associated thinning of the squamous part of the temporal bone (dashed arrow). (**b** and **c**) Anteroposterior and lateral DSA images confirm the transverse sinus stenosis (white arrow) and the presence of the diverticulum (dashed arrow). (**e** and **f**) Post-treatment anteroposterior DSA, unsubtracted and subtracted, shows successful stent placement restoring normal sinus caliber (black arrowhead) and coil embolization of the diverticulum (black arrow). *Abbreviations:* CTA = computed tomography angiography; DSA = digital subtraction angiography; PT = pulsatile tinnitus

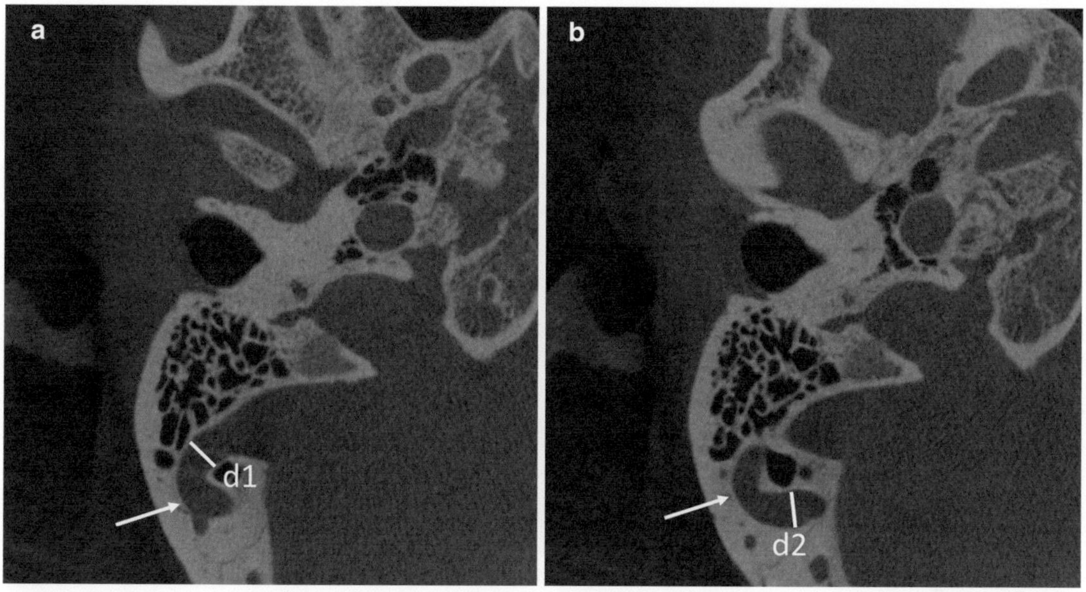

Fig. 12.14 Enlarged mastoid emissary vein (MEV). Emissary veins are valveless channels connecting intracranial venous sinuses, such as the sigmoid sinus and jugular bulb, to extracranial venous systems. Though typically small or vestigial, they are clinically significant as potential pathways for intracranial infection or tumor spread, and as structures vulnerable to hemorrhage during surgery. Enlarged emissary veins, particularly the MEV, have also been implicated in pulsatile tinnitus (PT) due to their proximity to middle ear structures, facilitating transmission of turbulent venous flow, above all when the bony wall is interrupted. The MEV connects the sigmoid sinus to the posterior auricular or occipital veins, with a variable diameter averaging approximately 3.5 mm [8]. (**a** and **b**) CBCT images show a prominent retromastoid emissary vein (arrow) measuring 4 mm (d1) and 5 mm (d2) in diameter. *Abbreviations:* CBCT = cone-beam computed tomography; MEV = mastoid emissary vein

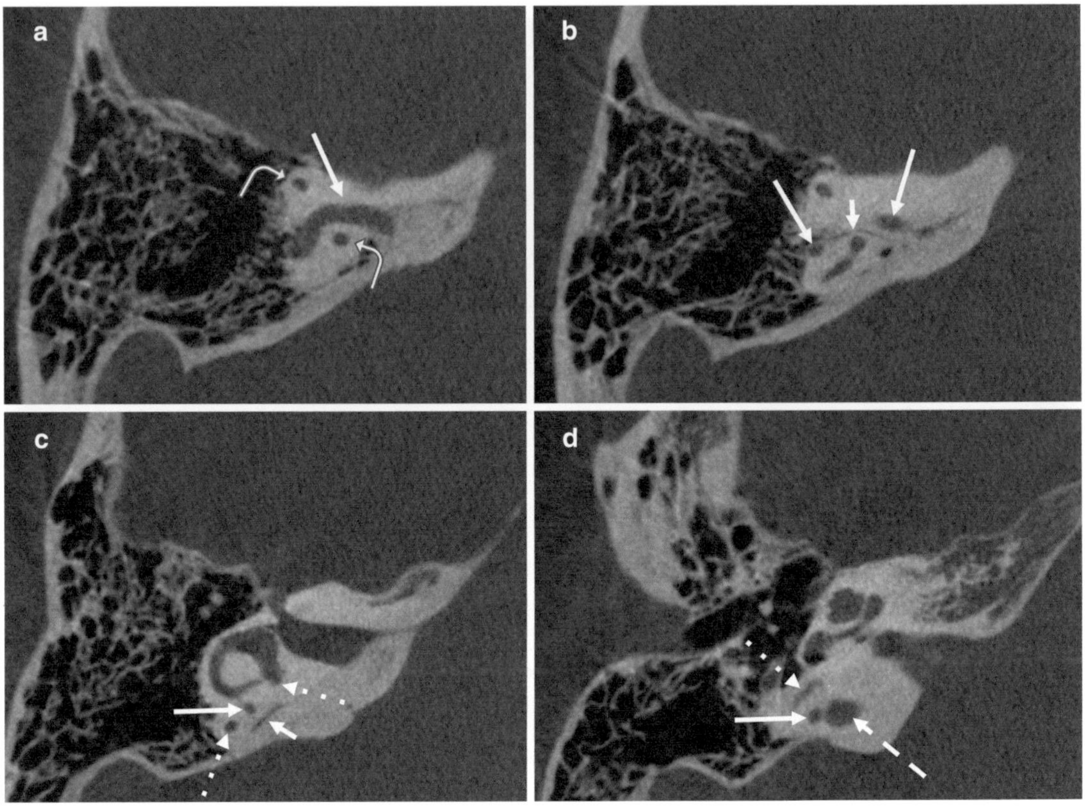

Fig. 12.15 Aberrant anastomotic vein between the superior petrous sinus and the jugular bulb. An aberrant vein arises from the superior petrous sinus, traverses the superior semicircular canal along the margin of the subarcuate (petromastoid) canal, then descends crossing the posterior semicircular canal before draining into a high-riding jugular bulb. (**a–d**) CBCT images in a rostral-to-caudal sequence depict: (**a**) Aberrant vein (arrow) crossing the superior semicircular canal (curved arrows); (**b**) Subarcuate canal (short arrow) located beneath the aberrant vein (arrows) at the level of the superior semicircular canal; (**c**) Aberrant vein (arrow) crossing the posterior semicircular canal (dotted arrows) and adjacent vestibular aqueduct (short); (**d**) Aberrant vein (arrow) draining into a high-riding jugular bulb (dashed arrow), with the inferior margin of the posterior semicircular canal also visible (dotted arrow). *Abbreviation:* CBCT = cone beam computed tomography

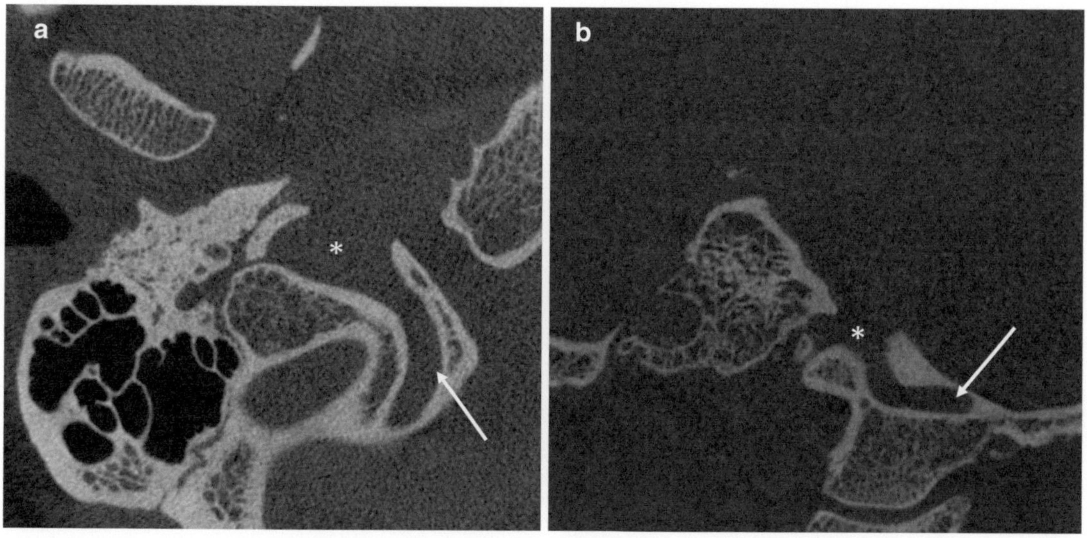

Fig. 12.16 Condylar vein. The anterior and posterior condylar veins are emissary anastomotic channels connecting the distal sigmoid sinus or proximal internal jugular vein with the suboccipital and deep cervical venous plexuses. When enlarged, these veins may exhibit increased turbulent blood flow that can transmit pulsations through the skull base to the middle ear's conductive structures, potentially causing PT. Notably, in cases of ipsilateral internal jugular vein stenosis or hypoplasia, these emissary veins may serve as critical compensatory outflow pathways and should be preserved during surgical or endovascular interventions. (**a** and **b**) Axial and sagittal reformatted CBCT images demonstrate a hypertrophic condylar vein (arrow) draining into the jugular bulb (asterisk). *Abbreviations:* CBCT = cone-beam computed tomography; PT = pulsatile tinnitus

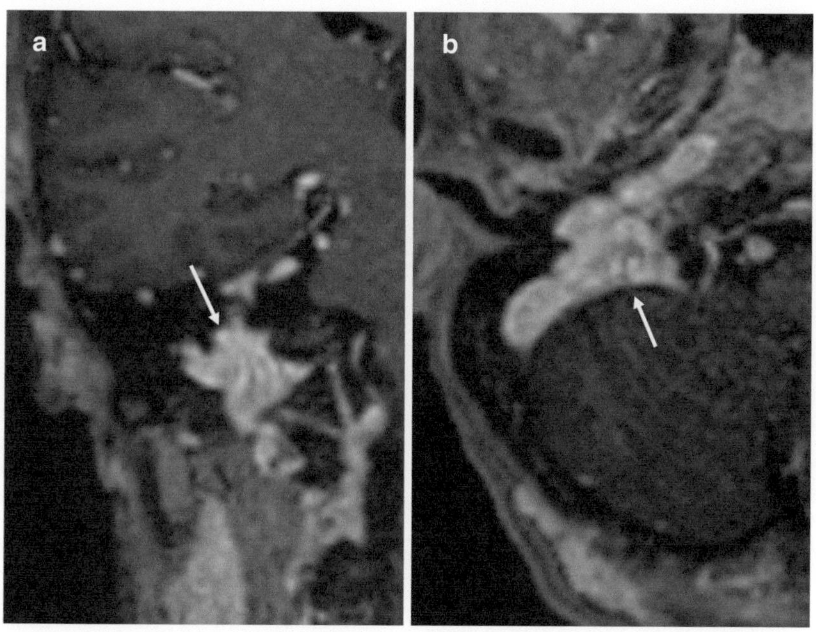

Fig. 12.17 High-riding jugular mega-bulb (HJB). HJB is an anatomical variant characterized by superior extension of the jugular bulb beyond its typical location beneath the hypotympanum. It is classified as high-riding when it reaches the level of the round window niche, sulcus tympani, basal turn of the cochlea, or lies within 2 mm of the inferior margin of the internal auditory canal. When significantly enlarged in cross-section, regardless of vertical position, it is termed a jugular megabulb. (**a** and **b**) Axial and coronal contrast-enhanced 3D FFE T1w without fat suppression images demonstrate a right-sided HJB ("megabulb") (arrows) protruding toward the hypotympanum. *Abbreviations:* HJB = high riding jugular bulb; FFE = fast field echo

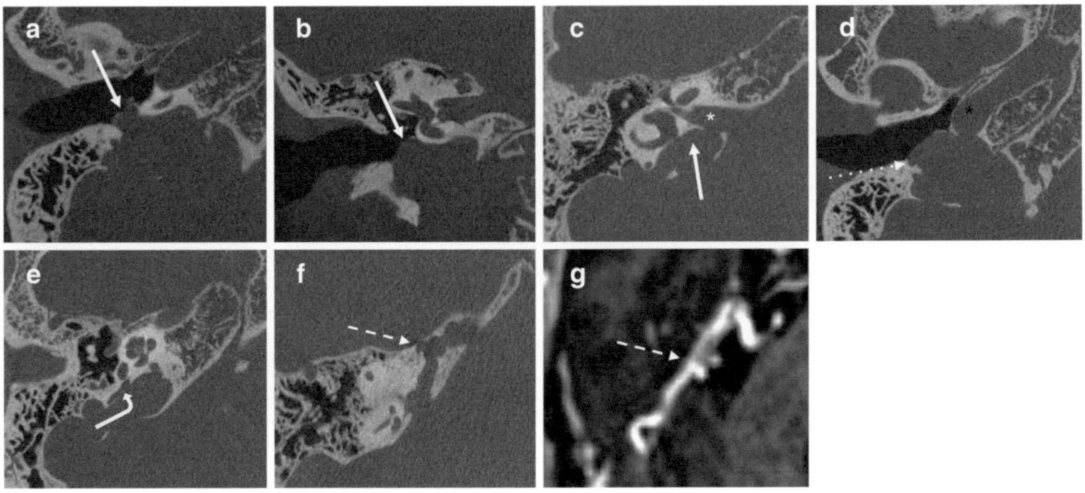

Fig. 12.18 High-riding jugular mega-bulb (HJB) (continued from Fig. 12.17). (**a** and **b**) Axial and coronal CBCT images reveal a HJB with bony wall dehiscence in the hypotympanum (arrow). (**c**) Axial CBCT image shows dehiscence of the HJB (arrow) extending into the IAC (asterisk). (**d**) Axial CBCT image demonstrates bony dehiscence of the carotid canal (black asterisk) and the mastoid segment of the facial nerve canal (dotted arrow). (**e**) Axial image depicts dehiscence of the HJB involving the posterior semicircular canal (curved arrow). (**f**) Axial image shows a tortuous, ectatic anomalous venous channel (dashed arrow), likely originating from the superior petrosal sinus, coursing along the superior surface of the petrous bone and draining caudally into the jugular bulb (not visualized). (**g**) Contrast-enhanced axial 3D FFE T1w without fat suppression MR image confirms the anomalous venous channel (dashed arrow) along the superior surface of the petrous bone. *Abbreviations:* CBCT = cone-beam computed tomography; HJB = high riding jugular bulb; FFE = fast field echo; IAC = internal auditory canal; MR = magnetic resonance

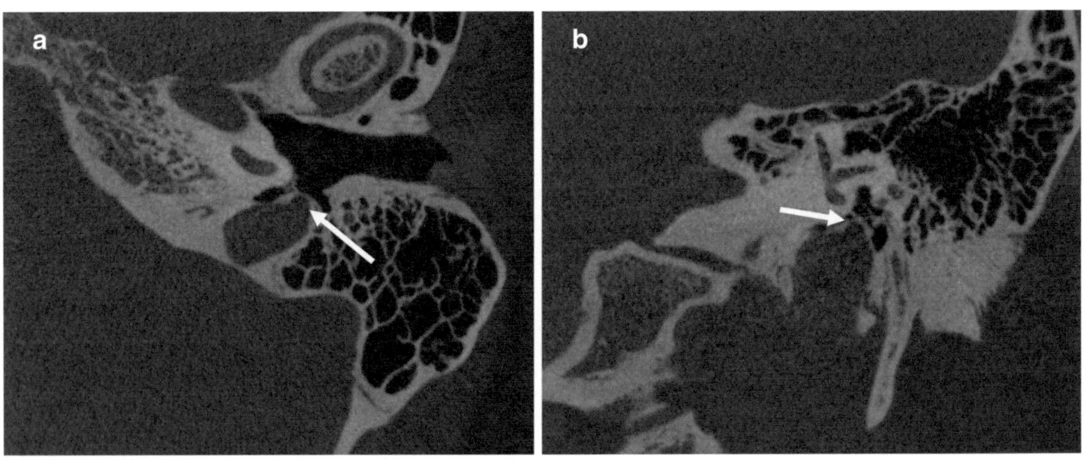

Fig. 12.19 High-riding jugular bulbs with small diverticula. A jugular bulb diverticulum is a focal, rounded, or oval outpouching arising from the jugular bulb, typically projecting superomedially into the petrous portion of the temporal bone. This anatomical variant has been linked to PT and other audiovestibular symptoms, including hearing loss and vertigo. (**a–b**) Axial and coronal CBCT images demonstrate a small diverticulum (arrow) extending toward the hypotympanum. *Abbreviations:* CBCT = cone-beam computed tomography; PT = pulsatile tinnitus

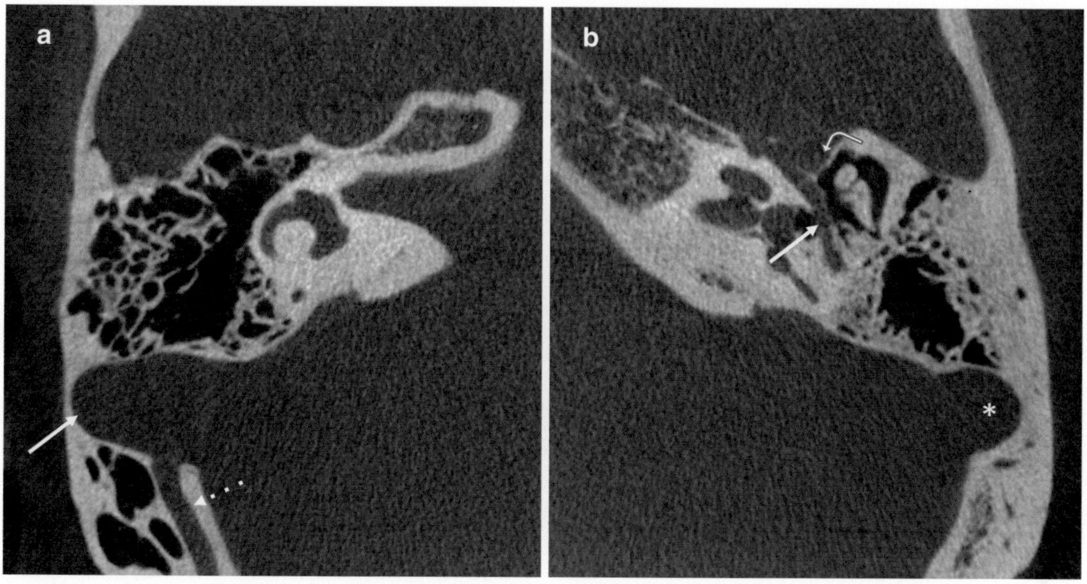

Fig. 12.20 Bilateral dehiscent sigmoid sinus, left petrous venous anomaly. A dehiscent or laterally positioned sigmoid sinus refers to a vascular variant in which the sinus wall is abnormally thin or absent and/or displaced toward the mastoid cavity, allowing direct transmission of venous flow pulsations to the middle ear, potentially resulting in venous pulsatile tinnitus. (**a**) axial CBCT of right side shows procident sigmoid sinus (arrow) and retromastoid emissary vein (dotted arrow). (**b**) axial CBCT shows a left procident sigmoid sinus (asterisk). A vascular groove is appreciable (probably venous, a tributary of middle superficial cerebral vein, curved arrow) along the anterior superior aspect of petrous bone, closely related to the tympanic tract of the facial nerve (arrow). *Abbreviation:* CBCT: cone beam computed tomography

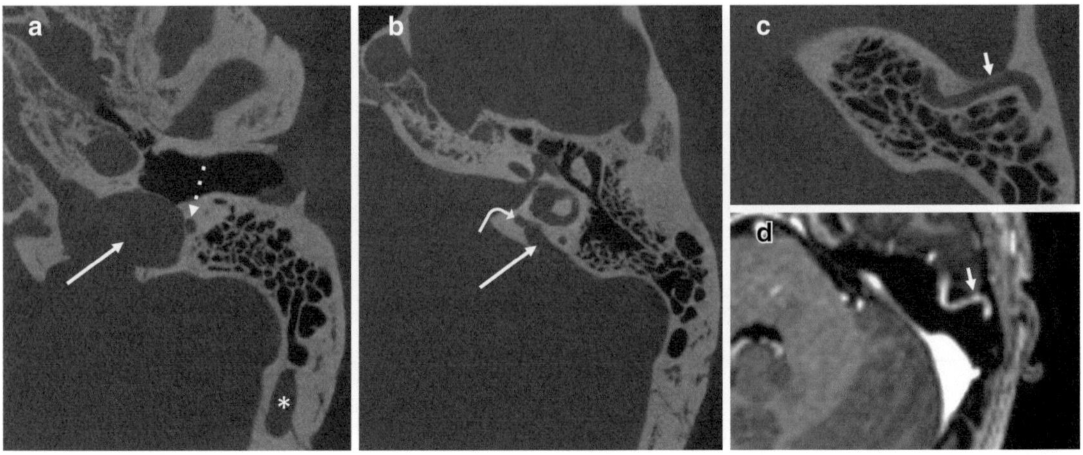

Fig. 12.21 Enlarged vestibular aqueduct (EVA) with internal jugular vein dehiscence and jugular bulb diverticula

EVA is defined by:

Valvassori criteria as a diameter >1.5 mm measured at the midpoint between the crus and the aperture on axial images;

Cincinnati criteria as a vestibular aqueduct width ≥2 mm at the operculum and/or ≥1 mm at the midpoint on axial images;

On the Pöschl plane (45° oblique), as a diameter >0.9 mm at the midpoint

(**a**) Axial CBCT image shows the jugular bulb (arrow), petrous segment of the ICA (arrow), and an enlarged retromastoid emissary vein (asterisk). (**b**) Axial CBCT image depicts an EVA measuring 2.1 mm (arrow), with dehiscence into a jugular bulb diverticulum (curved arrow); the posterior semicircular canal is also visible (dashed arrow). (**c** and **d**) Axial CBCT and contrast-enhanced 3D FFE T1w MR images demonstrate a venous canal along the tegmen antri, likely corresponding to a petrosquamous accessory vein (short arrow). *Abbreviations:* CBCT = cone-beam computed tomography; EVA = enlarged vestibular aqueduct; FFE = fast field echo

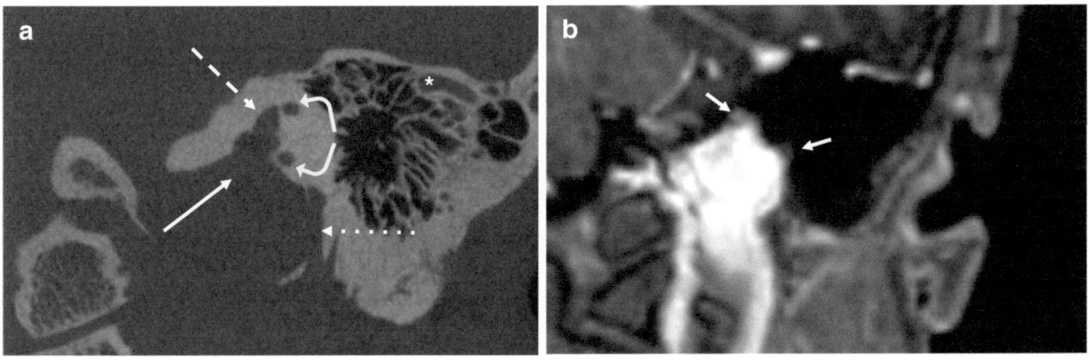

Fig. 12.22 Enlarged vestibular aqueduct with internal jugular vein dehiscence and jugular bulb diverticula (continued from Fig. 12.21). (**a**) Coronal CBCT image demonstrates an EVA measuring 2.1 mm (dashed arrow) with dehiscence into the jugular bulb (arrow). The posterior semicircular canal (curved arrows) and the mastoid segment of the facial nerve canal (dotted arrow) are adjacent to the jugular bulb, though dehiscence is not clearly evident. (**b**) Coronal contrast-enhanced 3D FFE T1w MR image reveals jugular bulb diverticula (short arrow). *Abbreviations:* CBCT = cone-beam computed tomography; EVA = enlarged vestibular acqueduct, FFE = fast field echo

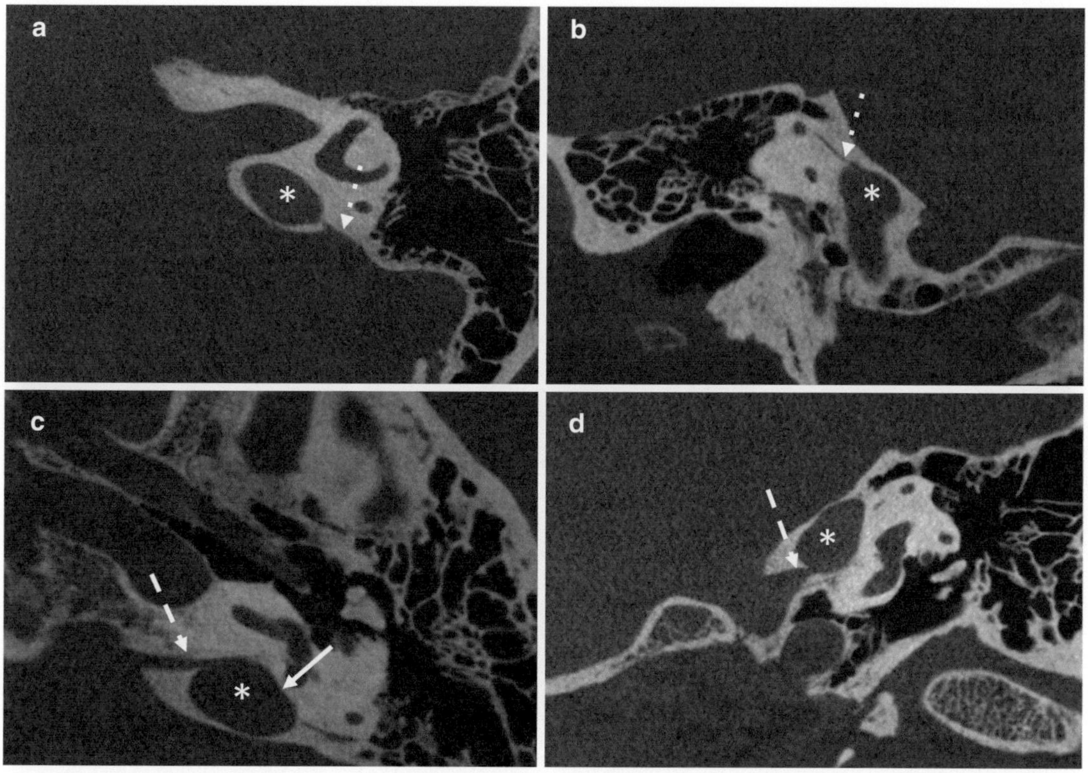

Fig. 12.23 Cochlear or vestibular aqueduct dehiscence into the high-riding jugular bulb. Dehiscence of the vestibular or cochlear aqueduct may lead to PT due to abnormal transmission of jugular venous pulsation into the inner ear causing aberrant transmitted signals to the vestibular and cochlear nerves or acting as a third mobile window and disrupting normal fluid dynamics. (**a**) axial and (**b**) Pöschl plane reformatted CBCT images show the vestibular aqueduct (dotted arrow) dehiscent into the HJB (asterisk). (**c**) axial and (**d**) oblique reformatted CBCT show cochlear aqueduct (dashed arrow) dehiscent into the high riding jugular bulb (asteriks). *Abbreviations:* CBCT = cone beam computed tomography; HJB = high riding jugular bulb; PT = pulsatile tinnitus

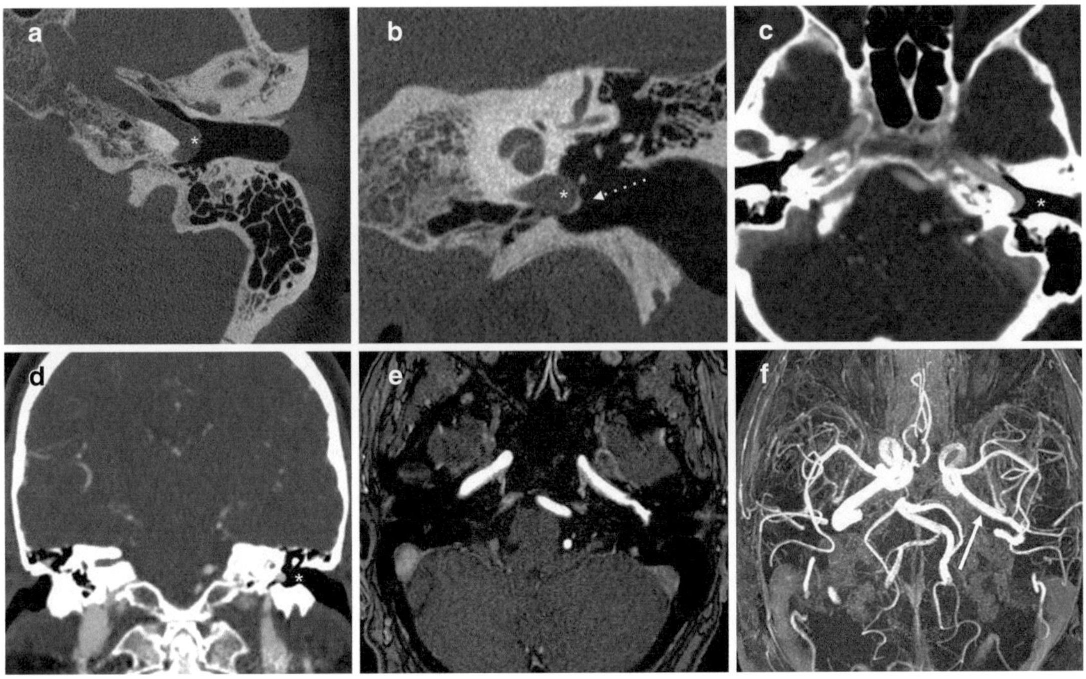

Fig. 12.24 Aberrant left internal carotid artery. Aberrant ICA is a rare congenital anomaly resulting from agenesis of the proximal embryonic ICA, with compensatory enlargement of the inferior tympanic branch of the ascending pharyngeal artery and the caroticotympanic branch. The aberrant ICA enters the tympanic cavity through an enlarged inferior tympanic canaliculus, courses through the hypotympanum, runs over the cochlear promontory, and rejoins the horizontal petrous ICA, often appearing narrowed and irregular at the point of confluence. This anomalous course leads the vessel to traverse the middle ear cavity, where it may appear as a pulsatile retrotympanic mass and represent a potential cause of PT. Recognition is crucial to avoid iatrogenic injury during otologic procedures. Aberrant ICA is associated with arterial PT, which, unlike venous PT, typically does not vary with internal jugular vein compression, head rotation or flexion, or during the Valsalva maneuver. (**a**) Axial and (**b**) coronal CBCT images demonstrate the aberrant course of the left ICA (asterisk), which protrudes into the tympanic cavity. A thin residual bony plate (dotted arrow) is visibile. (**c**) axial and (**d**) coronal CTA image confirms the laterally displaced and aberrant course of the left ICA (asterisk) within the tympanic cavity. (**e**) axial MRA and (**f**) corresponding MIP reconstruction show diffusely reduced and irregular caliber of the left aberrant ICA (arrow) compared to the contralateral side. *Abbreviations*: CBCT: cone beam computed tomography; CTA: computed tomography angiography; ICA: internal carotid artery; MIP: maximum intensity projection; MRA = magnetic resonance angiography; PT: pulsatile tinnitus

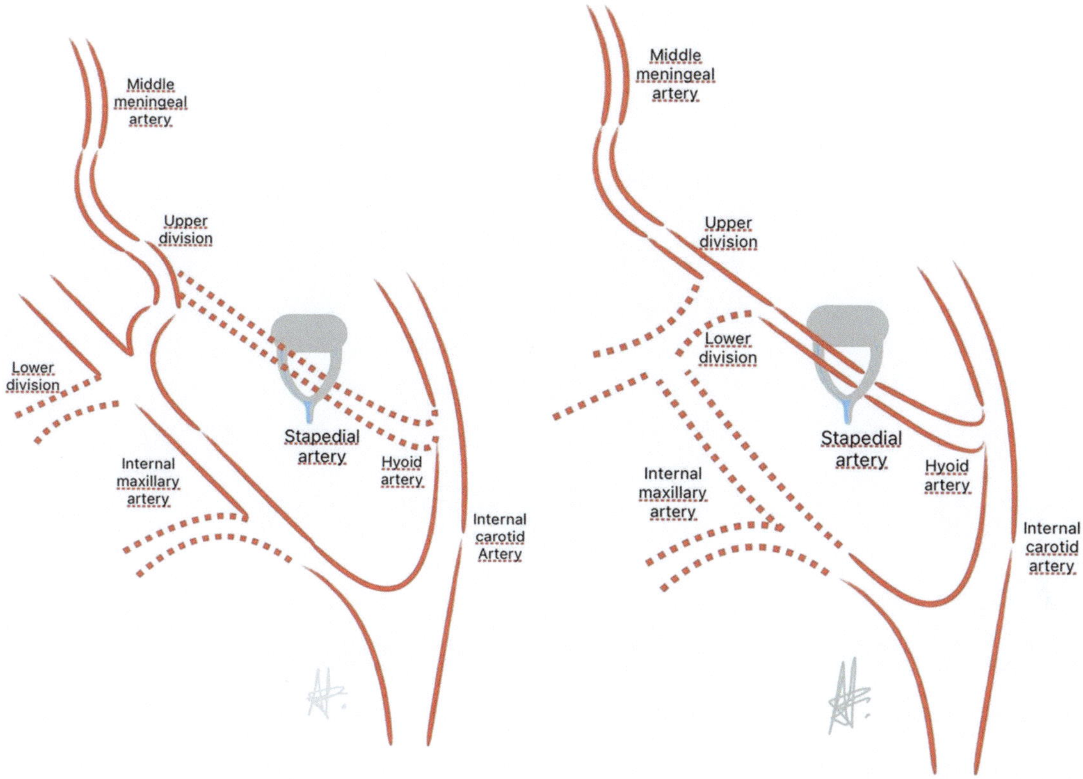

Fig. 12.25 Persistent right stapedial artery. The PSA is a rare embryological vascular anomaly resulting from the failure of involution of the hyoid artery, a branch of the second aortic arch. In this condition, an enlarged carotico-tympanic artery—a remnant of the embryonic hyoid artery stem—originates from the petrous segment of the internal carotid artery and courses through the carotico-tympanic canaliculus. This vascular channel is termed the persistent hyoidostapedial artery. Schematic illustrations depicting (a) normal anatomy and the (b) persistent stapedial artery variant. *Abbreviation:* PSA = persistent stapedial artery

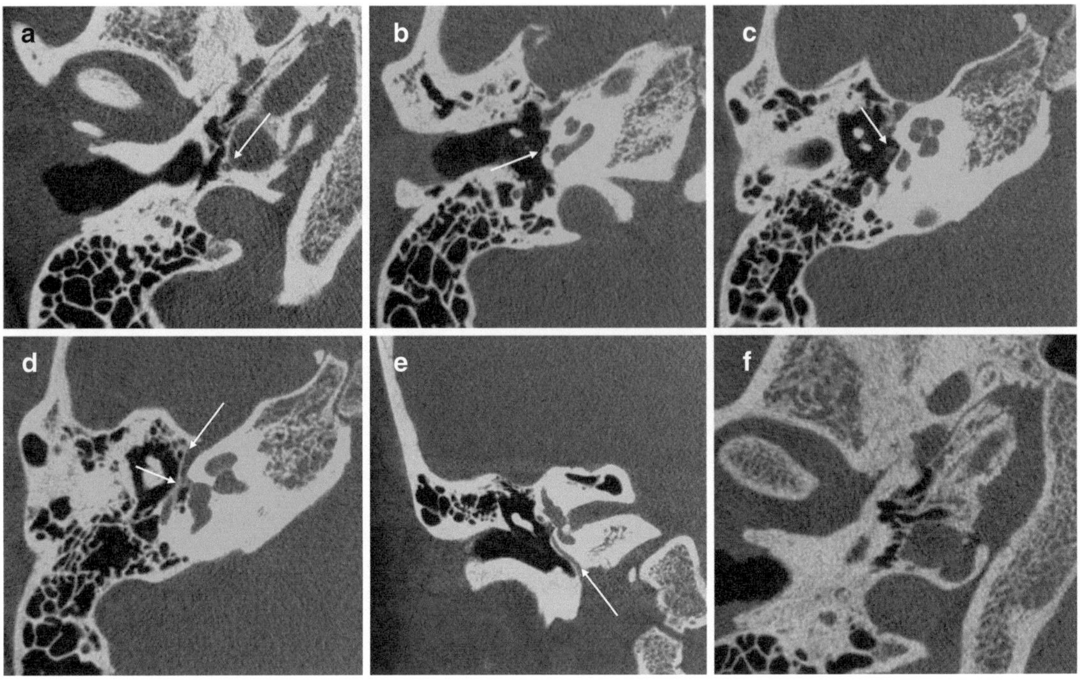

Fig. 12.26 Persistent right hyoido-stapedial artery. A PSA can cause pulsatile tinnitus with arterial features due to its intratympanic course and close proximity to the ossicular chain. (**a–d, f**) Axial and (**e**) coronal CBCT images illustrate the course of the persistent hyoido-stapedial artery (arrow): originating from the petrous segment of the internal carotid artery (**a**), crossing the cochlear promontory (**b**), passing through the stapes (**c**), and entering the tympanic segment of the facial nerve canal (**d-e**). (**f**) Axial CBCT image demonstrates absence of the foramen spinosum. *Abbreviations:* CBCT: cone-beam computed tomography; PSA = persistent stapedial artery

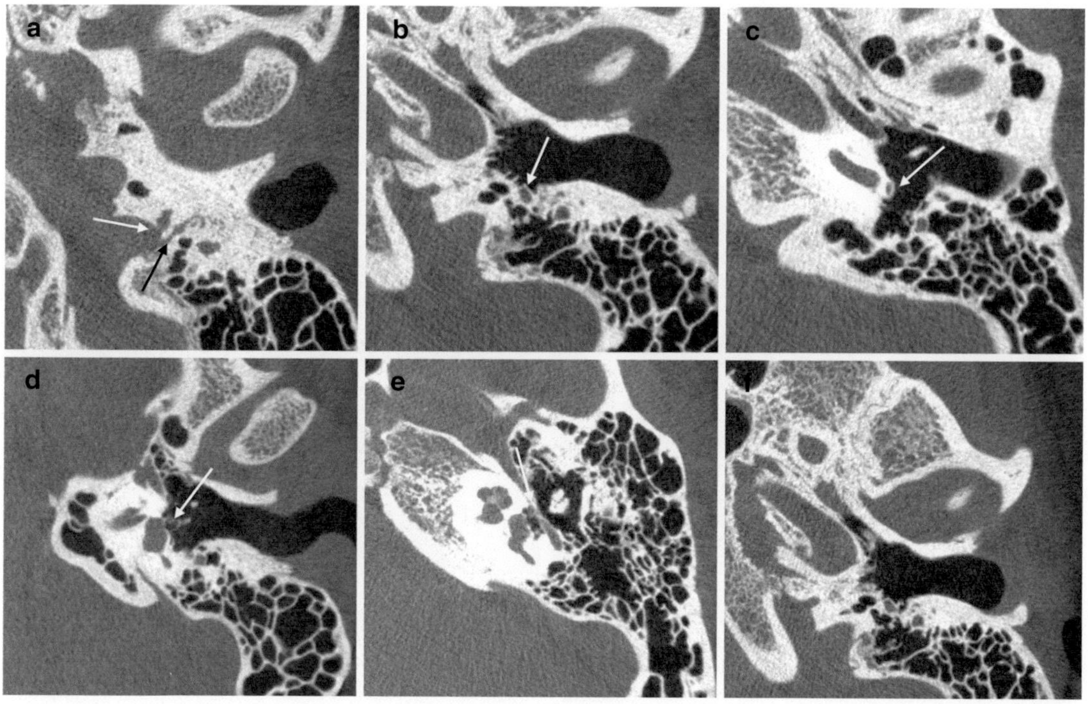

Fig. 12.27 Persistent left pharyngo-stapedial artery. In this variant, the PSA is supplied by an enlarged inferior tympanic artery, a branch of the ascending pharyngeal artery. This artery travels through the inferior tympanic canaliculus into the middle ear, where it anastomoses with the embryonic hyoid artery. (**a**–**f**) Axial CBCT images depict the course of the PPhSA (arrow). A dilated Jacobson's canal (black arrow) originates near the jugular foramen adjacent to the PSA (**a**). The artery crosses the hypotympanic recess (**b**), runs along the promontory (**c**), passes between the two crura of the stapes into the tympanic cavity (**d**), and continues into the tympanic segment of the facial nerve canal (**e**). The foramen spinosum is absent, reflecting middle meningeal artery supply via the persistent stapedial artery (**f**). *Abbreviations:* CBCT = cone-beam computed tomography; PSA = persistent stapedial artery; PPhSA = persistent pharyngo-stapedial artery

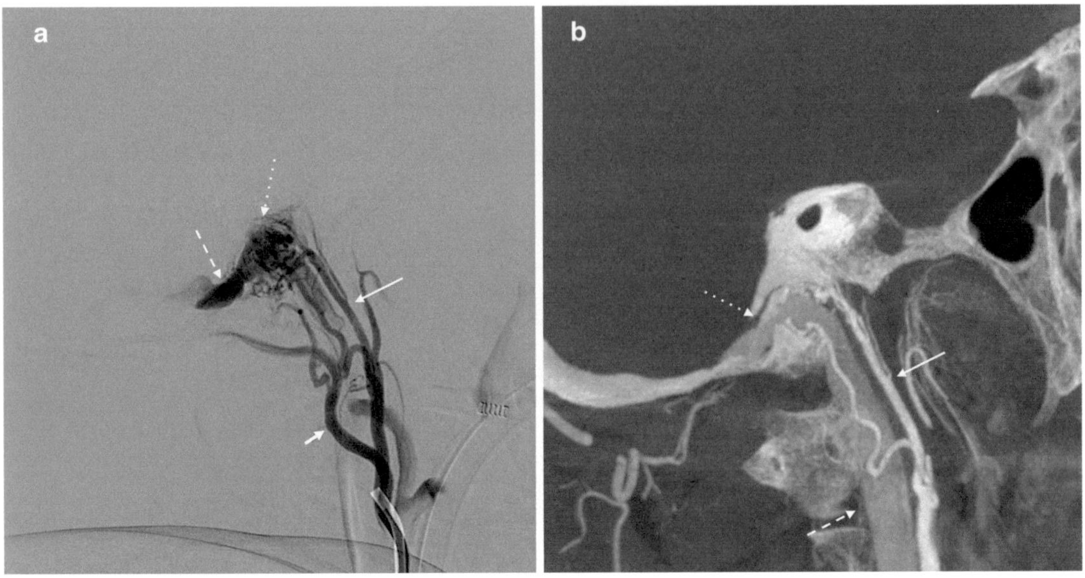

Fig. 12.28 Type I dAVF (Cognard's classification) of the left transverse-sigmoid sinus. A dAVF is an acquired vascular malformation characterized by a direct pathological shunt between dural arteries and dural venous sinuses or cortical veins, lacking an intervening capillary network or nidus, distinguishing it from AVMs. These lesions often arise secondary to venous sinus thrombosis, trauma, surgery, or infection. Unlike AVMs, which are supplied by cerebral arteries, dAVFs are primarily vascularized by dural arteries, typically meningeal branches of the external carotid artery. The Cognard classification stratifies dAVFs based on venous drainage patterns, flow direction, and presence of venous ectasia, correlating with clinical prognosis and hemorrhage risk. Type I dAVFs exhibit antegrade drainage into a dural venous sinus without cortical venous reflux and may present clinically with pulsatile tinnitus of arterial character. (**a**) DSA, lateral projection with selective catheterization of the external carotid artery, reveals a vascular nidus (dotted nidus) near the transverse-sigmoid sinus junction (dashed arrow), supplied by branches of the ascending pharyngeal artery (arrow) and occipital artery (short arrow). (**b**) MIP reformatted CBCT image demonstrates an enlarged ascending pharyngeal artery (arrow) contributing to the fistula's arterial supply, alongside branches of the occipital, middle meningeal, and auricular arteries (not shown). Early opacification of the transverse-sigmoid sinus junction (dotted arrow) and jugular vein (dashed arrow) is also observed. *Abbreviations:* AVM = arteriovenous malformation; CBCT = cone beam computed tomography; dAVF = dural arteriovenous fistula; DSA = digital subtraction angiography; MIP = maximum intensity projection; PT: pulsatile tinnitus

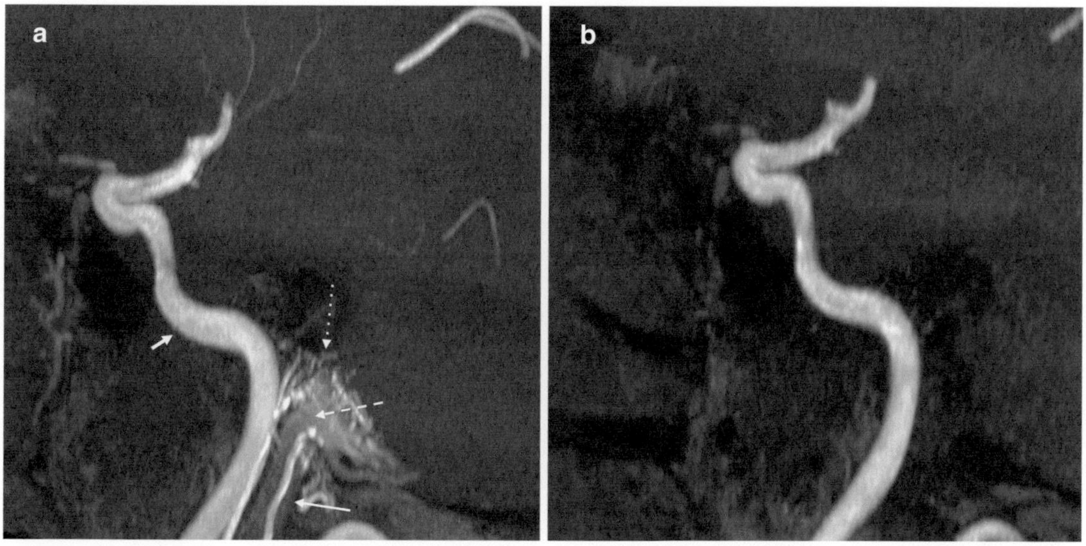

Fig. 12.29 Type I dAVF (Cognard's classification) of the left transverse-sigmoid sinus (continuation from Fig. 12.28). (**a**) Oblique sagittal reformatted MRA demonstrates an enlarged ascending pharyngeal artery (arrow) and a cluster of vessels near the transverse-sigmoid sinus junction (dotted arrows). A subtle flow signal is also noted within the transverse-sigmoid sinus region (dashed arrow). The internal carotid artery is visible (short arrow). (**b**) Post-embolization oblique sagittal MRA reveals complete resolution of the fistula with disappearance of the abnormal flow signals. *Abbreviations:* dAVF = dural arteriovenous fistula; MIP: maximum intensity projection; MRA = magnetic resonance angiography

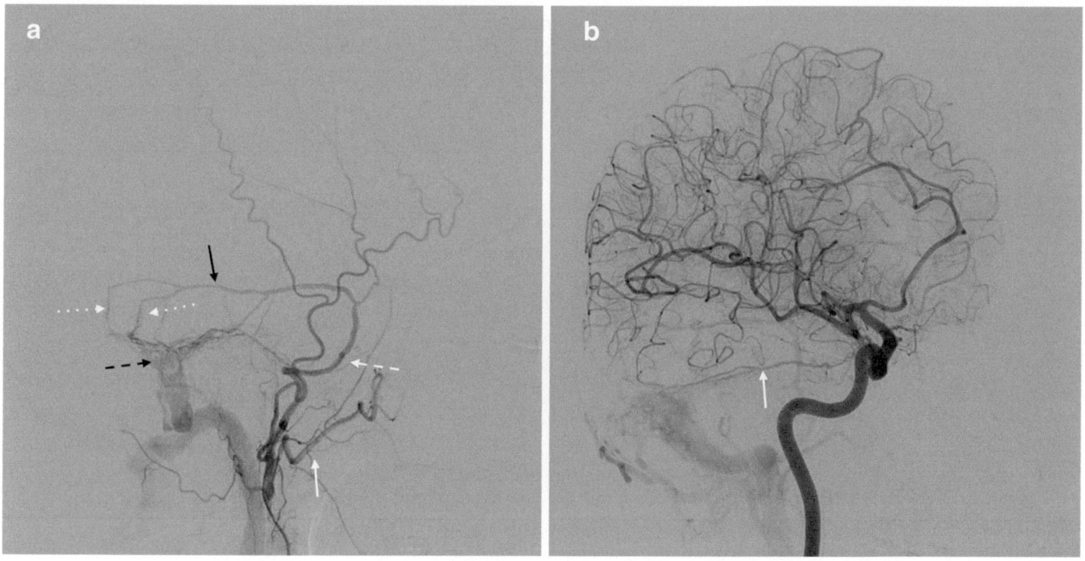

Fig. 12.30 Type I dAVF (Cognard classification) of the left transvers-sigmoid sinus. (**a**) Lateral projection DSA image with selective injection of the left ECA demonstrates a fistulous connection at the sigmoid-transverse sinus junction (dashed black arrow). The fistula is supplied by distal branches (dotted arrows) of the petrosquamous branch (black arrow) arising from the MMA (dashed white arrow). (**b**) Oblique projection DSA image with selective injection of the ICA reveals additional arterial supply to the fistula via the Bernasconi's artery (arrow). *Abbreviations:* dAVF: dural arteriovenous fistula; DSA: digital subtraction angiography; ECA: external carotid artery; ICA: internal carotid artery; MMA = middle meningeal artery

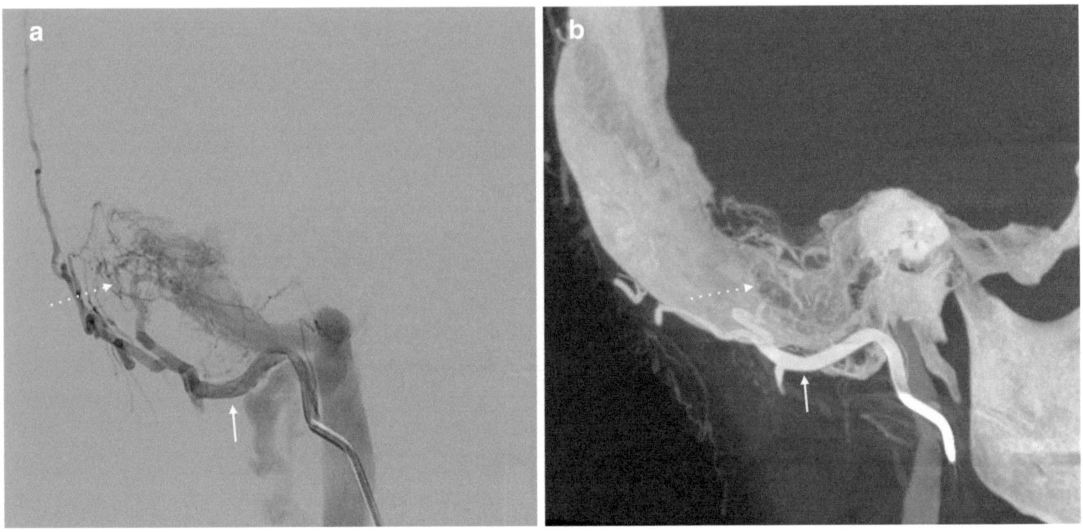

Fig. 12.31 Type I dAVF (Cognard's classification) of the transvers-sigmoid sinus. (**a**) Lateral projection DSA image with selective injection of the occipital artery demonstrates multiple small trans-diploic branches (dotted arrow) supplying the fistula from the occipital artery (arrow). (**b**) Sagittal reformatted MIP image from intra-arterial CBCT, acquired after selective occipital artery injection (arrow), clearly depicts the trans-diploic branches (dotted arrow) vascularizing the fistula. *Abbreviations:* CBCT: cone-beam computed tomography; dAVF = dural arteriovenous fistula; DSA: digital subtraction angiography

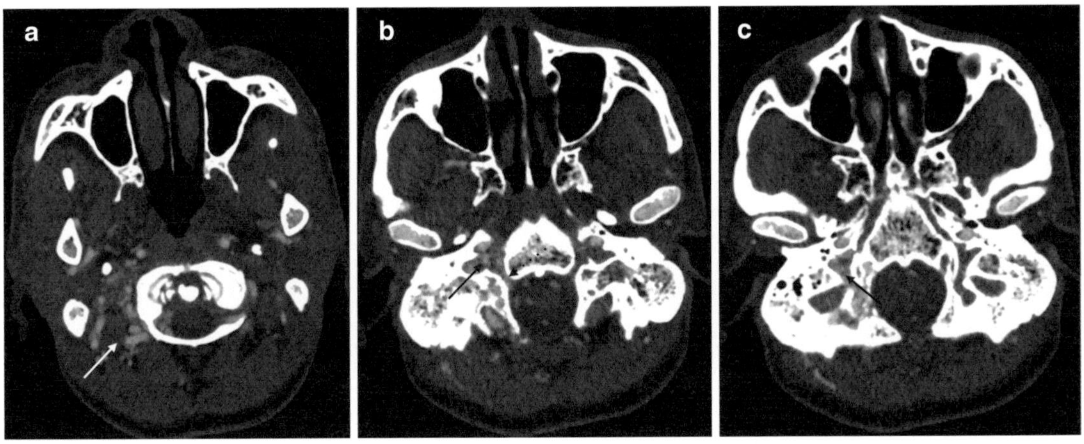

Fig. 12.32 dAVF of the right condylar region, with fistula point at the level of the intercondylar vein. The patient complained of a PT in the right ear with arterial characteristics. (a, b, c) CT angiography in the arterial phase shows the early opacification of abundant veins on the right side of C1-C2 (white arrow), of the anterior condylar confluence (black arrow) and anterior condylar vein in the hypoglossal canal (black dotted arrow). These findings in association with the clinical finding of PT raise the suspicion of a dAVF. *Abbreviations*: CT: computed tomography; dAVF: dura arteriovenous fistula; PT: pulsatile tinnitus

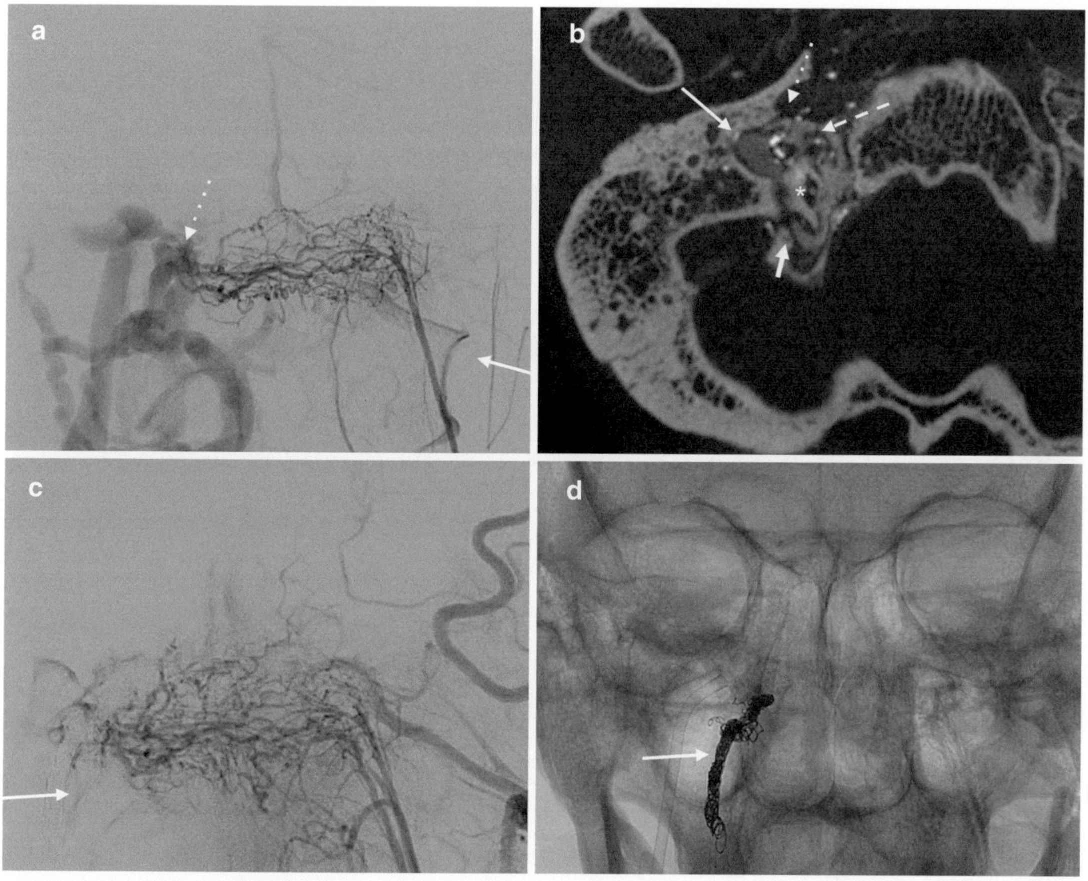

Fig. 12.33 dAVF of the right condylar region with the fistula point at the intercondylar vein (continues from Fig. 12.32). (**a**) Antero-posterior DSA projection with selective injection of the left ascending pharyngeal artery (arrow) demonstrating the right condylar sinus dAVF and early opacification of venous structures (dotted arrow). (**b**) Post-contrast CBCT during injection in the ascending pharyngeal artery reveals the vascular anatomy of the condylar region opacified during the arterial phase due to the dAVF: anterior condylar vein within the hypoglossal canal (dashed arrow), anterior condylar confluence (dotted arrow), internal jugular bulb (arrow), posterior condylar vein (short arrow), and intercondylar vein (asterisk). The intercondylar vein shows the greatest opacification, consistent with the fistula site. (**c** and **d**) Post-treatment DSA images after coil embolization of the condylar vein (arrow) demonstrate successful fistula occlusion. *Abbreviations:* CBCT = cone beam computed tomography; dAVF = dural arteriovenous fistula; DSA = digital subtraction angiography

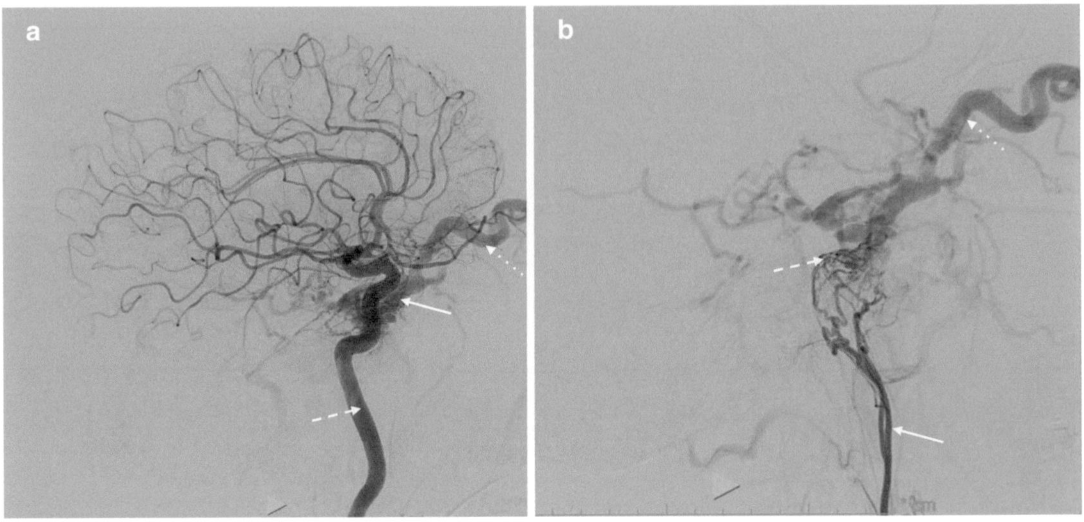

Fig. 12.34 dAVF of the right cavernous sinus region causing PT. dAVFs in the cavernous sinus cause PT with arterial characteristics due to abnormal arteriovenous shunting within the dura mater, allowing high-pressure arterial blood to flow directly into the venous system. This creates turbulent flow near the auditory apparatus, transmitting pulsatile sounds perceived as PT. (**a**) Lateral DSA with selective injection of the right internal carotid artery (dashed arrow) demonstrates early arterial-phase opacification of the right cavernous sinus region (arrow) and drainage via an enlarged ophthalmic vein (dotted arrow). (**b**) Lateral DSA with selective injection of the right ascending pharyngeal artery (arrow) shows dural branches (dashed arrow) supplying the fistula, with drainage through an enlarged ophthalmic vein (dotted arrow). *Abbreviations:* dAVF: dural arteriovenous fistula; DSA: Digital Subtraction Angiography; PT: pulsatile tinnitus

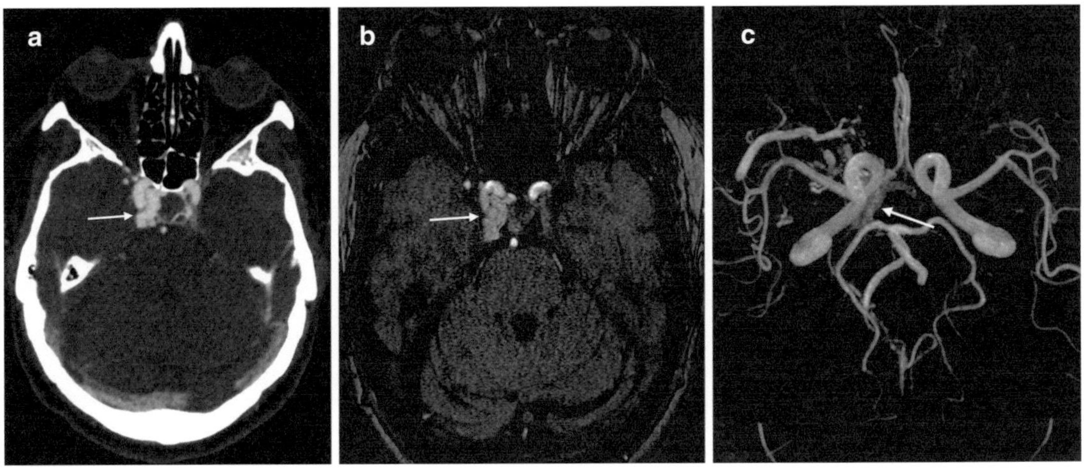

Fig. 12.35 dAVF of the right cavernous sinus region presenting with PT with arterial characteristics. (**a**) Axial CTA in the arterial phase shows early opacification of the right cavernous sinus region (arrow), raising suspicion for a dAVF. (**b** and **c**) MRA and corresponding MIP reconstruction demonstrate arterial signal within the cavernous sinus (arrow). *Abbreviations:* CTA: computed tomography angiography; dAVF: dural arteriovenous fistula; MIP: maximum intensity projection; MRA: magnetic resonance angiography

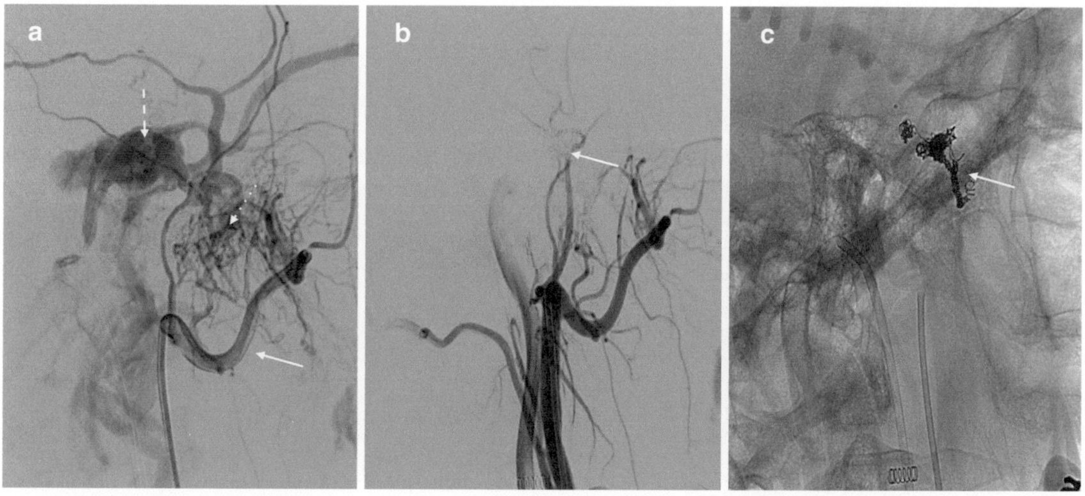

Fig. 12.36 dAVF of the right cavernous sinus region (continuation from Fig. 12.35). (**a**) Lateral DSA with selective injection from the ECA (arrow) demonstrates the dural fistula involving the cavernous sinus region (dashed arrow), with arterial feeders from branches of the internal maxillary artery (dotted arrow). (**b** and **c**) Post-embolization DSA images with selective injection from the ECA show coils deployed in the antero-inferior portion of the cavernous sinus (arrow), confirming successful treatment of the dAVF. *Abbreviations:* dAVF = dural arteriovenous fistula; DSA = digital subtraction angiography; ECA = external carotid artery

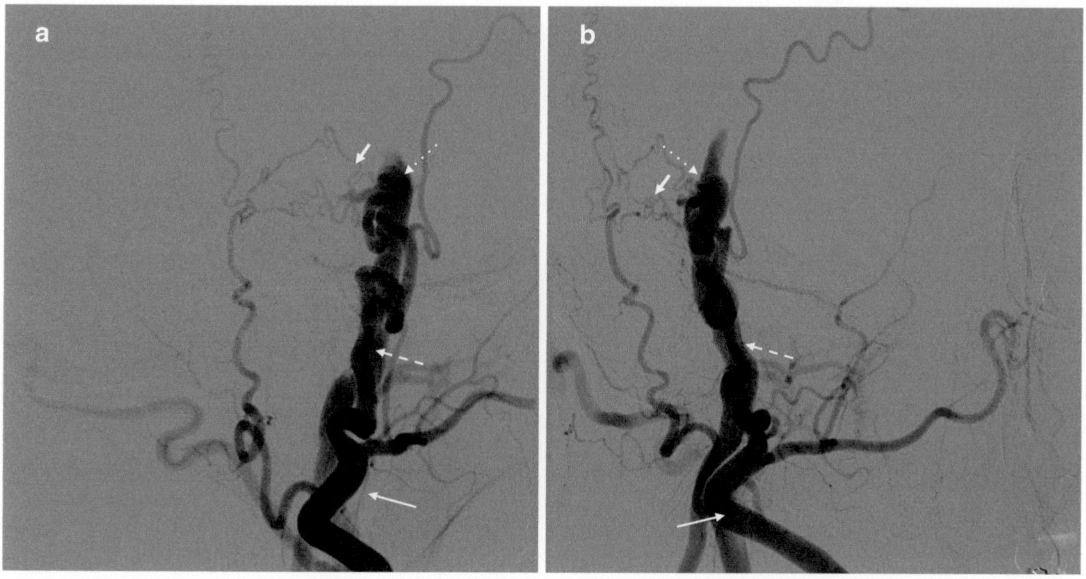

Fig. 12.37 Post-traumatic extracranial arteriovenous fistula of the right peri-auricular region in a patient presenting with PT. (**a**) Lateral and (**b**) anteroposterior DSA images with selective injection from the external carotid artery (arrow) demonstrate an arteriovenous fistula involving the superficial temporal vein (dotted arrow). The arterial supply includes the superficial temporal artery (dashed arrow) and small branches from the posterior auricular artery (short arrow). *Abbreviations:* DSA = digital subtraction angiography; PT = pulsatile tinnitus

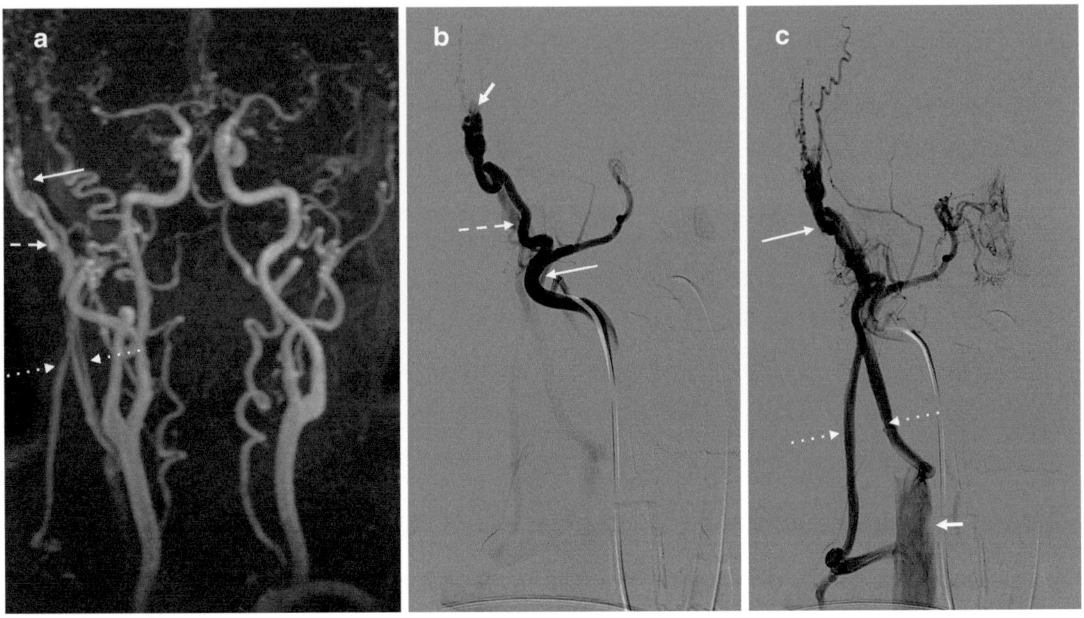

Fig. 12.38 Post-traumatic extracranial arteriovenous fistula of the right peri-auricular region in a patient presenting with PT. (Continues from Fig. 12.37). (**a**) Post-contrast time-resolved 4D MRA sequence shows early arterial phase enhancement of a venous vessel cluster in the right periauricular region (arrow), including the superficial temporal vein (dashed arrow) and the external jugular vein (dotted arrow). (**b** and **c**) Anteroposterior DSA with selective injection from the ECA (arrow) demonstrates increased caliber of the STA (dashed arrow). The fistulous point is identified at the STV(short arrow), which drains through the external jugular vein (dotted arrows) and internal jugular vein (arrowhead). *Abbreviations:* DSA: digital subtraction angiography; ECA = external carotid artery; MRA = magnetic resonance angiography; STA = superficial temporal artery; STV = superficial temporal vein

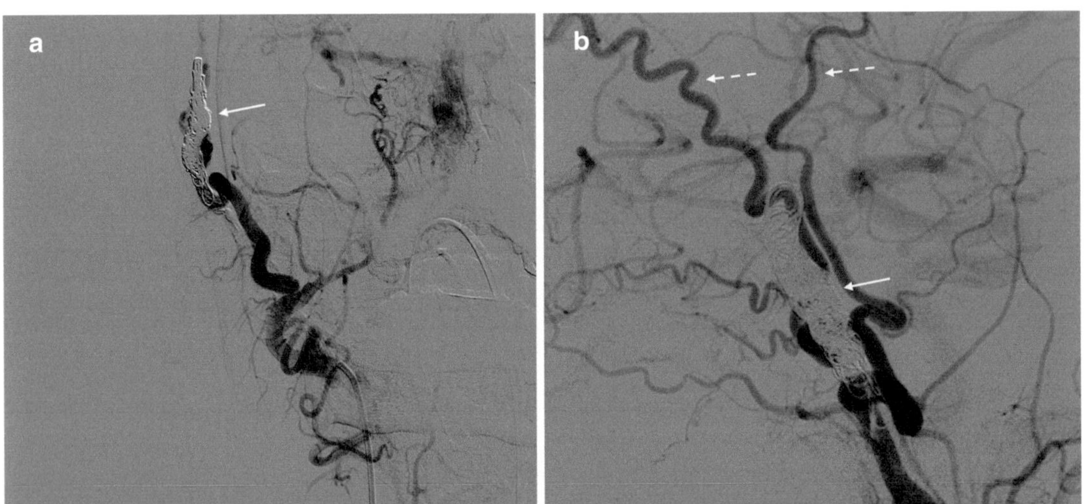

Fig. 12.39 Post-traumatic extracranial arteriovenous fistula of the right peri-auricular region in a patient with PT. (Continues from Fig. 12.38). (**a**) Anteroposterior and (**b**) lateral DSA images with selective injection of the external carotid artery following transvenous coiling of the superficial temporal vein (arrow). Distal branches of the superficial temporal artery are now visible (dashed arrows). *Abbreviations:* DSA = digital subtraction angiography; PT = pulsatile tinnitus

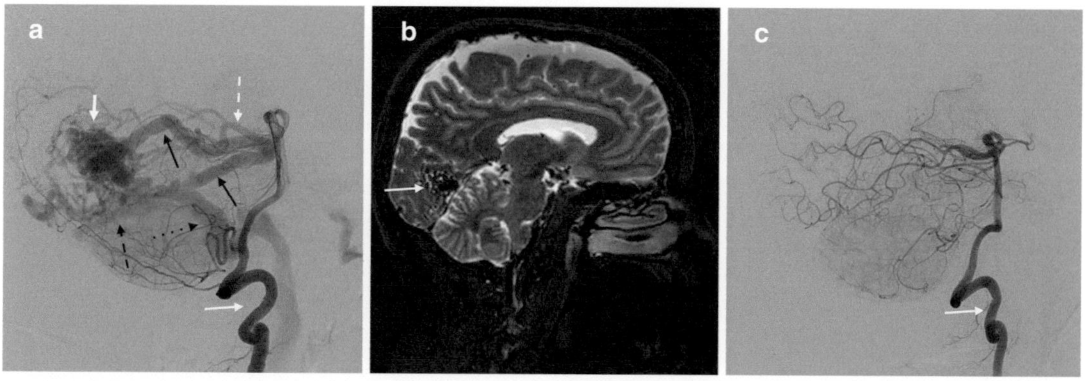

Fig. 12.40 AVM of the left occipital lobe in a patient complaining of PT. Brain AVM is a vascular anomaly characterized by a direct connection between cerebral arteries and veins, bypassing the normal capillary network. This creates a high-flow shunt that may result in various neurological symptoms, depending on the lesion's location, size, and angioarchitecture. The AVM comprises three main components: (1) *Feeding arteries*, often arising from pial branches of cerebral vessels. (2) *Nidus*, a compact cluster of dysplastic vessels where the arteriovenous connections occur. (3) *Draining veins*, which are frequently dilated and shunt blood directly from the nidus to the superficial or deep venous systems. When located near the temporal bone, posterior fossa, or dural venous sinuses—particularly the transverse or sigmoid sinuses—AVMs can present with PT of arterial origin. (**a**) Lateral DSA following selective injection of the left vertebral artery (arrow) reveals a malformative nidus (short arrow) in the left occipital lobe, supplied by arterial feeders from the posterior cerebral artery (white dashed arrow). The lesion drains via dilated venous outflow (black arrows) into the transverse (black dashed arrow) and sigmoid sinuses (black dotted arrow). (**b**) 3D FFE T2w with fat suppression MRI demonstrates the AVM nidus (white arrow) adjacent to the calcarine cortex in the left occipital lobe. (**c**) Postoperative DSA with left vertebral artery injection (white arrow) confirms complete obliteration of the AVM. *Abbreviations:* AVM = arteriovebous malformation; DSA = digital subtraction angiography; FFE = fast field echo; PT = pulsatile tinnitus

References

1. Grevin P, Ohresser M, Kossowski M, et al. Current understanding of subjective tinnitus in adults: epidemiology, mechanisms, evaluation and treatment. Eur Arch Otorrinolaringol. 2024;281(9):4507–17.
2. McCormack A, Edmondson-Jones M, Somerset S, Hall D. A systematic review of the reporting of tinnitus prevalence and severity. Hear Res. 2016;337:70–9.
3. Baguley D, McFerran D, Hall D. Tinnitus. Lancet. 2013;382(9904):1600–7.
4. Park SN, Jin SG, Yeo SW, et al. Clinical characteristics and therapeutic response of objective tinnitus due to middle ear myoclonus: a large case series. Laryngoscope. 2013;123(10):2516–20.
5. Abdalkader M, Nguyen TN, Norbash AN, Raz E, Shapiro M, Lenck S, Brinjikji W, Weber P, Sakai O. State of the art: venous causes of pulsatile tinnitus and diagnostic considerations guiding endovascular therapy. Radiology. 2021;300(1):2–16. https://doi.org/10.1148/radiol.2021202584.
6. Duvvuri M, Ali H, Amans MB. Non-invasive imaging modalities for diagnosing pulsatile tinnitus: a comprehensive review and recommended imaging algorithm. J Neurointerv Surg. 2025;17:916.
7. Alkhatib SG, Kandregula S, Flesher K, Choudhri OA, Brant JA, Mohan S. Imaging of pulsatile tinnitus. Radiographics. 2024;44(10):e240030.
8. Louis RG Jr, Loukas M, Wartmann CT, Tubbs RS, Apaydin N, Gupta AA, Spentzouris G, Ysique JR. Clinical anatomy of the mastoid and occipital emissary veins in a large series. Surg Radiol Anat. 2009;31(2):139–44. https://doi.org/10.1007/s00276-008-0423-5. PMID: 1897491.

Miscellanea 13

Elisa Massullo, Antonia Valentina Genovese, Silvia Casale, Elena Caloro, Eleonora Piccin, Lorenzo Maria Gaini, Diego Zanetti, Lorenzo Pinelli, Fabio Triulzi, Giorgio Conte, and Elisa Scola

The following chapter will address conditions and diseases that were not covered in previous chapters. An anatomical order will be followed starting from the apex of the petrous bone and moving from the center to the periphery of the skull to pathologies involving the skull base

Anatomical variants and pathologies involving the petrous bone apex such as asymmetry of pneumatization, effusion, meningocele, mucocele, cholesteatoma, and cholesterol granuloma [1–7] will be illustrated in figures along with lesions of the geniculate fossa such as arachnoid cyst, schwannoma, and venous vascular malformations [8, 9]. Infectious conditions and complications related to radiotherapy affecting the skull base will also be described [10–13]. Finally, tumors involving petrous bone will be listed: chondrosarcoma, metastasis, and tumor of the endolymphatic sac [14–16]. Each figure caption will provide a concise description of the corresponding condition.

In the following Table 13.1 the conditions that are shown in figures are listed.

E. Massullo · A. V. Genovese · S. Casale · E. Piccin
E. Scola (✉)
Neuroradiology Unit, Fondazione IRCCS Ca' Granda Ospedale Maggiore Policlinico, Milan, Italy
e-mail: elisa.massullo@policlinico.mi.it; valentina.genovese@policlinico.mi.it; silvia.casale@policlinico.mi.it; eleonora.piccin@policlinico.mi.it; elisa.scola@policlinico.mi.it

E. Caloro
Postgraduation School in Radiodiagnostics, Università Degli Studi di Milano, Milan, Italy
e-mail: elena.caloro@unimi.it

L. M. Gaini
Department of Otolaryngology and Head and Neck Surgery, Fondazione IRCCS Ca' Granda Ospedale Maggiore Policlinico, Milan, Italy

Department of Clinical Sciences and Community Health, Università Degli Studi di Milano, Milan, Italy
e-mail: lorenzo.gaini@policlinico.mi.ti

D. Zanetti
Department of Clinical Sciences and Community Health, Università Degli Studi di Milano, Milan, Italy

Audiology Unit, Fondazione IRCCS Ca' Granda Ospedale Maggiore Policlinico, Milan, Italy
e-mail: diego.zanetti@policlinico.mi.it

L. Pinelli
Neuroradiology Unit, Pediatric Neuroradiology Section, ASST Spedali Civili of Brescia, Brescia, Italy
e-mail: lorenzo.pinelli@asst-spedalicivili.it

F. Triulzi · G. Conte
Neuroradiology Unit, Fondazione IRCCS Ca' Granda Ospedale Maggiore Policlinico, Milan, Italy

Department of Pathophysiology and Transplantation, University of Milan, Milan, Italy
e-mail: fabio.triulzi@policlinico.mi.it; giorgio.conte@policlinico.mi.it

G. Conte et al. (eds.), *Atlas of Normal and Pathological Findings in Otoneuroradiology*,
https://doi.org/10.1007/978-3-032-08232-9_13

Table 13.1 The conditions that are illustrated in the figures of the chapter are listed in the table with the corresponding figure number

Miscellanea		Figures
Petrous bone apex	Asymmetry of pneumatization	Fig. 13.1
	Effusion	Fig. 13.2
	Meningocele	Fig. 13.3
	Mucocele	Fig. 13.4
	Cholesteatoma	Fig. 13.5
	Cholesterol granuloma	Fig. 13.6
	Venous malformation	Fig. 13.7
	Apicitis	Fig. 13.16
Geniculate fossa	Arachnoid cyst and granulation	Figs. 13.8, 13.9, 13.10, and 13.11
	Schwannoma	Figs. 13.12, 13.13, and 13.14
	Facial nerve venous vascular malformation (previously referred to as hemangioma)	Fig. 13.15
Skull base	Osteomyelitis	Figs. 13.16, 13.17, 13.18, 13.19, 13.20, 13.21, and 13.22
	Osteoradionecrosis	Figs. 13.23 and 13.24
	Chondrosarcomas	Fig. 13.25
	Metastasis	Fig. 13.26
Endolymphatic sac	Tumor of the endolymphatic sac	Figs. 13.27 and 13.28

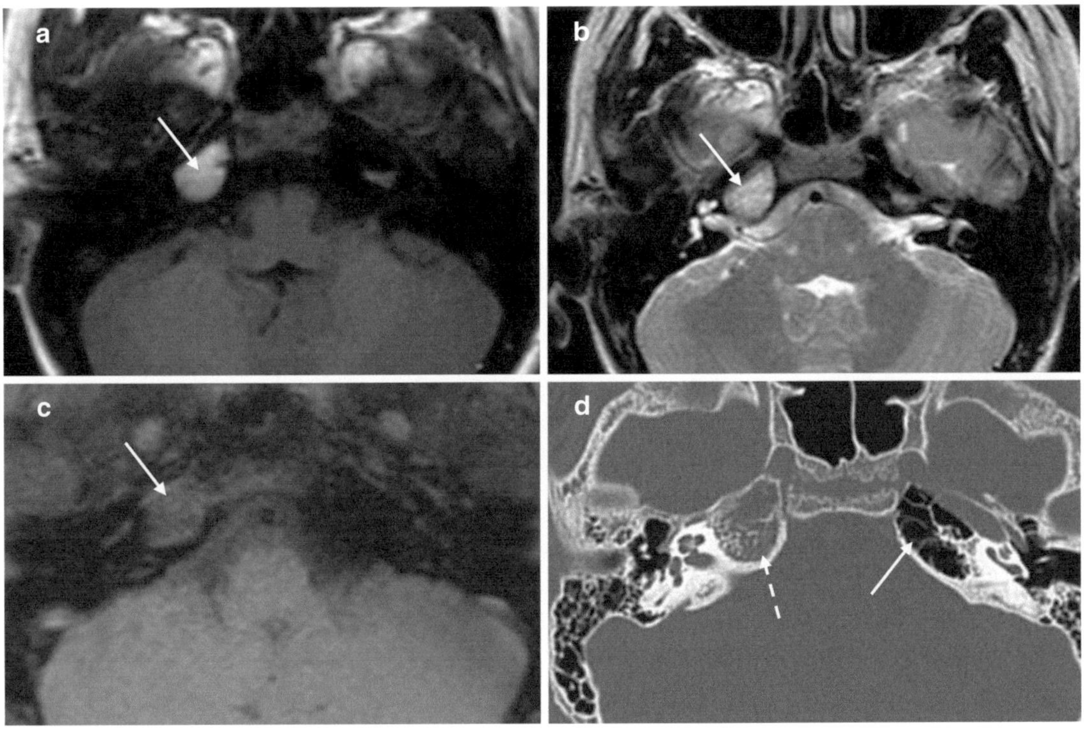

Fig. 13.1 Asymmetric pneumatization of the petrous bone apices. This anatomical variant, together with petrous bone apex effusion, can mimic a lesion of the petrous apex. (**a**) Axial TSE-T1W; (**b**) Axial TSE-T2W; (**c**) Axial fat-saturated TSE-T1W; (**d**) Axial MDCT scan. The images demonstrate asymmetrical pneumatization of the petrous apices, with absence of pneumatization on the right side. The right petrous apex appears hyperintense on both T1- and T2-weighted images (arrows in **a** and **b**), and shows signal suppression on fat-saturated T1W image (arrow in **c**), consistent with yellow bone marrow. On MDCT (**d**), air cells are visible on the left (arrow) but absent on the right (dashed arrow). A possible differential diagnosis may occur when a cholesterol granuloma is suspected: in this case, the T1W sequence with saturation of the fat tissue signal would show the persistence of T1 hyperintensity. *Abbreviations:* TSE = turbo spin echo, MDCT = multidetector computed tomography

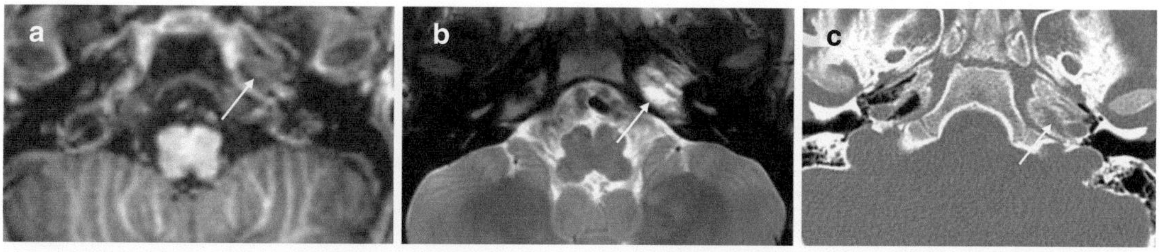

Fig. 13.2 **Left petrous apex air cell effusion.** This condition is a common incidental finding and can mimic a lesion of the petrous apex. Persistent fluid in petrous apex air cells may occur in conjunction with and after otitis media, even despite the resolution of inflammatory process. This is due to fibrosis along communicating air channels between petrous bone apex air cells and middle ear. Nevertheless the "trapped effusion" has no clinical relevance as microbiological analyses have shown that the fluid is not nonpurulent and does not contain microorganisms. (**a**) Axial 3D FFE-T1W; (**b**) Axial TSE-T2W MRI; (**c**) Axial MDCT. MRI demonstrates a fluid collection within the left petrous apex, appearing as a low signal on T1-weighted imaging (arrow in **a**) and high signal on T2-weighted imaging (arrow in **b**), consistent with simple fluid. MDCT is complementary to MRI and shows fluid attenuation (arrow in **c**) within the left petrous apex air cells, without bony erosion or expansion, confirming the presence of air cells effusion. *Abbreviations:* MRI= magnetic resonance imaging, FFE= fast field echo, TSE = turbo spin echo, MDCT = multidetector computed tomography

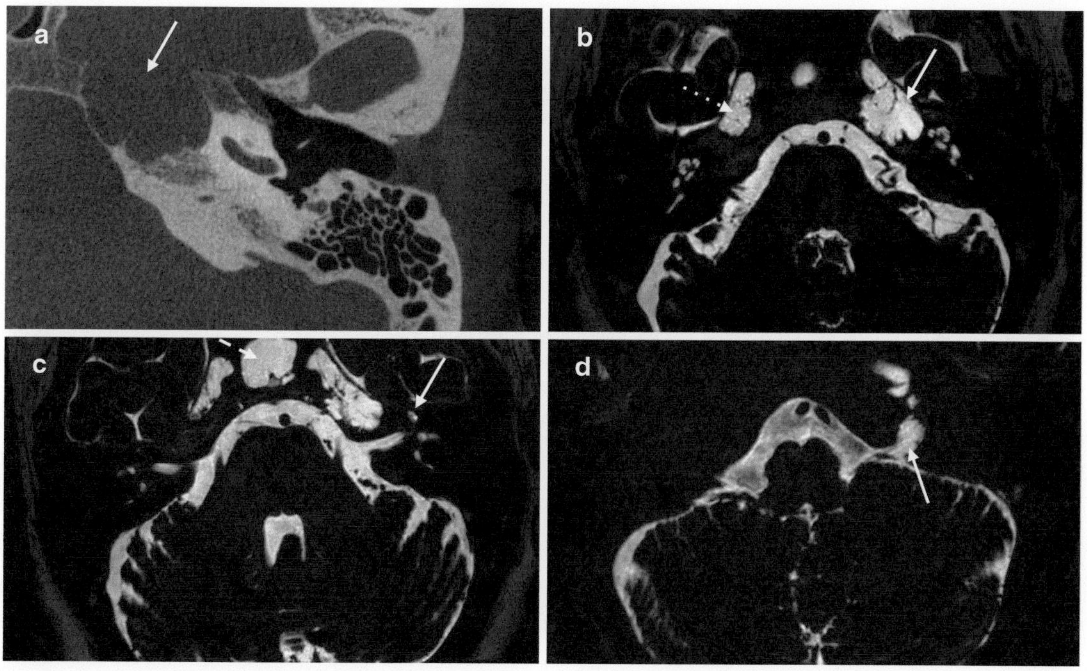

Fig. 13.3 **Meckel's cave meningocele in the setting of idiopathic intracranial hypertension.** Meningoceles are herniations of the meninges and CSF that occur through a bony defect or weak areas in the bony structure of the skull base or calvaria. They are typically classified into three types: congenital, which are present from birth and are the most frequently observed; iatrogenic, which arise as a result of surgical procedures such as craniotomy or sinus surgery; and spontaneous, which occur without a clear external cause but are often linked to elevated intracranial pressure usually in the setting of spontaneous intracranial hypertension. (**a**) Axial CBCT; (**b–d**) Axial 3D TSE-T2W. The images show a well-defined, lobulated, expansive lesion within the left petrous apex (arrow in **a**), showing CSF-like signal intensity on TSE T2-weighted images (arrow in **b**), findings consistent with a Meckel's cave meningocele. Additional imaging features are consistent with idiopathic intracranial hypertension: enlarged right Meckel's cave (dotted arrow in **b**), a millimetric arachnoid cyst at the level of the left geniculate ganglion (arrow in **c**), CSF-filled enlarged pituitary fossa consistent with empty sella (dashed arrow in **c**) and CSF-filled meningeal ectasia within the left jugular foramen (arrow in **d**). *Abbreviations:* CSF = cerebrospinal fluid, CBCT = cone beam computed tomography, TSE = turbo spin echo, MPR = multiplanar reconstruction

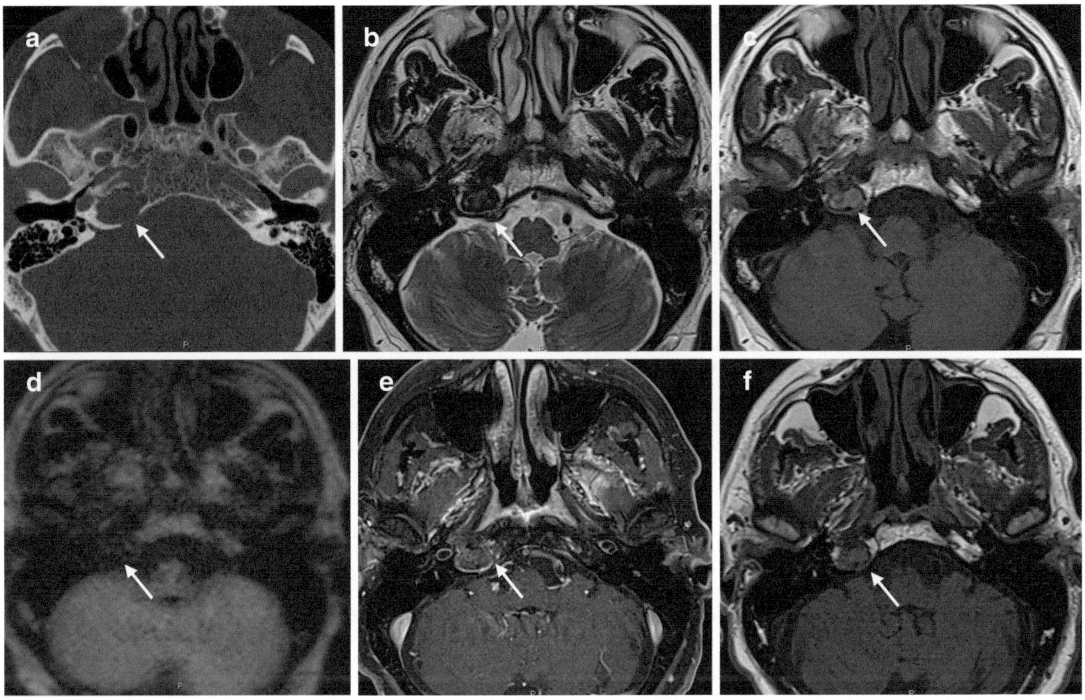

Fig. 13.4 **Petrous apex mucocele**. Petrous apex mucocele (incidentally discovered at paranasal sinuses MDCT performed for nasal obstruction). (**a**) axial MDCT scan, bone image; (**b**) axial TSE-T2W; (**c**) axial 3D FFE-T1W; (**d**) TSE DWI; and **e**) contrast-enhanced 3D FFE-T1We; (**f**) seven year MRI follow-up, axial 3D FFE-T1W image. Expansile osteolytic lesion of the right petrous apex causing focal bone defect in the posterior margin of the petrous pyramid (white arrow in **a**). At MRI, the content of the lesion shows low signal on T2 weighted image (arrow in **b**), iso-hyperintense signal on T1 weighted image (arrow in **c**) and no diffusion restriction at DWI (arrow in **d**); after contrast medium administration a thin linear enhancement is seen along the posterior margin of the lesion, likely due to mucosal enhancement of the enlarged petrous apex (arrow in **e**). At 7 year MRI follow-up, axial T1 weighted image, the lesion is unchanged (arrow in **f**). (Courtesy of Dr. Lorenzo Pinelli Neuroradiology Unit ASST Spedali Civili of Brescia, Italy). *Abbreviations:* MDCT = multi-detector computed tomography, MRI = magnetic resonance imaging; EPI-DWI = Echo Planar Imaging - Diffusion Weighted Imaging

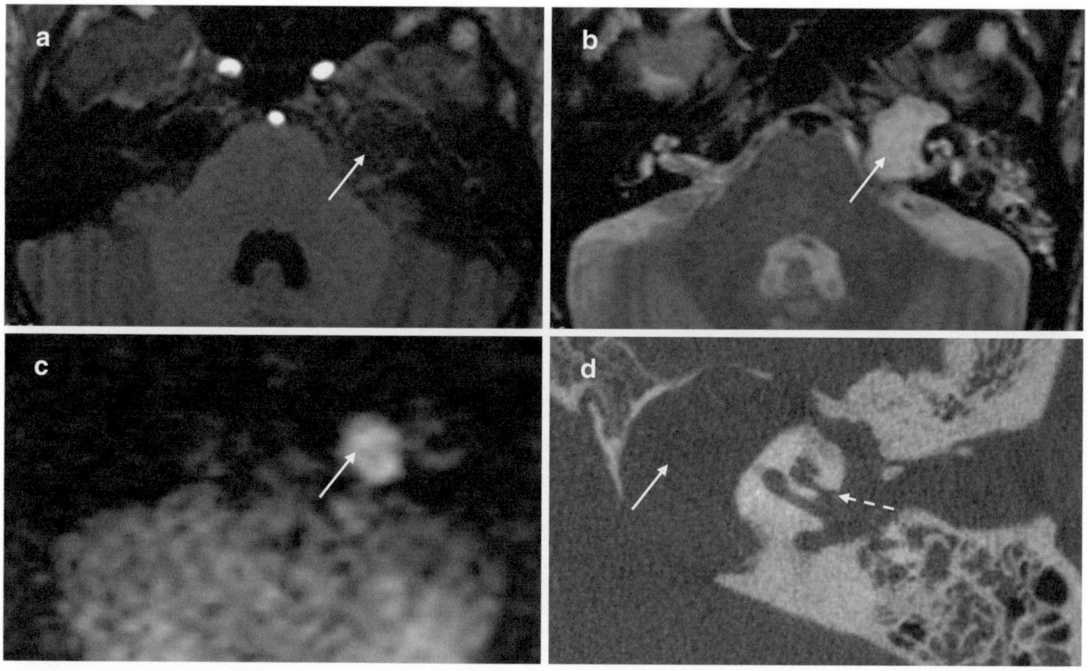

Fig. 13.5 **Cholesteatoma of the petrous apex.** Petrous apex cholesteatomas are rare lesions, typically congenital in origin, arising from ectopic embryologic rests of stratified squamous epithelium. Acquired form may occur as a result of secondary extension from adjacent structures. Like other cholesteatomas, they are characterized by restricted diffusion due to their keratinized debris content. (**a**) Axial TSE T1W; (**b**) Axial TSE T2W; (**c**) Axial TSE DWI; (**d**) Axial MDCT scan. The images show an expansile cholesteatoma of the left petrous apex, appearing with low signal on T1-weighted imaging (arrow in **a**), high signal on T2-weighted imaging (arrow in **b**), and exhibiting diffusion restriction on DWI (arrow in **c**). The corresponding CBCT image (**d**) demonstrates erosion and remodeling of the petrous bone (arrow), with evidence of perilymphatic fistula involving cochlear turns (dashed arr ow). *Abbreviations:* TSE = turbo spin echo, MDCT = multidetector computed tomography, CBCT = cone-beam computed tomography, DWI = diffusion-weighted imaging, EPI = echo-planar imaging

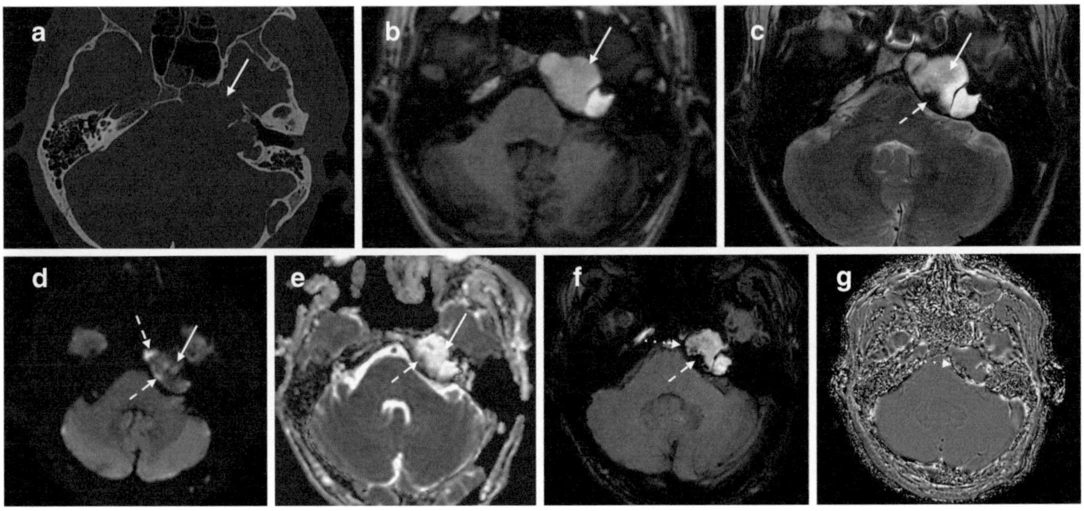

Fig. 13.6 Left petrous apex cholesterol granuloma. Cholesterol granulomas are cyst-like lesions that commonly occur in the petrous apex of the temporal bone; however, they can develop in any air-filled part of the temporal bone. These lesions often affect individuals in their teens to middle age and are frequently associated with a history of chronic middle otitis. Although their exact cause remains debated, two main theories have been proposed: the obstruction-vacuum theory, which suggests that poor function of the eustachian tube leads to negative pressure in the middle ear, resulting in mucosal swelling and repeated hemorrhages, or the exposed marrow theory. According to the latter theory the mucosal lining grows into the bone, exposing bone marrow and causing bleeding. In both models, the accumulated blood products break down and trigger a chronic inflammatory response. When cholesterol granulomas cause symptoms, surgical removal is usually recommended. Complete excision should include the cyst wall to prevent recurrence. (**a**) Axial MDCT scan, (**b**) axial 3D FFE-T1W (**c**) axial TSE-T2W, (**d**) axial TSE DWI, (**e**) ADC map, (**f**) axial SWI magnitude image, (**g**) SWI phase image. The images show a large, oval-shaped lesion within the left petrous apex causing bone expansion without evidence of destruction (arrow in **a**). The lesion shows a high signal on T1-weighted images (arrow in **b**), consistent with cholesterol and methemoglobin content, and a variable but predominantly high signal on T2-weighted images (arrow in **c**). On DWI the lesion displays overall low signal intensity (arrow in **d**) with corresponding high ADC values (arrow in **e**), indicating increased diffusion compared to normal brain tissue. Along the outer edge of the lesion, there are small areas showing restricted diffusion (dashed arrows in **d** and **e**). These areas correspond to low signal periferic spot on T2-weighted images (dashed arrow in **c**) and SWI sequences (dashed arrow in **f**), reflecting methemoglobin at different stages of breakdown. A peripheral rim of hemosiderin is visible, best seen on SWI and phase images (dotted arrows in **f** and **g**). These features are typical of a cholesterol granuloma. *Abbreviations:* MDCT = multidetector computed tomography, FFE = fast field echo, TSE = turbo spin echo, DWI = diffusion weighted imaging, ADC = apparent diffusion coefficient, SWI = susceptibility weighted imaging

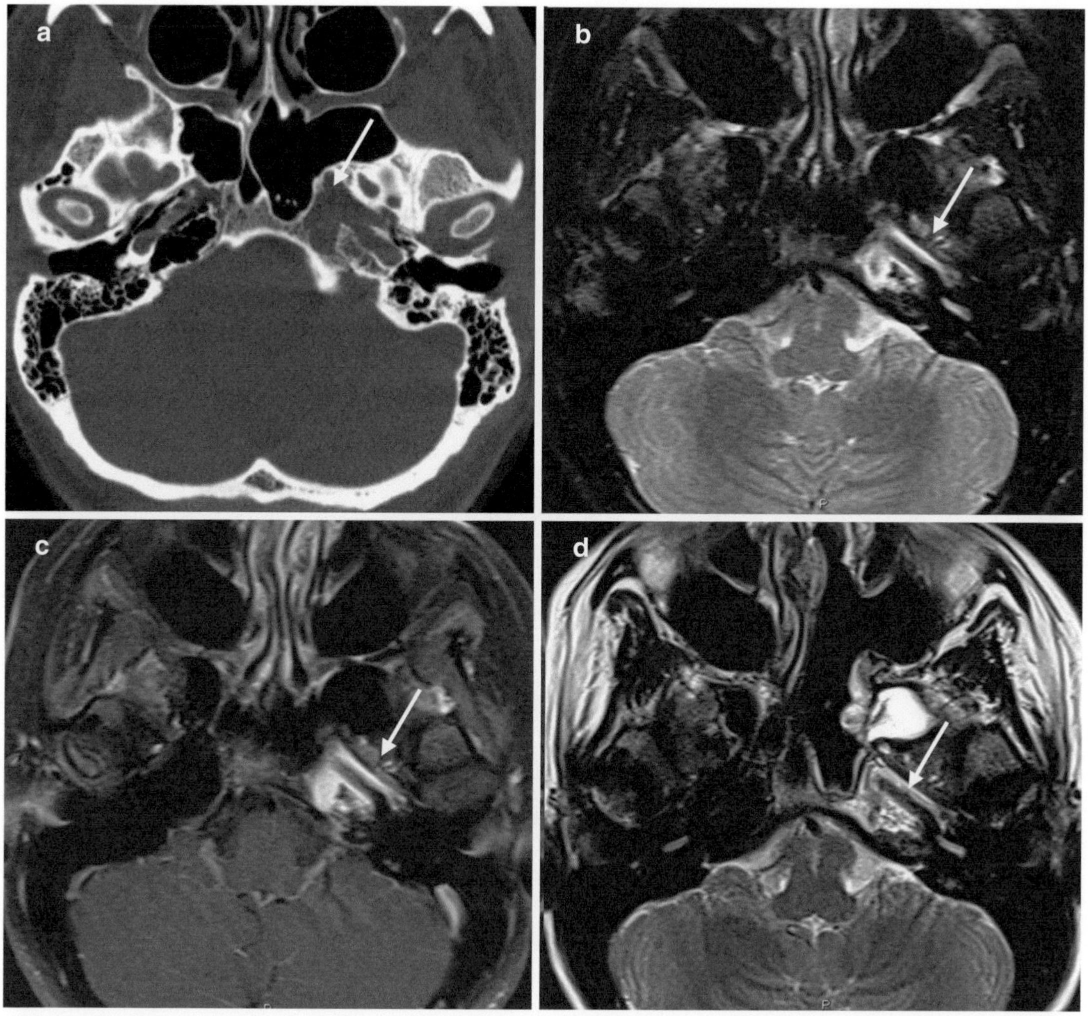

Fig. 13.7 Petrous apex venous malformation. Petrous apex venous malformation (improperly called "hemangioma"). (**a**) axial MDCT scan, bone image; (**b**) axial TSE-T2W with fat suppression and (**c**) contrast-enhanced 3D FFE-T1W with fat suppression; (**d**) axial TSE-T2W, two year MRI follow-up. MDCT shows an osteolytic lesion of the left petrous apex (arrow in **a**) with sharp margins; no internal trabeculae nor calcifications are visible. MRI shows marked high signal of the left petrous apex (arrow in **b**) on T2-weighted image, also surrounding the carotid canal, with intense contrast enhancement (arrow in **c**). Due to the concern of malignant lesion (likely a chondrosarcoma), the lesion was biopsied, and histology showed an intraosseous venous malformation. At the 2-year follow-up MRI (**d**) the lesion (arrow) is unchanged. In (**d**) anterior to the lesion, mucosal thickening of the left lateral recess of the sphenoid sinus appeared. (Courtesy of Dr. Lorenzo Pinelli Neuroradiology Unit ASST Spedali Civili of Brescia, Italy). *Abbreviations:* TSE = turbo spin echo, FFE = fast field echo, MDCT = multi-detector computed tomography, MRI = magnetic resonance imaging

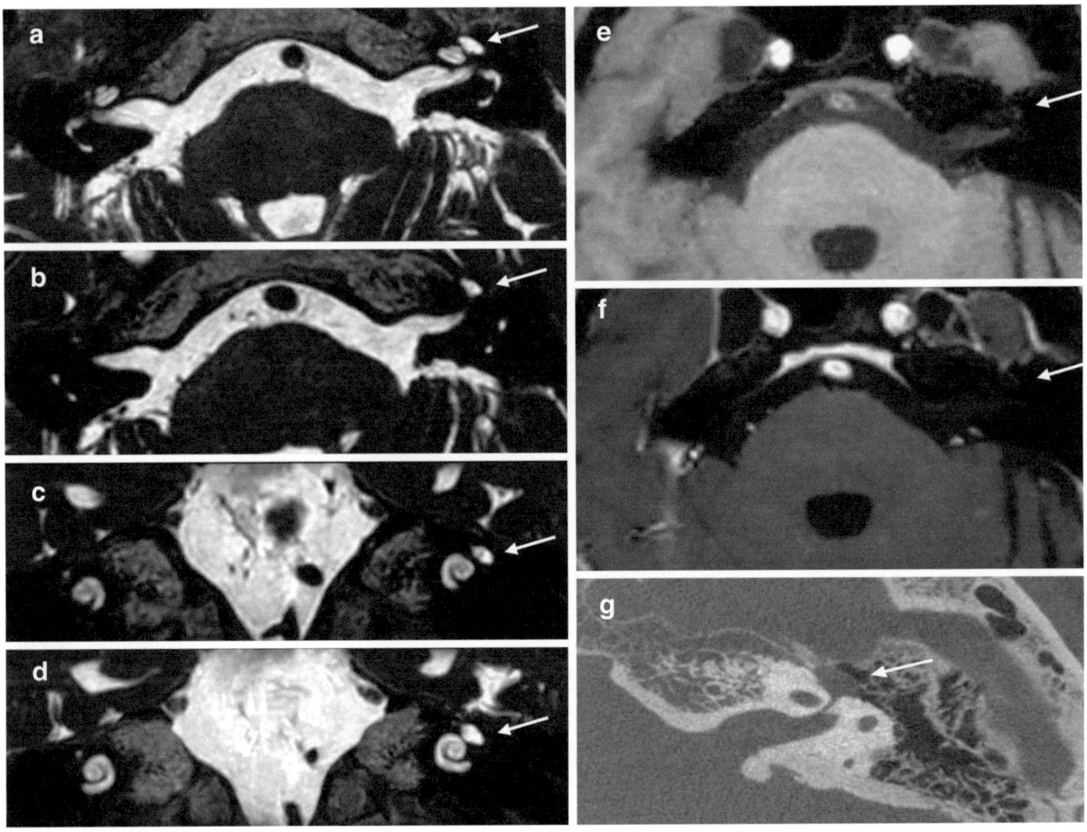

Fig. 13.8 Geniculate fossa arachnoid cyst. Arachnoid cysts of the geniculate fossa are rare. As the facial nerve passes through the lateral meatus of the internal auditory canal into the labyrinthine segment of the facial nerve canal, a fibrous ring tightly seals the nerve to prevent CSF from leaking into the peripheral nerve sheath. The arachnoid may extend distally to the meatal foramen in a variable manner thus leading to the possible development of arachnoid cyst in the geniculate fossa and possible risk of CSF leakage. (**a** and **b**) Axial 3D TSE T2W, (**c** and **d**) coronal MIP TSE T2W, (**e**) axial TSE T1W with fat suppression, (**f**) axial contrast-enhanced TSE T1W with fat suppression, (**g**) axial CBCT. A small cyst is observed at the level of the left geniculate fossa with CSF-like signal on both T2-weighted (arrow in **a**–**d**) and T1-weighted image (arrow in **e**), without contrast-enhancement (arrow in **f**). The CTCB study shows an enlargement of the geniculate fossa (arrow in **g**). *Abbreviations:* CSF = cerebrospinal fluid, TSE = turbo spin echo, MIP = maximum intensity projection, CBCT = cone beam computed tomography

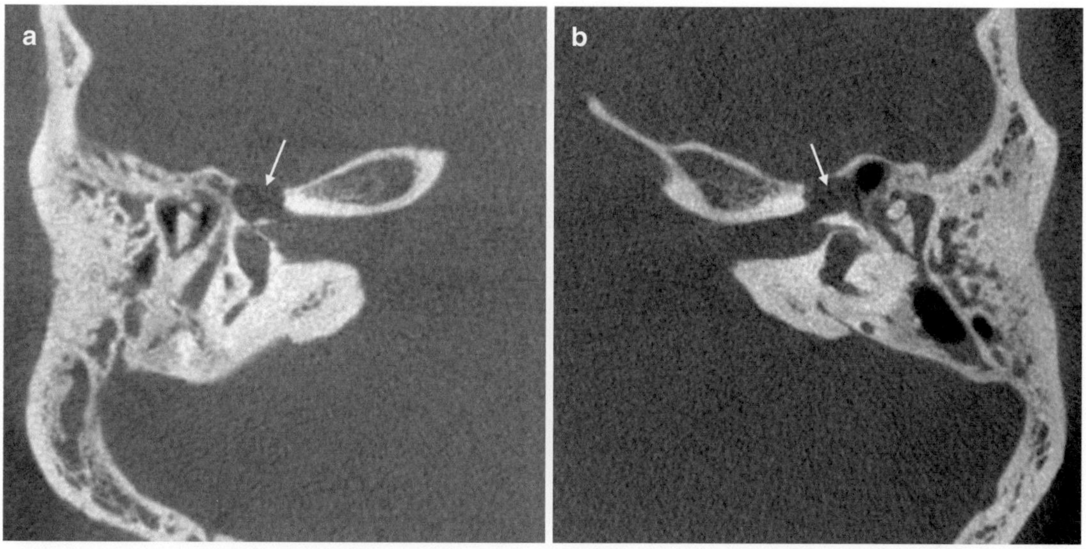

Fig. 13.9 Bilateral geniculate fossa arachnoid cysts. (**a** and **b**) axial CBCT of right and left petrous bone show bilateral enlargement of geniculate fossa (arrow in **a** and **b**) in a patient with suspected intracranial pressure. Arachnoid cysts in the geniculate fossa may be due to raise in the intracranial pressure. It is known that sites at which cranial nerves pierce the meninges to exit the skull base can be location of meningocele formation when the intracranial pressure raises chronically. *Abbreviation:* CBCT = cone beam computed tomography

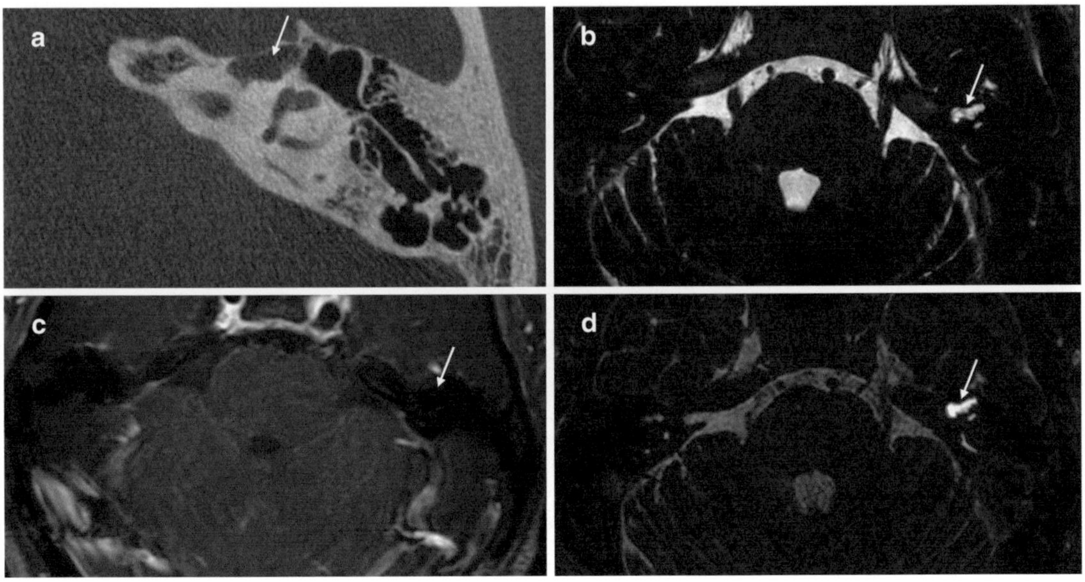

Fig. 13.10 **Aberrant left Pacchioni granulation in the left geniculate fossa in a patient with left vestibular schwannoma.** Arachnoid granulations are small protrusions of the arachnoid membrane that extend into the dural venous sinuses. Their main function is to enable cerebrospinal fluid to be absorbed from the subarachnoid space into the bloodstream. Aberrant arachnoid granulations, also known as arachnoid pits, are structures that penetrate the dura but do not communicate with the venous sinuses. They are most often found in the greater wing of the sphenoid bone and have been associated with idiopathic intracranial hypertension. (**a**) Axial CBCT, (**b**) Axial 3D TSE T2W, (**c**) Axial contrast-enhanced 3D FFE-T1W with fat suppression, (**d**) 4-hour delayed contrast-enhanced 3D FLAIR. The images show a right osteolytic lesion centered in the geniculate fossa (arrow in **a**), with high signal on the T2-weighted sequence (arrow in **b**) and no contrast enhancement (arrow in **c**). On the delayed contrast-enhanced FLAIR sequence, the lesion demonstrates signal intensity similar to the perilymphatic fluid (arrow in **d**). Given these imaging characteristics, the most likely diagnosis is an aberrant arachnoid granulation, possibly related to altered perilymphatic–subarachnoid pressure dynamics caused by the vestibular schwannoma. The delayed enhancement observed in sequence (**d**) is probably due to the arachnoid granulation slowly retaining contrast agent, similar to the behavior of perilymph. *Abbreviations:* CBCT= cone beam computed tomography, TSE = turbo spin echo, FFE= fast field echo FLAIR = fluid attenuated inversion recovery

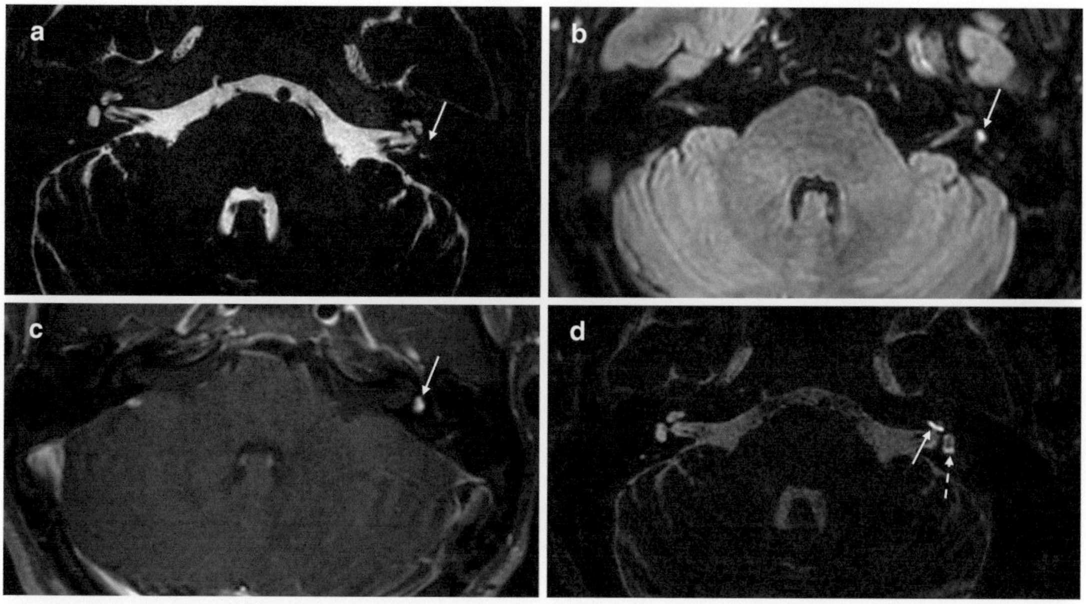

Fig. 13.11 **Aberrant left Pacchioni granulation in the left geniculate fossa in a patient with left vestibular schwannoma** (continues from Fig. 13.10). (**a**) Axial 3D TSE-T2W, (**b**) Axial 3D FLAIR, and (**c**) Axial contrast-enhanced 3D FFE-T1W with fat suppression sequences show a millimetric lesion in the left vestibule (arrows in **a**–**c**), as loss of the normal T2 signal in the left vestibule (arrow in **a**) and with high signal on FLAIR sequence (arrow in **b**). After contrast administration, the lesion demonstrates marked enhancement (arrow in **c**). Axial 4-hour delayed contrast-enhanced 3D FLAIR shows blood-labyrinth barrier breakdown in the middle turn of the cochlea (arrow in **d**) and in the posterior portion of the vestibule (dashed arrow in **d**), likely due to abnormal perilymphatic dynamics. *Abbreviations:* TSE = turbo spin echo, FLAIR = fluid attenuated inversion recovery, FFE = fast field echo

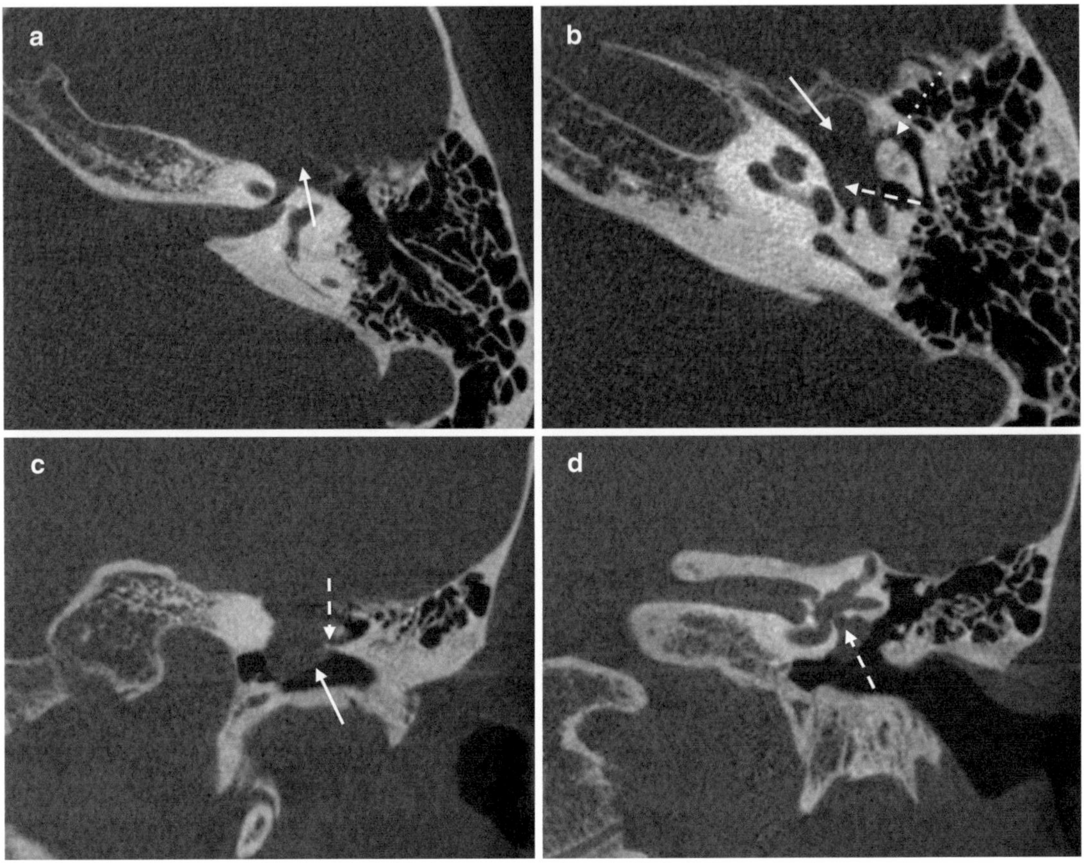

Fig. 13.12 **Left geniculate fossa schwannoma.** Axial (**a** and **b**) and coronal (**c** and **d**) reformatted CBCT images show a mass centered in the left geniculate fossa (arrow in **a**), extending into the anterior epitympanum and mesotympanum (arrow in **b and c**). The mass is indistinguishable from the tympanic segment of the osseous facial nerve canal (dashed arrow in **b**) and completely obliterates the oval window (dashed arrow in **d**). The scutum remains intact (dashed arrow in **c**), and the head of the malleus is preserved (dotted arrow in **b**). *Abbreviation:* CBCT = cone beam computed tomography

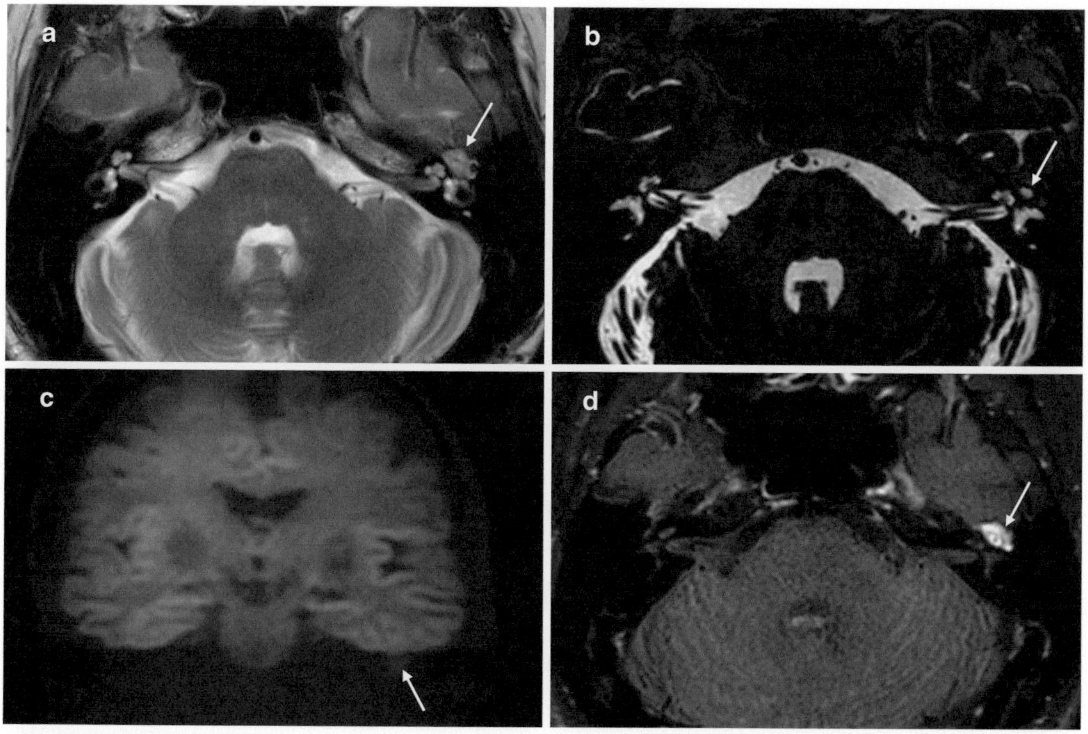

Fig. 13.13 **Left geniculate fossa schwannoma** (continues from Fig. 13.12). (**a**) Axial TSE T2W, (**b**) Axial 3D TSE T2W, (**c**) Coronal TSE DWI, (**d**) Axial contrast enhanced 3D TSE T1W BB. A millimetric mass is seen centered in the left geniculate ganglion with high signal on the T2-weighted sequence (arrow in **a**) and with internal cystic degeneration (arrow in **b**). The mass does not demonstrate restricted diffusion (arrow in **c**). Following contrast administration, the lesion shows vivid enhancement (arrow in **d**). The imaging characteristics are consistent with a right geniculate ganglion schwannoma. *Abbreviations:* TSE = turbo spin echo, EPI-DWI = echo planar imaging diffusion weighted imaging, BB= black blood

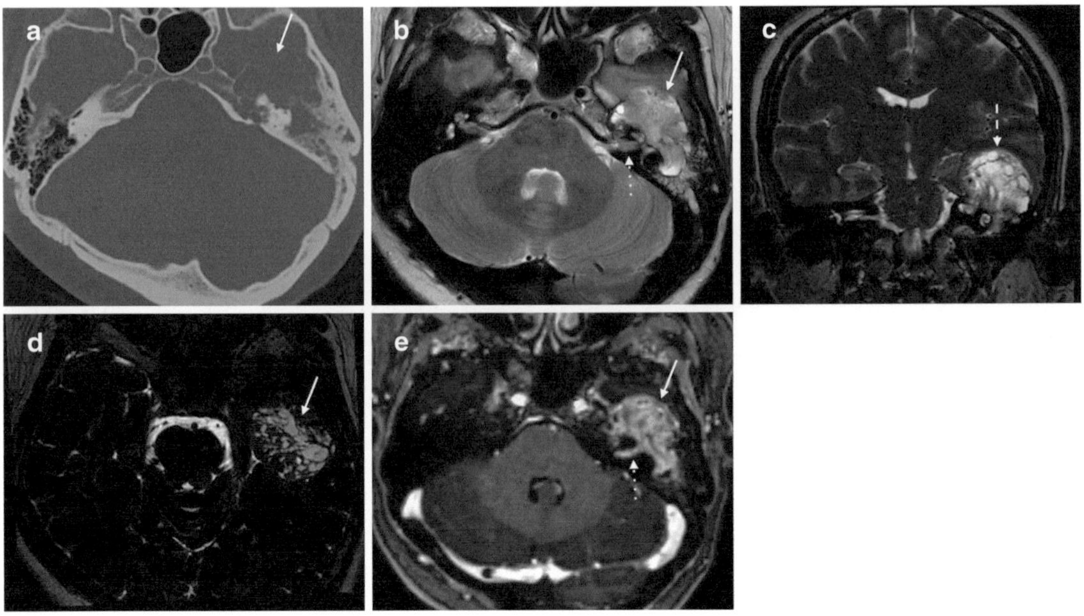

Fig. 13.14 Left geniculate fossa schwannoma. (**a**) Axial MDCT, (**b**) Axial TSE T2W, (**c**) Coronal TSE T2W, (**d**) Axial 3D TSE T2W, and (**e**) Axial contrast-enhanced 3D FFE-T1W with fat suppression. The MRI sequences show a voluminous mass centered in the left geniculate fossa (arrows in **a**, **b**, **d**, and **e**), with high signal intensity on T2-weighted sequences (arrow in **b** and dashed arrow in **c**) and areas of internal cystic degeneration (arrow in **d**). The mass shows vivid contrast enhancement (arrow **e**) and extends into the internal auditory canal (dotted arrow in **b** and **e**) and dislocates the adjacent brain parenchyma (dashed arrow in **c**). After contrast administration, the lesion shows marked enhancement (arrow in **e**). The imaging features are consistent with a geniculate fossa schwannoma. *Abbreviations:* MDCT = multidetector computed tomography, TSE = turbo spin echo, FFE = fast field echo, MRI = magnetic resonance imaging

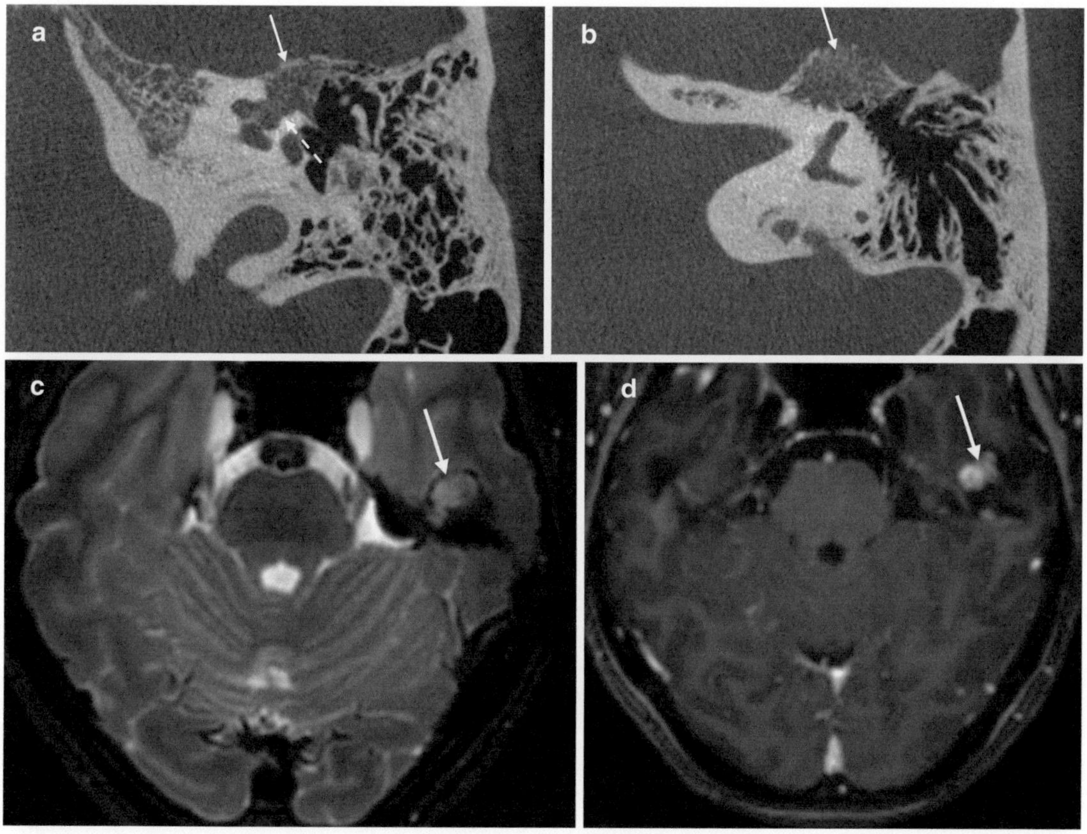

Fig. 13.15 Left geniculate fossa venous malformation (facial nerve hemangioma). Venous vascular malformations involving the facial nerve, previously referred to as facial nerve hemangiomas, are uncommon benign vascular lesions. These malformations typically present with facial nerve dysfunction, most often in the form of facial paralysis. Despite they generally have small size, they often cause significant clinical symptoms. This is in contrast with facial nerve schwannomas, which can grow to a larger size while remaining relatively asymptomatic. Additional symptoms may include sensorineural hearing loss and tinnitus. These malformations are most frequently located in the geniculate ganglion region of the facial nerve. (**a** and **b**) Axial CBCT; (**c**) 3D TSE T2W; (**d**) Contrast-enhanced 3D FFE-T1W images show a medium-sized expansile lytic lesion situated at the expected anatomical site of the left geniculate ganglion of the facial nerve. On the CBCT the lesion displays a characteristic multiloculated or "honeycomb-like" appearance, which is a recognized imaging feature of facial nerve venous malformation (arrows in **a** and **b**). There is involvement of the otic capsule, with the lesion appearing to merge with or be inseparable from the middle turn of the cochlea (dashed arrow in **a**). The lesion shows high signal intensity on T2-weighted image (arrow in **c**), and marked enhancement after contrast administration on T1-weighted image (arrow in **d**). The imaging findings are consistent with a facial nerve venous malformation, previously referred to as a facial nerve hemangioma. *Abbreviations:* CBCT = cone beam computed tomography, TSE = turbo spin echo, FFE = fast field echo

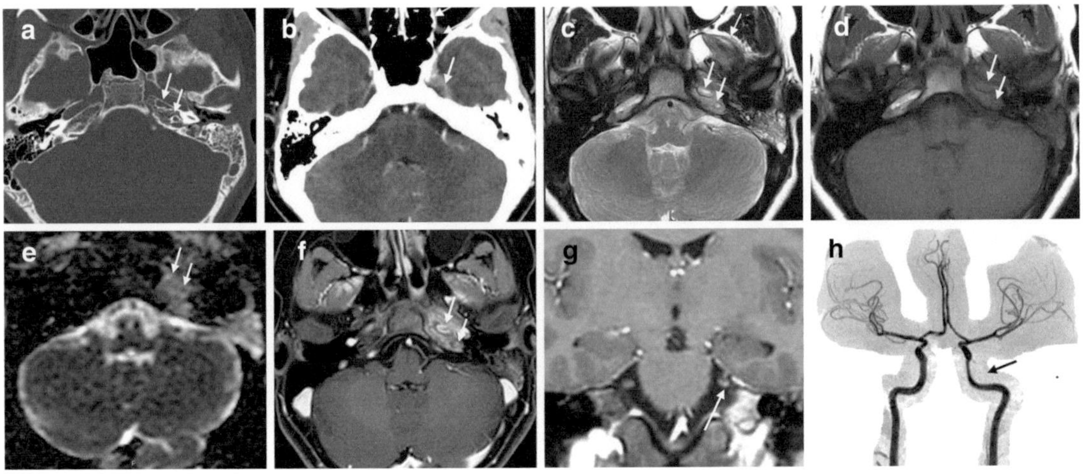

Fig. 13.16 Petrous apicitis/osteomyelitis. Twelve-year-old boy with fever, left sided otalgia, facial pain, and acute strabismus due to VI cranial nerve deficit (Gradenigo syndrome). (**a**) axial MDCT scan, bone and (**b**) soft tissue images; (**c**) axial TSE-T2W MR image, (**d**) SE-T1W MR image, (**e**) DWI ADC map; (**f**) contrast-enhanced 3D FFE-T1W with fat suppression; (**g**) coronal contrast-enhanced 3D FFE-T1W with fat suppression and (**h**) MIP reconstruction from 3D TOF MR-angiography. The MDCT scan shows opacification of left mastoid cells, middle ear cavity, external acoustic canal and partially pneumatized petrous apex (arrows in **a**); there is no intercellular septa erosion. The contrast-enhanced MDCT image shows increased enhancement along the lateral wall of the ipsilateral Meckel's cave (arrow in **b**), consistent with pachymeningitis adjacent to the infected petrous apex. MRI shows fluid collection in the left petrous apex cells (arrows in **c** and **d**) and diffuse signal abnormality in the adjacent marrow spaces of the petrous apex, with reduced diffusion on ADC map (arrows in **e**) and diffuse contrast enhancement (arrows in **f**). Mild enhancement of the cisternal segment of the left V cranial nerve (arrow in **g**) is consistent with neuritis of the trigeminal nerve, due to spread of the infection from the Meckel's cave. Arteritis of the distal petrous and cavernous portion of the left internal carotid artery is responsible for the ICA stenosis at MRA (black arrow in **h**). (Courtesy of Dr. Lorenzo Pinelli Neuroradiology Unit ASST Spedali Civili of Brescia, Italy). *Abbreviations:* MDCT = multidetector computed tomography, TSE= turbo spin echo, SE= spin echo, FFE= fast field echo, MR= magnetic resonance, MIP= maximum intensity projection, DWI = Diffusion Weighted Imaging, TOF = time of flight, ADC = apparent diffusion coefficient, ICA = internal carotid artery, MRA = magnetic resonance angiography

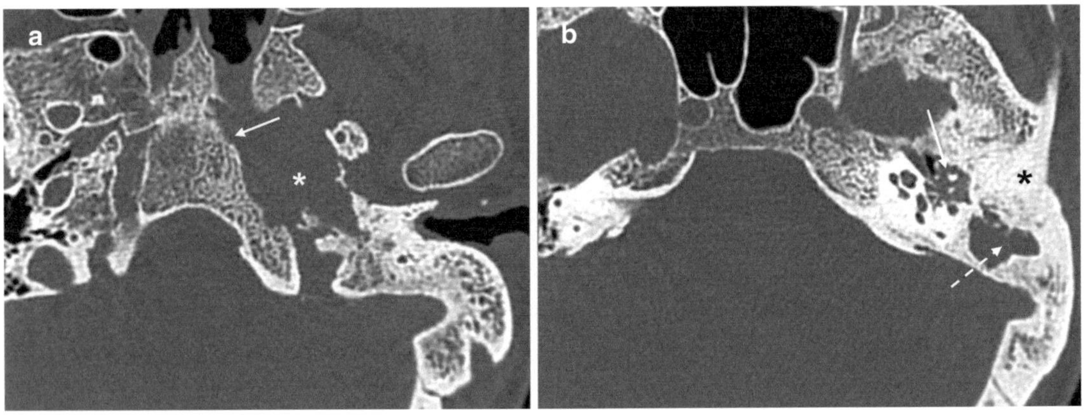

Fig. 13.17 Left Skull Base Osteomyelitis. Skull base osteomyelitis is an infection affecting the temporal, sphenoid, or occipital bones, commonly resulting from inadequately treated otogenic or sinonasal infections. It primarily occurs in elderly patients with diabetes or those who are immunocompromised. Diagnostic imaging options include non-contrast and contrast-enhanced MDCT, contrast-enhanced MRI and nuclear imaging. MDCT is the preferred modality for evaluating bone erosion and demineralization; MDCT is valuable in emergency settings. (**a**) MDCT image demonstrates osteolytic changes with bone demineralization and cortical disruption involving the left half of the clivus (arrow) and the apex of the left petrous temporal bone (asterisk). (**b**) MDCT shows sclerotic changes of the mastoid secondary to chronic otomastoiditis (black asterisk). Inflammatory material is present within the mastoid antrum (dashed arrow), mesotympanum, and epitympanum, with encasement of the ossicular chain, which remains intact (arrow). *Abbreviation:* MDCT = multidetector computed tomography

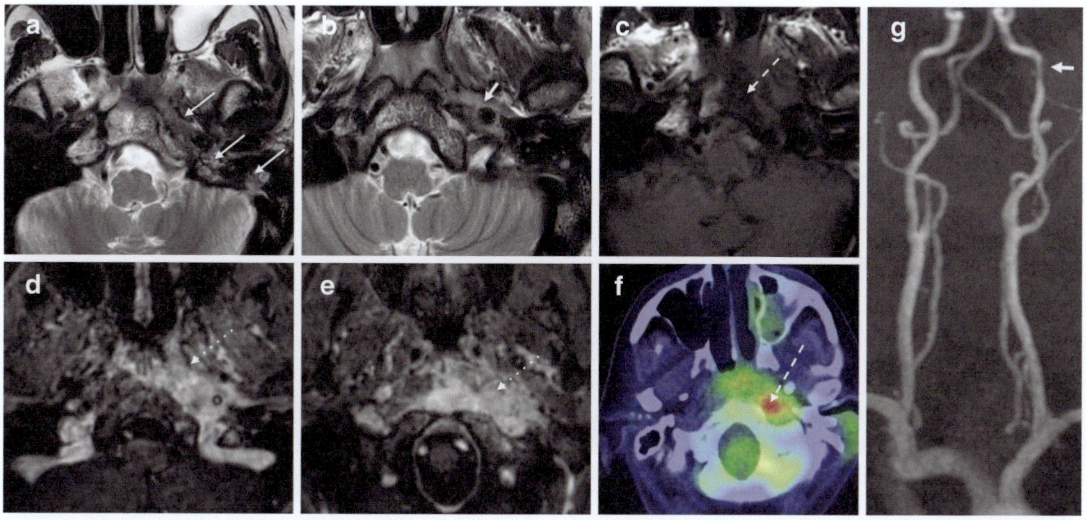

Fig. 13.18 **Left skull base osteomyelitis** (continues from Fig. 13.17). MRI plays a key role in evaluating the location and extent of skull base osteomyelitis. On contrast-enhanced T1-weighted images, skull base osteomyelitis typically appears as an enhancing soft-tissue with an infiltrative pattern. MRI can also reveal bone marrow involvement—seen as low signal on T1-weighted images with contrast medium enhancement—as well as adjacent soft-tissue edema, loss of fat planes, and possible intracranial or perineural spread, or vascular involvement such as venous sinus thrombosis, arterial pseudoaneurysm, or ischemic infarction. DWI is valuable in identifying inflammatory tissue, which usually shows restricted diffusion (high signal on DWI and low signal on ADC maps) and in detecting abscesses. Nuclear imaging techniques such as PET/CT with FDG can further aid in detecting increased metabolic activity, supporting the diagnosis and monitoring of infection. (**a** and **b**) axial TSE-T2W MR image shows extensive high signal inflammatory tissue involving the left middle ear, mastoid cells and antrum and petrous apex (arrows in **a**) and extending into the cervical vascular compartment with encasement of the carotid artery (arrow in **b**). (**c**) axial TSE-T1W MR image shows low signal tissue involving the clivus (dashed arrow). (**d** and **e**) contrast-enhanced axial 3D FFE-T1W images reveal vivid contrast enhancement involving the left retro-pharyngeal, parapharingeal and vascular spaces (dotted arrows). (**f**) axial PET/TC image shows increased tracer uptake corresponding to the inflammatory tissue (dashed arrow). (**g**) 4D track imaging demonstrates luminal narrowing of the left carotid artery (arrow). The osteomyelitis was due to Aspergillus flavus infection in a patient with HIV and diabetes. *Abbreviations:* MRI= magnetic resonance imaging, DWI = Diffusion-weighted imaging, ADC = apparent diffusion coefficient, PET-CT = positron emission tomography computed tomography, FDG = fluorodeoxyglucose, TSE = turbo spin echo, FFE = fast field echo

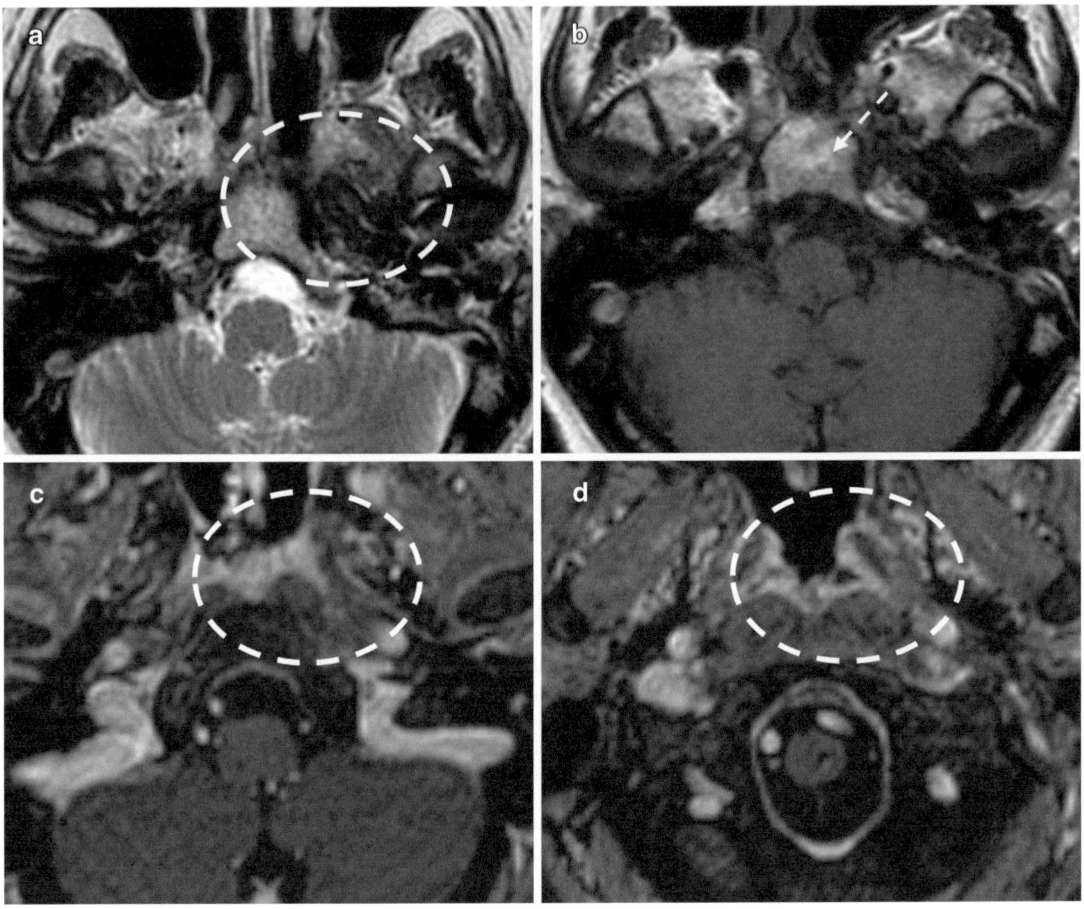

Fig. 13.19 Left skull base osteomyelitis (continues from Fig. 13.17). Two-years follow up after therapy. (**a**) axial TSE-T2W MR image, (**b**) axial TSE-T1W, (**c** and **d**) contrast-enhanced axial FFE-T1W with fat suppression images show the resolution of the inflammatory process with disappearance of pathological soft tissue previously observed in the left parapharyngeal, retropharyngeal and vascular spaces (dashed circles), normal yellow bone marrow signal is visible within the clivus (dashed arrow in **b**). *Abbreviations:* TSE = turbo spin echo, MR = magnetic resonance, FFE = fast field echo

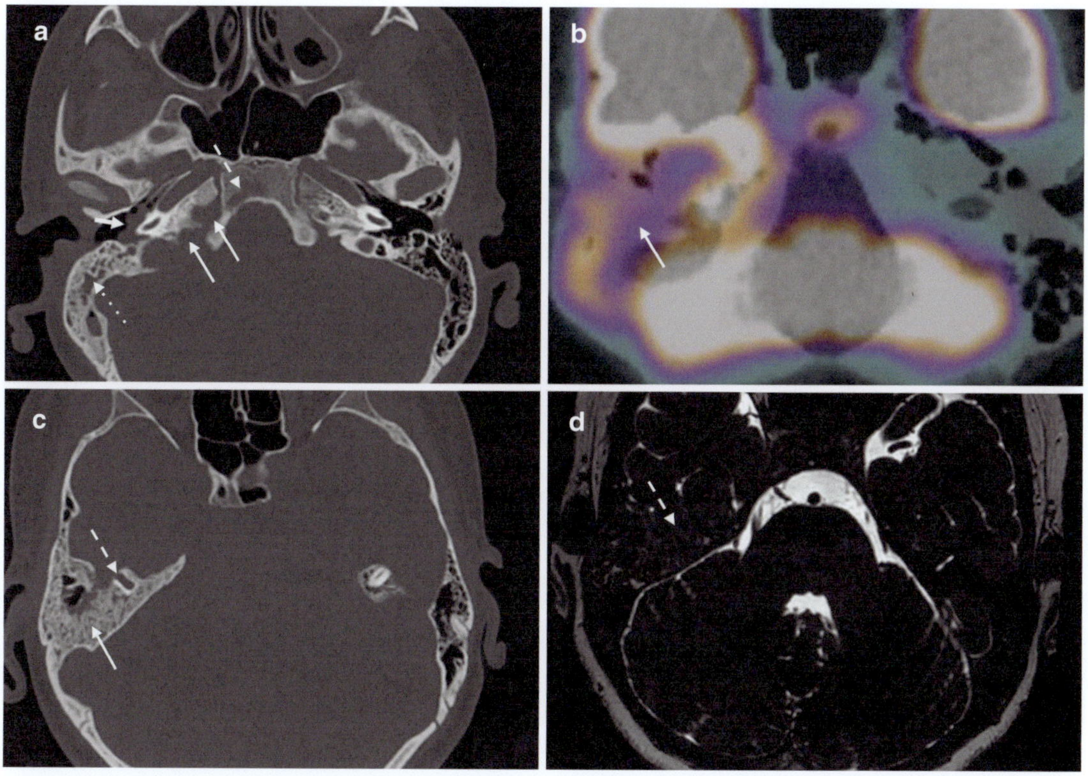

Fig. 13.20 Right skull base tuberculosis osteomyelitis. (**a** and **c**) Axial MDCT bone scans; (**b**) Axial PET-CT image fusion, (**d**) Axial 3D TSE-T2-W image. MDCT image (**a**) show multiple osteolytic, destructive lesions in the right petrous apex (arrows) and the right portion of the clivus (dashed arrow), opacification of the right mastoid (dotted arrow) and mesotympanum (short arrow). The PET-CT (**b**) image demonstrates increased FDG uptake in the right mastoid (arrow). MDCT image (**c**) shows sclerotic changes in the right mastoid air cells (arrow), consistent with a chronic inflammatory process, and pathological enlargement of the right superior semicircular canal (dashed arrow), with corresponding loss of normal high T2 signal (dashed arrow in **d**), likely due to the presence of infected fluid. *Abbreviations:* MDCT= mutidetector computer tomography, PET-CT = positron emission tomography computed tomography, TSE = turbo spin echo, FDG = Fluorodeoxyglucose

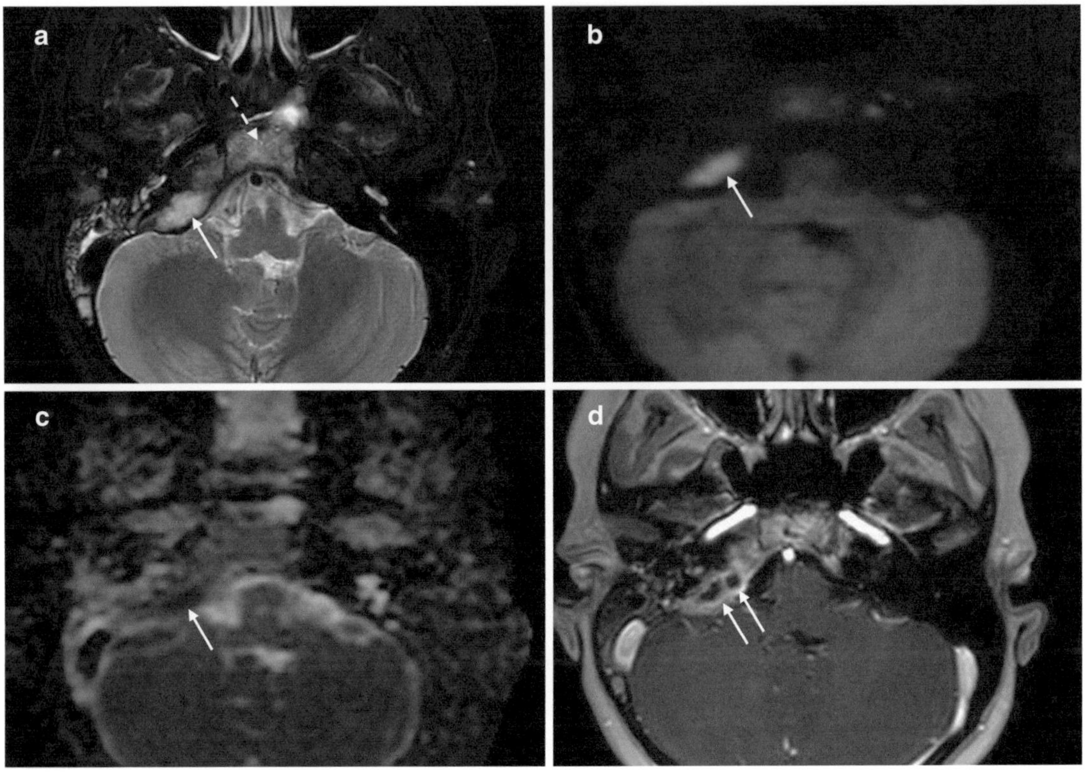

Fig. 13.21 **Right skull base tuberculosis osteomyelitis** (continues from Fig. 13.20). (**a**) Axial TSE-T2W; (**b**) Axial DWI; (**c**) ADC map; (**d**) Axial contrast-enhanced 3D FFE-T1W with fat suppression. MRI shows a lesion with high signal intensity on T2-weighted imaging (arrow in **a**), suggestive of a necrotic component, and high signal of the clivus (dashed arrow in **a**). The lesion has high signal on DWI (arrow in **b**) with corresponding low ADC values (arrow in **c**), approximately 0.5×10^{-3} mm^2/s, indicating marked diffusion restriction. Post-contrast T1-weighted imaging demonstrates peripheral ring enhancement (arrows in **d**). These imaging findings are consistent with liquefactive ossifluent abscess. Tuberculous osteomyelitis was suspected. PCR testing for *Mycobacterium tuberculosis* in the blood was negative, while PCR performed on sputum was positive. *Abbreviations:* TSE = turbo spin echo, DWI = diffusion weighted imaging, ADC = apparent diffusion coefficient, FFE = fast field echo, MRI = magnetic resonance imaging; PCR = polymerase chain reaction

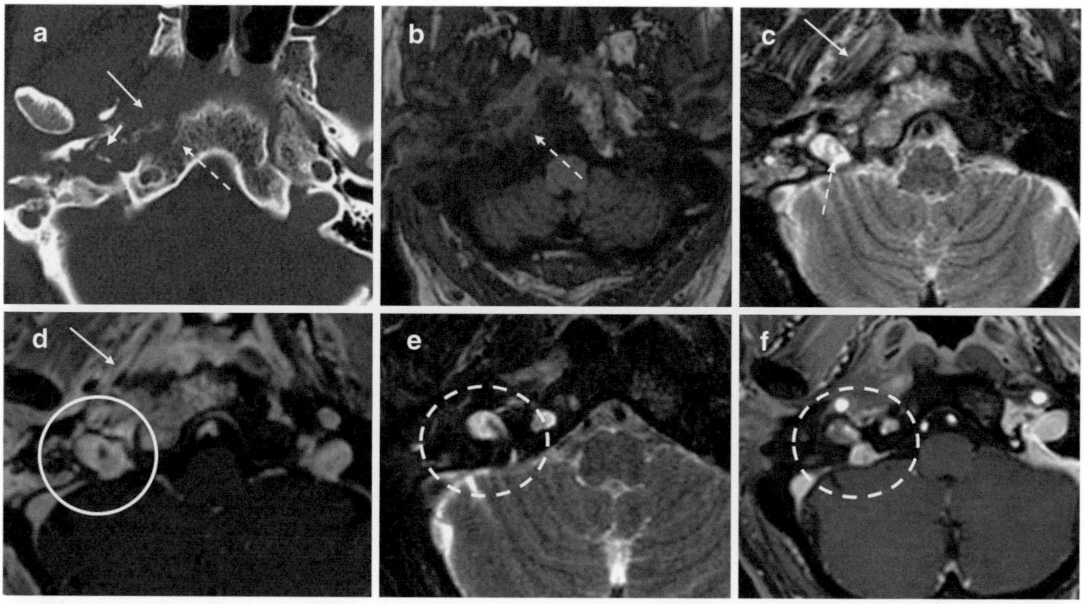

Fig. 13.22 Skull base osteomyelitis with venous thrombosis. Venous thrombosis is a possible complication of osteomyelitis. It is diagnosed using contrast-enhanced MDCT and MRI, which typically reveal filling defects known as the "empty delta sign," often accompanied by venous dilation. The thrombosis can involve multiple venous sinuses and may lead to cerebral venous infarctions. (**a**) Axial MDCT shows bony erosion of the apex of the petrous bone (arrow), in the region of the jugular foramen (short arrow), and irregularities of the cortical bone in the right margin of the clivus (dashed arrow). (**b**) Axial FFE-T1W MR image shows involvement of the right half of the clivus, which demonstrates low signal (dashed arrow). (**c**) Axial TSE-T2W reveals an high signal alteration of the mastoid, middle ear, preauricular region, extending into the posterolateral portion (*pars vascularis*) of the right jugular foramen (dashed arrow) and to the median and paramedian soft tissues of right prevertebral and masticatory space (arrow). (**d**) axial post contrast 3D FFE-T1 with fat soppression sequence MR image shows thrombosis of the ipsilateral jugular vein (white circle in **d**), encased by the inflammatory tissue which demonstrates strong contrast-enhancement and involves also the masticatory space (arrow). (**e** and **f**) 3 months follow-up MRI: axial TSE-T2W and post contrast FFE-T1W with fat suppression show chronic thrombosis of the internal jugular vein (dotted circles). *Abbreviations:* MDCT = multidetector computed tomography, MRI = magnetic resonance imaging, FFE = fast field echo, TSE = turbo spin echo

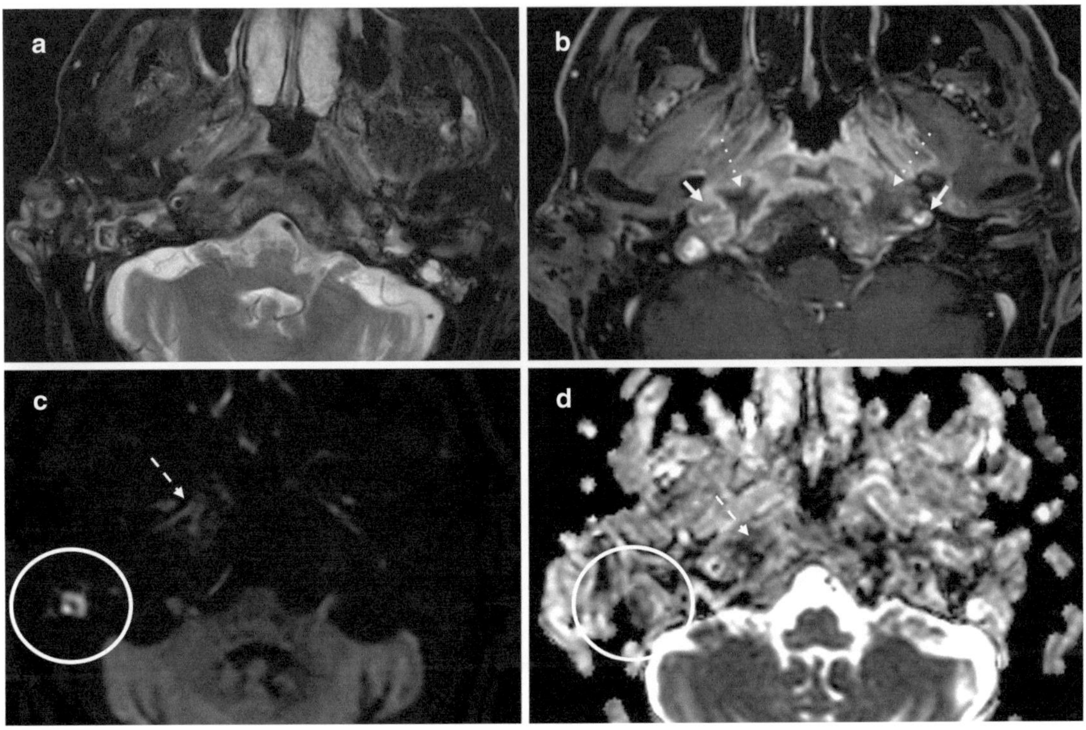

Fig. 13.23 **Skull Base Osteoradionecrosis** in a patient treated for squamous cell carcinoma of the external auditory canal. ORN is an uncommon but serious complication of RT, resulting from vascular damage that impairs blood supply and leads to tissue and bone necrosis. Bones with naturally limited vascularization, such as the skull base, are particularly susceptible. ORN may involve the anterior, central, and lateral skull base regions along with adjacent soft tissues. RT can also cause injury to the surrounding brain tissue. (**a** and **b**) Axial TSE-T2W with fat-suppression and contrast-enhanced 3D FFE-T1W with fat suppression MR images reveal diffuse soft tissue alterations in the retrolateral pharyngeal spaces with necrotic and liquefactive areas (dotted arrows in **b**), consistent with an inflammatory process. The involvement extends to the vascular compartments, showing encasement of the carotid arteries (short arrows). (**c** and **d**) Axial DWI and ADC maps demonstrate mild diffusion restriction within the necrotic area of the skull base soft tissues (dashed arrow), and moderate restriction of the residual tumor lesion surrounding the right external auditory canal (white circles). *Abbreviations:* ORN = osteoradionecrosis, RT = radiotherapy, TSE = turbo spin echo, FFE = fast field echo, DWI = Diffusion-Weighted Imaging, ADC = Apparent Diffusion Coefficient

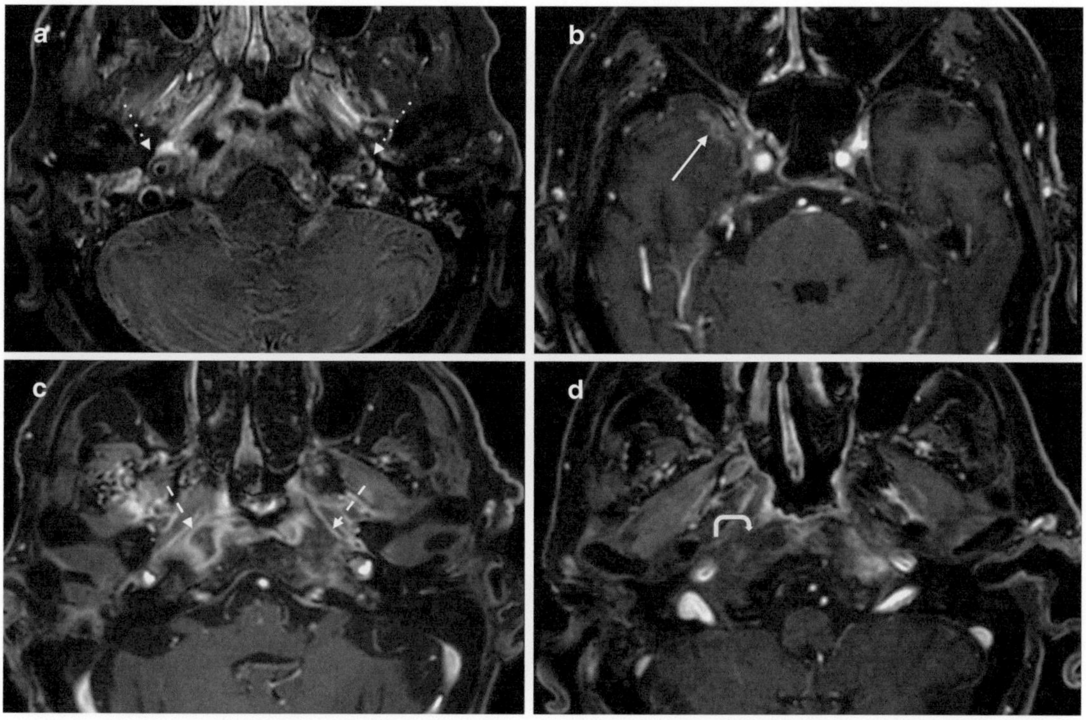

Fig. 13.24 Skull Base Osteoradionecrosis in a patient treated for squamous cell carcinoma of the external auditory canal (continues from Fig. 13.23). (**a**) Axial contrast-enhanced 3D FFE-T1WMR image demonstrates focal narrowing of the internal carotid arteries with associated intimal enhancement (dotted arrows). Perifocal soft tissue enhancement is also evident surrounding the right internal carotid artery. (**b**) Same sequence as in a passing through a more cranial plane shows right mesial temporal enhancement (arrow) consistent with radionecrosis within brain tissue. (**c** and **d**) Follow-up MRI scans reveal progressive reduction of skull base soft tissue enhancement (dashed arrow in **c**), with gradual replacement by fibrous tissue (curved arrow in **d**)

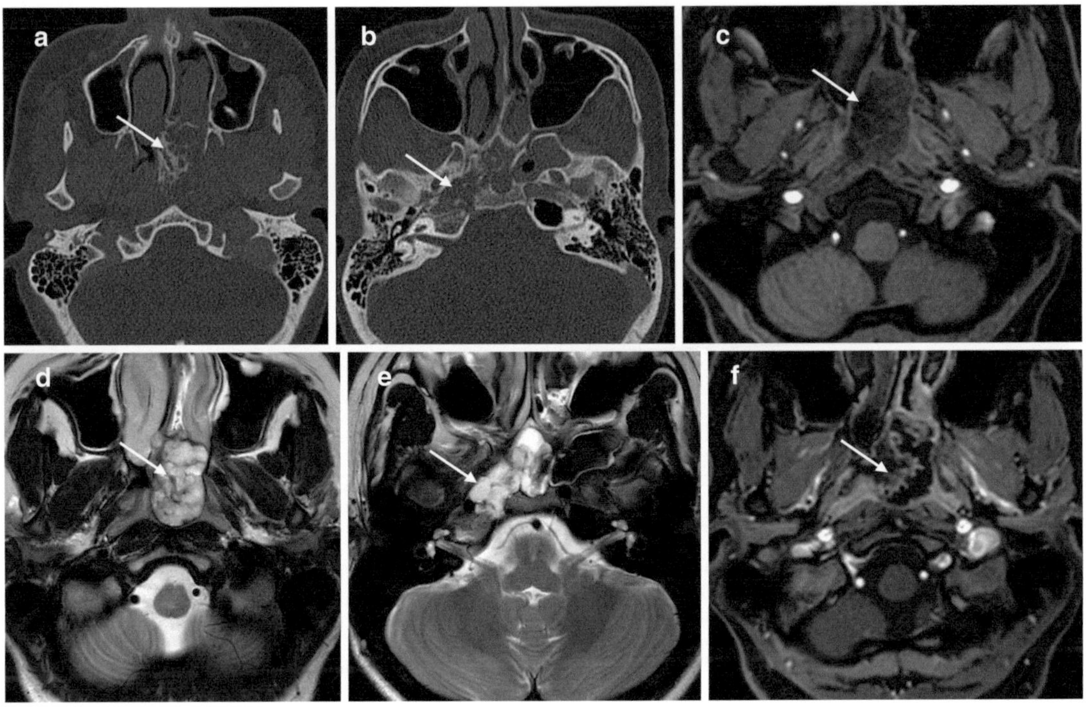

Fig. 13.25 Nasopharynx chondrosarcoma. Chondrosarcomas of the skull base can originate from cartilaginous remnants of the petro-occipital fissure and then commonly spread to invade the cavernous sinus, the petrous segment of the carotid artery, and the clivus. Notably, they have a strong propensity to extend laterally and downward, affecting the petrous apex and the foramen lacerum. They are slow-growing tumors that can cause symptoms from involvement of associated cranial nerves, (usually the VI cranial nerve). MDCT scan evaluates bony erosive aspects and foraminal involvement. Since chondrosarcomas are composed of a chondroid matrix their calcifications typically appear as so-called "arches and whorls", which are variously oriented, rounded or curvilinear calcifications, an appearance observed in about 50 % of cases. The lesion may have a lobular appearance with a "cauliflower" shape. MRI is useful in the diagnosis because chondrosarcomas tipically show hyperintensityon T2-weighted images, with hypointense foci due to the presence of calcifications, isoipointense signal at T1-weighted images and can show significant heterogeneous or uniform contrast enhancement. The main treatment of chondrosarcoma is surgical resection and radiotherapy. (**a** and **b**) Axial MDCT bone scans; (**c**) Axial 3D FFE-T1W with fat suppression; (**d** and **e**) Axial TSE-T2W; (**f**) Axial contrast-enhanced FFE-T1W with fat suppression. The images show an extra-axial calcified mass centered in the nasopharynx (arrow in **a**, **c**, **d**, **f**), with posterolateral extension toward the right petrous apex (arrow in **b** and **e**). The calcifications display the characteristic ring-and-arc pattern (arrow in **a** and **b**), consistent with a chondroid matrix. The lesion demonstrates a heterogeneous signal, with predominantly high signal on T2-weighted images (arrow in **d** and **e**), low signal on T1-weighted images (arrow in **c**), and loculated or bubbly internal enhancement following contrast administration (arrow in **f**).These imaging findings are suggestive of chondrosarcoma. *Abbreviations*: MDCT= multidetector computed tomography, MRI= magnetic resonance imaging, FFE = fast field echo, TSE = turbo spin echo

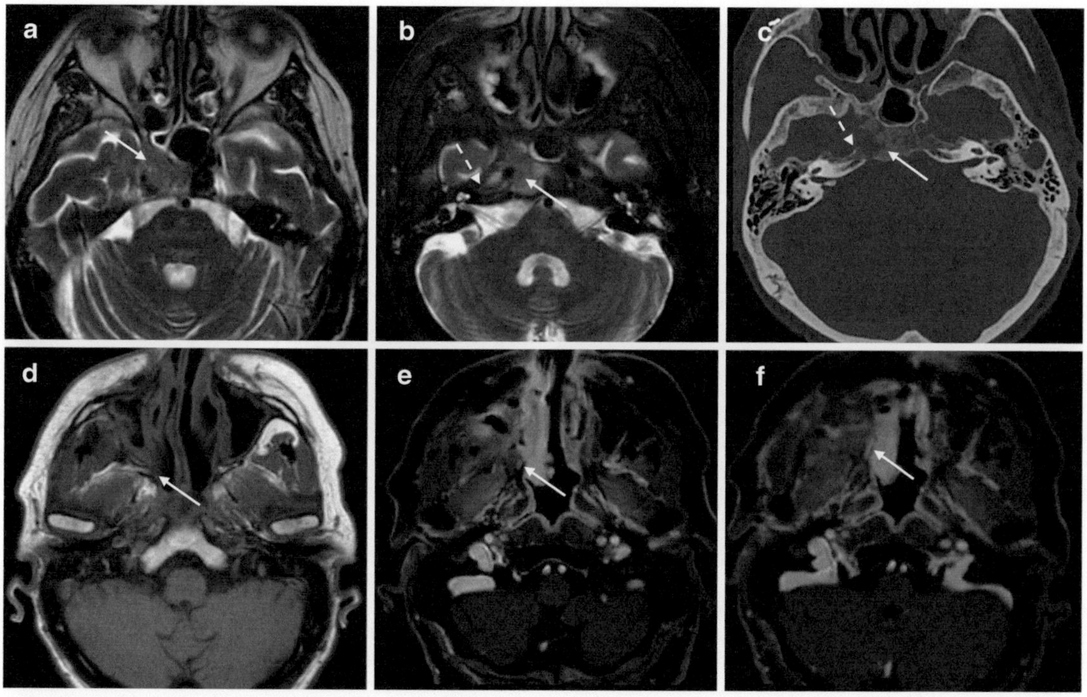

Fig. 13.26 **Squamous cell carcinoma of the right alveolar maxillary ridge** with perineural spread. PNS refers to the extension of tumor cells along the sheaths of cranial nerves, typically through the perineurium and endoneurium. PNS allows malignant cells to travel far from the primary lesion, often reaching the skull base or intracranial compartment. PNS is not simply direct invasion but rather a distinct biological pathway of tumor dissemination. Perineural spread occurs most frequently in head and neck malignancies, especially : adenoid cystic carcinoma of the salivary gland, squamous cell carcinoma of the skin and mucosal surfaces, and lymphoma. Clinically, PNS may be silent or present with neuropathic pain, paresthesia, or motor deficits depending on the affected nerve. MRI is the modality of choice, key findings include nerve enlargement and abnormal enhancement along its course, loss of normal fat signal in neural foramina or surrounding spaces, and denervation changes in the muscles supplied by the involved nerve. MDCT is also useful because it can show foraminal widening and asymmetry. (**a** and **b**) Axial TSE-T2W; (**c**) Axial MDCT bone scan; (**d**) Axial TSE-T1W; (**e** and **f**) Axial contrast-enhanced MIP reformatted 3D FFE-T1W with fat suppression. The images show an extra-axial mass centered in the right cavernous sinus (arrow in **a**), with posterolateral extension to the clivus (arrow in **b** and **c**) and the right petrous apex (dashed arrow in **b** and **c**), associated with bone erosion. On the T1-weighted image (**d**), there is obliteration of the sphenopalatine foramen (arrow in **d**). Post-contrast images reveal slight enlargement of the greater palatine foramen (arrow in **e**) and mild contrast enhancement of the greater palatine nerve (arrow in **e** and **f**). These imaging findings are consistent with perineural spread of previously diagnosed squamous cell carcinoma of the maxillary ridge, extending along the right greater palatine nerve to the cavernous sinus, with subsequent involvement of the right petrous apex. *Abbreviations:* PNS = perineural spread, MDCT = multidetector computed tomography, TSE = turbo spin echo, MIP = maximum intensity projection, FFE = fast field echo

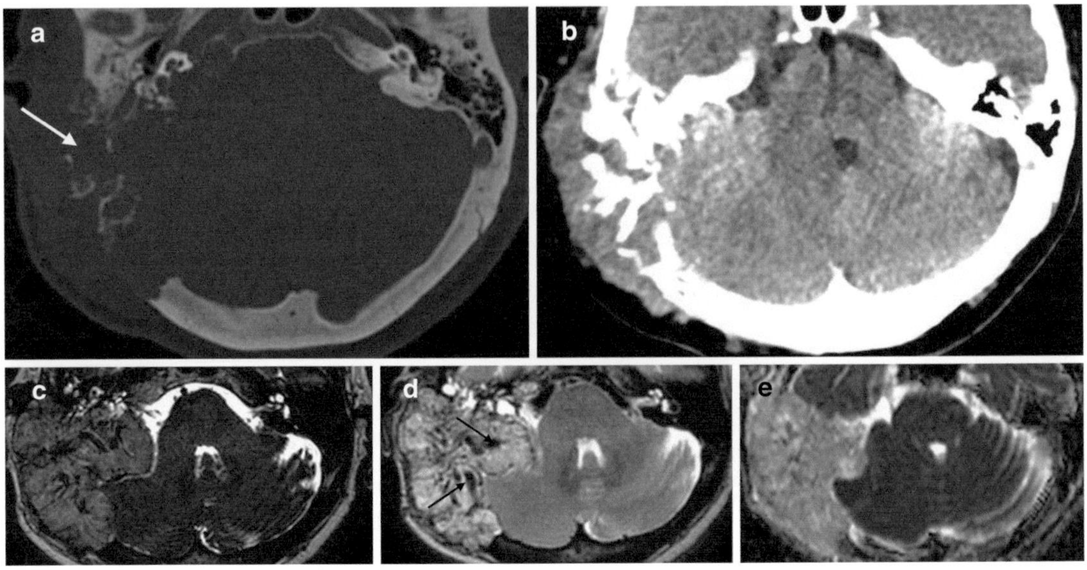

Fig. 13.27 Endolymphatic sac tumor. ELST are rare and usually occur in the fourth or fifth decade with a wide age range. They may occur sporadically but can be associated with von Hippel-Lindau syndrome and in this case are bilateral. They are indolent low-grade adenocarcinoma that usually became locally aggressive causing bone erosion. They arise from the posterior petrous ridge and may cause sensorineural hearing loss, tinnitus and facial-nerve dysfunction due to tumor progression and invasion of adjacent tissues. The treatment is surgical or, in case of residual disease or unresectable tumor, with radiotherapy or radiosurgery. (**a** and **b**) MDCT bone and soft tissue images, (**c**) Axial 3D TSE-T2W, (**d**) Axial TSE-T2W, (**e**) ADC map. The images show a large lobulated, heterogeneous lesions with well-defined margins of the right petrous and temporal bones extending to posterior cranial fossa and extracranial tissues. The lesion shows diffuse bone erosion on MDCT (arrow in **a**), intermediate signal on T2-weighted images and high ADC values due to low cellularity. On T2-weighted images vascular flow voids are depicted (black arrows in **d**). (Courtesy of Dr. Giuseppe Vaccaro Neuroradiology Unit Sant'Elia Hospital, Caltanissetta, Italy). *Abbreviations:* ELST = endolymphatic sac tumor, MDCT = multidetector computed tomography, TSE = turbo spin echo, ADC = apparent diffusion coefficient

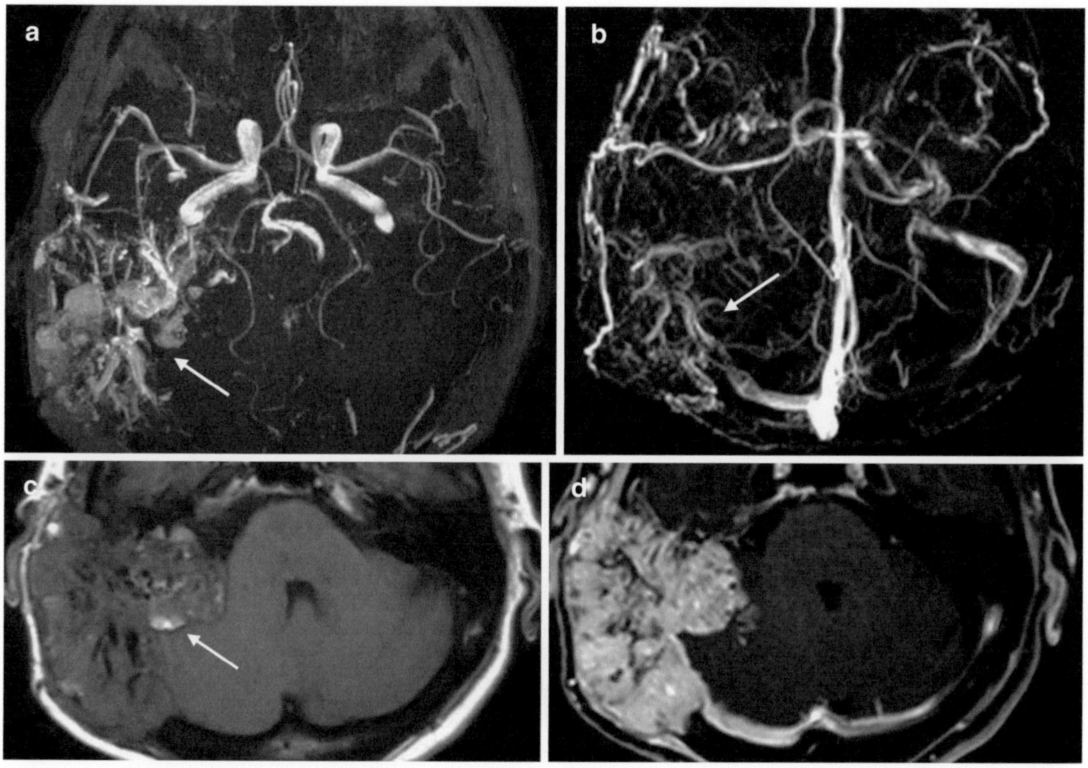

Fig. 13.28 **Endolymphatic sac tumor** (continues from Fig. 13.27). (**a**) 3D-TOF MRA; (**b**) PC MRA; (**c**) axial TSE-T1W image; (**d**) Axial contrast-enhanced 3D FFE-T1W sequences. ELST is highly vascular tumor as shown in (**a**) and (**b**) (arrows). Some areas of hyperintensity are present on T1 weighted image (arrow in **c**) suggestive of small foci of haemorrhage. The lesion has significant heterogeneous enhancement (**d**). (Courtesy of Dr. Giuseppe Vaccaro Neuroradiology Unit Sant'Elia Hospital, Caltanissetta, Italy) *Abbreviations:* TOF = time of flight, MRA = magnetic resonance angiogram, PC = phase contrast, TSE = turbo spin echo, ELST = endolymphatic sac tumor

References

1. Moore KR, Harnsberger HR, Shelton C, Davidson HC. 'Leave me alone' lesions of the petrous apex. AJNR. 1998;19:733–8.
2. Settecase F, Harnsberger HR, Michel MA, Chapman P, Glastonbury CM. Spontaneous lateral sphenoid cephaloceles: anatomic factors contributing to pathogenesis and proposed classification. AJNR Am J Neuroradiol. 2014;35(4):784–9. https://doi.org/10.3174/ajnr.A3744. Epub 2013 Oct 3. PMID: 24091443; PMCID: PMC7965830.
3. Bialer OY, Rueda MP, Bruce BB, Newman NJ, Biousse V, Saindane AM. Meningoceles in idiopathic intracranial hypertension. AJR Am J Roentgenol. 2014;202(3):608–13. https://doi.org/10.2214/AJR.13.10874. PMID: 24555598; PMCID: PMC4041691.
4. Watane GV, Patel B, Brown D, Taheri MR. The significance of arachnoid granulation in patients with idiopathic intracranial hypertension. J Comput Assist Tomogr. 2018;42(2):282–5. https://doi.org/10.1097/RCT.0000000000000668. PMID: 28937488.
5. Sadé J, Halévy A, Klajman A, Mualem T. Cholesterol granuloma. Acta Otolaryngol. 1980;89(3–4):233–9. https://doi.org/10.3109/00016488009127133. PMID: 6156569.
6. Jackler RK, Cho M. A new theory to explain the genesis of petrous apex cholesterol granuloma. Otol Neurotol. 2003;24(1):96–106; discussion 106. doi:https://doi.org/10.1097/00129492-200301000-00020. PMID: 12544037.
7. Hoa M, House JW, Linthicum FH Jr. Petrous apex cholesterol granuloma: maintenance of drainage pathway, the histopathology of surgical management and histopathologic evidence for the exposed marrow theory. Otol Neurotol. 2012;33(6):1059–65. https://

doi.org/10.1097/MAO.0b013e31825d63ea. PMID: 22710556; PMCID: PMC3846394.

8. Lee EE, Andresen NS, McKenzie B, Sharon JD, Francis HW, Sun DQ. Perigeniculate arachnoid cysts and CSF fistulae of the fallopian canal: histopathologic correlates of a rare clinical entity. World J Otorhinolaryngol Head Neck Surg. 2021;7(2):71–81. https://doi.org/10.1016/j.wjorl.2020.12.005. PMID: 33997715; PMCID: PMC8103539.
9. Benoit MM, North PE, McKenna MJ, Mihm MC, Johnson MM, Cunningham MJ. Facial nerve hemangiomas: vascular tumors or malformations? Otolaryngol Head Neck Surg. 2010 Jan;142(1):108–14. https://doi.org/10.1016/j.otohns.2009.10.007.
10. Chapman PR, Choudhary G, Singhal A. Skull base osteomyelitis: a comprehensive imaging review. AJNR Am J Neuroradiol. 2021;42(3):404–13. https://doi.org/10.3174/ajnr.A7015. PMID: 33478944; PMCID: PMC7959418.
11. Van Kroonenburgh AMJL, van der Meer WL, Bothof RJP, van Tilburg M, van Tongeren J, Postma AA. Advanced imaging techniques in skull base osteomyelitis due to malignant otitis externa. Curr Radiol Rep. 2018;6(1):3. https://doi.org/10.1007/s40134-018-0263-y. PMID: 29416952; PMCID: PMC5778178.
12. Ahmed S, Gupta N, Hamilton JD, Garden AS, Gidley PW, Ginsberg LE. CT findings in temporal bone osteoradionecrosis. J Comput Assist Tomogr. 2014;38(5):662. Available from: https://pmc.ncbi.nlm.nih.gov/articles/PMC4186743/
13. Raghavan P, Witek ME, Morales RE. Imaging of complications of chemoradiation. Neuroimaging Clin N Am. 2022;32(1):93–109. https://doi.org/10.1016/j.nic.2021.08.012.
14. Pamir MN, Ozduman K. Analysis of radiological features relative to histopathology in 42 skull-base chordomas and chondrosarcomas. Eur J Radiol. 2006;58:461–70.
15. Isaacson B, Kutz JW, Roland PS. Lesions of the petrous apex: diagnosis and management. Otolaryngol Clin N Am. 2007;40:479–519. viii.
16. Mukherji SK, Albernaz VS, Lo WW, et al. Papillary endolymphatic sac tumors: CT, MR imaging, and angiographic findings in 20 patients. Radiology. 1997;202:801–8.

MIX
Papier aus verantwortungsvollen Quellen
Paper from responsible sources
FSC® C105338

If you have any concerns about our products,
you can contact us on
ProductSafety@springernature.com

In case Publisher is established outside the EU,
the EU authorized representative is:
Springer Nature Customer Service Center GmbH
Europaplatz 3, 69115 Heidelberg, Germany

Printed by Libri Plureos GmbH
in Hamburg, Germany